Pathology Informatics

Editor

ANIL V. PARWANI

SURGICAL PATHOLOGY CLINICS

www.surgpath.theclinics.com

Consulting Editor

JOHN R. GOLDBLUM

June 2015 • Volume 8 • Number 2

ELSEVIER

1600 John F. Kennedy Boulevard • Suite 1800 • Philadelphia, Pennsylvania, 19103-2899

http://www.theclinics.com

SURGICAL PATHOLOGY CLINICS Volume 8, Number 2
June 2015 ISSN 1875-9181, ISBN-13: 978-0-323-35667-1

Editor: Joanne Husovski
Developmental Editor: Donald Mumford

Surgical Pathology Clinics (ISSN 1875-9181) is published quarterly by Elsevier Inc., 360 Park Avenue South, New York, NY 10010. Months of issue are March, June, September, and December. Business and Editorial Office: Elsevier Inc., 1600 John F. Kennedy Blvd., Ste. 1800, Philadelphia, PA 19103-2899. Accounting and Circulation Offices: Elsevier Inc., 3251 Riverport Lane, Maryland Heights, MO 63043. Periodicals postage paid at New York, NY and at additional mailing offices. Subscription prices are $200.00 per year (US individuals), $233.00 per year (US institutions), $100.00 per year (US students/residents), $250.00 per year (Canadian individuals), $266.00 per year (Canadian Institutions), $250.00 per year (foreign individuals), $266.00 per year (foreign institutions), and $120.00 per year (international & Canadian students/residents). Foreign air speed delivery is included in all *Clinics'* subscription prices. All prices are subject to change without notice. **POSTMASTER:** Send address changes to *Surgical Pathology Clinics*, Elsevier, 3251 Riverport Lane, Maryland Heights, MO 63043. **Customer Service: 1-800-654-2452 (US). From outside the United States, call 1-314-447-8871. Fax: 1-314-447-8029. E-mail: JournalsCustomerServiceusa@elsevier.com (for print support)** and **JournalsOnlineSupport-usa@elsevier.com (for online support).**

Reprints. For copies of 100 or more, of articles in this publication, please contact the Commercial Reprints Department, Elsevier Inc., 360 Park Avenue South, New York, NY 10010-1710. Tel. 212-633-3874; Fax: 212-633-3820; E-mail: reprints@elsevier.com.

Surgical Pathology Clinics of North America is covered in *MEDLINE/PubMed (Index Medicus)*.

Contributors

CONSULTING EDITOR

JOHN R. GOLDBLUM, MD
Chairman, Department of Anatomic Pathology,
Professor of Pathology; Cleveland Clinic
Lerner College of Medicine, Cleveland Clinic,
Cleveland, Ohio

EDITOR

ANIL V. PARWANI, MD, PhD, MBA
Director of Pathology Informatics, Department
of Pathology, University of Pittsburgh Medical
Center, Pittsburgh, Pennsylvania

AUTHORS

MILON AMIN, MD
Staff Pathologist, Affiliated Pathologists
Medical Group, Torrance, California

DAVID R. ARTZ, MD
Medical Director, Information Systems,
Memorial Sloan Kettering Cancer Center,
New York, New York

KENNETH E. BLICK, PhD
Professor, Department of Pathology, University
of Oklahoma Health Sciences Center,
Oklahoma City, Oklahoma

DONAVAN T. CHENG, PhD
Assistant Attending, Memorial Sloan Kettering
Cancer Center, New York, New York

IOAN C. CUCORANU, MD
Assistant Professor and Director of
Informatics, Department of Pathology and
Laboratory Medicine, University of Florida
College of Medicine - Jacksonville,
Jacksonville, Florida

BRYAN DANGOTT, MD
Associate Professor, Director of Pathology
Informatics, East Carolina University,
Greenville, North Carolina

RAJIV DHIR, MBBS, MBA
Chief of Pathology, University of Pittsburgh
Medical Center Shadyside Hospital,
Pittsburgh, Pennsylvania

NAVID FARAHANI, MD
Department of Pathology and Laboratory
Medicine, Cedars-Sinai Medical Center,
Los Angeles, California

JEFFREY L. FINE, MD
Assistant Professor; Director, Subdivision of
Advanced Imaging and Image Analysis
(Pathology Informatics) Department of
Pathology, University of Pittsburgh School of
Medicine, Pittsburgh, Pennsylvania

JIANJIONG GAO, PhD
Postdoctoral Research Fellow, Memorial
Sloan Kettering Cancer Center, New York,
New York

ERIC F. GLASSY, MD, FCAP
Medical Director, Affiliated Pathologists
Medical Group, Torrance, California

MATTHEW G. HANNA, MD
Department of Pathology, The Mount Sinai
Hospital, New York, New York

DOUGLAS J. HARTMAN, MD
Assistant Professor, Department of
Anatomic Pathology, University of
Pittsburgh Medical Center, Pittsburgh,
Pennsylvania

LEWIS ALLEN HASSELL, MD
Professor, Department of Pathology, University
of Oklahoma Health Sciences Center,
Oklahoma City, Oklahoma

WALTER H. HENRICKS, MD
Medical Director, Center for Pathology
Informatics; Staff Pathologist, Pathology and
Laboratory Medicine Institute, Cleveland
Clinic, Cleveland, Ohio

KEITH J. KAPLAN, MD
Publisher, tissuepathology.com; Pathologist
and Laboratory Medical Director; Charlotte,
North Carolina

BRUCE LEVY, MD, CPE
Associate Professor of Pathology,
Department of Pathology, University of
Illinois at Chicago; Associate Chief Health
Information Officer, University of Illinois
Hospital and Health Sciences System,
Chicago, Illinois

RAOUF E. NAKHLEH, MD
Professor of Pathology, Department of
laboratory Medicine and Pathology, Mayo
Clinic Florida, Jacksonville, Florida

LIRON PANTANOWITZ, MD
Department of Pathology, University of
Pittsburgh Medical Center, Pittsburgh,
Pennsylvania

B. ALAN RAMPY, DO, PhD, FCAP
Assistant Professor of Pathology, University
of Texas Medical Branch, Galveston, Texas

LUIGI K.F. RAO, MD, MS
Director of Pathology Informatics and
Attending Pathologist, Department of
Pathology, Walter Reed National Military
Medical Center, Bethesda, Maryland

MICHAEL RIBEN, MD
Associate Professor, Department of
Pathology, Medical Director, Laboratory
Informatics, University of Texas MD
Anderson Cancer Center, Houston,
Texas

SOMAK ROY, MD
Assistant Professor; Director of Genetic
Services and Molecular Informatics,
Department of Pathology, Molecular and
Genomic Pathology, University of
Pittsburgh Medical Center, Pittsburgh,
Pennsylvania

NIKOLAUS SCHULTZ, PhD
Associate Attending, Memorial Sloan
Kettering Cancer Center, New York,
New York

S. JOSEPH SIRINTRAPUN, MD
Assistant Attending/Director of Pathology
Informatics, Department of Pathology,
Memorial Sloan Kettering Cancer Center,
New York, New York

AIJAZUDDIN SYED, MS
Bioinformatics Engineer, Memorial Sloan
Kettering Cancer Center, New York,
New York

AHMET ZEHIR, PhD
Bioinformatics Engineer, Memorial Sloan
Kettering Cancer Center, New York,
New York

Contents

Laboratory information systems (LISs) supply mission-critical capabilities for the vast array of information-processing needs of modern laboratories. LIS architectures include mainframe, client-server, and thin client configurations. The LIS database software manages a laboratory's data. LIS dictionaries are database tables that a laboratory uses to tailor an LIS to the unique needs of that laboratory. Anatomic pathology LIS (APLIS) functions play key roles throughout the pathology workflow, and laboratories rely on LIS management reports to monitor operations. This article describes the structure and functions of APLISs, with emphasis on their roles in laboratory operations and their relevance to pathologists.

The immense volume of cases signed out by surgical pathologists on a daily basis gives little time to think about exactly how data are stored. An understanding of the basics of data representation has implications that affect a pathologist's daily practice. This article covers the basics of data representation and its importance in the design of electronic medical record systems. Coding in surgical pathology is also discussed. Finally, a summary of communication standards in surgical pathology is presented, including suggested resources that establish standards for select aspects of pathology reporting.

Bar coding and specimen tracking are intricately linked to pathology workflow and efficiency. In the pathology laboratory, bar coding facilitates many laboratory practices, including specimen tracking, automation, and quality management. Data obtained from bar coding can be used to identify, locate, standardize, and audit specimens to achieve maximal laboratory efficiency and patient safety. Variables that need to be considered when implementing and maintaining a bar coding and tracking system include assets to be labeled, bar code symbologies, hardware, software, workflow, and laboratory and information technology infrastructure as well as interoperability with the laboratory information system. This article addresses these issues, primarily focusing on surgical pathology.

Optimizing pathologist workflow can be difficult because it is affected by many variables. Surgical pathologists must complete many tasks that culminate in a final pathology report. Several software systems can be used to enhance/improve pathologist workflow. These include voice recognition software, pre–sign-out quality assurance, image utilization, and computerized provider order entry. Recent changes in the diagnostic coding and the more prominent role of centralized electronic health records represent potential areas for increased ways to enhance/improve the workflow for surgical pathologists. Additional unforeseen changes to the pathologist workflow may accompany the introduction of whole-slide imaging technology to the routine diagnostic work.

Some laboratories or laboratory sections have unique needs that traditional anatomic and clinical pathology systems may not address. A specialized laboratory information system (LIS), which is designed to perform a limited number of functions, may perform well in areas where a traditional LIS falls short. Opportunities for specialized LISs continue to evolve with the introduction of new testing methodologies. These systems may take many forms, including stand-alone architecture, a module integrated with an existing LIS, a separate vendor-supplied module, and customized software. This article addresses the concepts underlying specialized LISs, their characteristics, and in what settings they are found.

The main mission of a laboratory information system (LIS) is to manage workflow and deliver accurate results for clinical management. Successful selection and implementation of an anatomic pathology LIS is not complete unless it is complemented by specialized information technology support and maintenance. LIS is required to remain continuously operational with minimal or no downtime and the LIS team has to ensure that all operations are compliant with the mandated rules and regulations.

Many health care providers believe that the autopsy is no longer relevant in high-technology medicine era. This has fueled a decline in the hospital autopsy rate. Although it seems that advanced diagnostic tests answer all clinical questions, studies repeatedly demonstrate that an autopsy uncovers as many undiagnosed conditions today as in the past. The forensic autopsy rate has also declined, although not as precipitously. Pathologists are still performing a nineteenth century autopsy procedure that remains essentially unchanged. Informatics offers several potential answers that will evolve the low-tech autopsy into the high-tech autopsy.

The practice of surgical pathology is under constant pressure to deliver the highest quality of service, reduce errors, increase throughput, and decrease turnaround time while at the same time dealing with an aging workforce, increasing financial constraints, and economic uncertainty. Although not able to implement total laboratory automation, great progress continues to be made in workstation automation in all areas of the pathology laboratory. This report highlights the benefits and challenges of pathology automation, reviews middleware and its use to facilitate automation, and reviews the progress so far in the anatomic pathology laboratory.

Molecular informatics (MI) is an evolving discipline that will support the dynamic landscape of molecular pathology and personalized medicine. MI provides a fertile ground for development of clinical solutions to bridge the gap between clinical informatics and bioinformatics. Rapid adoption of next generation sequencing (NGS) in the clinical arena has triggered major endeavors in MI that are expected to bring a paradigm shift in the practice of pathology. This brief review presents a broad overview of various aspects of MI, particularly in the context of NGS based testing.

The underutilized practice of photographing anatomic pathology specimens from surgical pathology and autopsies is an invaluable benefit to patients, clinicians, pathologists, and students. Photographic documentation of clinical specimens is essential for the effective practice of pathology. When considering what specimens to photograph, all grossly evident pathology, absent yet expected pathologic features, and gross-only specimens should be thoroughly documented. Specimen preparation prior to photography includes proper lighting and background, wiping surfaces of blood, removing material such as tubes or bandages, orienting the specimen in a logical fashion, framing the specimen to fill the screen, positioning of probes, and using the right-sized scale.

Advanced imaging refers to direct microscopic imaging of tissue, without the need for traditional hematoxylin-eosin (H&E) microscopy, including microscope slides or whole-slide images. A detailed example is presented of optical coherence tomography (OCT), an imaging technique based on reflected light. Experience and example images are discussed in the larger context of the evolving relationship of surgical pathology to clinical patient care providers. Although these techniques are diagnostically promising, it is unlikely that they will directly supplant H&E histopathology. It is likely that OCT and related technologies will provide narrow, targeted diagnosis in a variety of in vivo (patient) and ex vivo (specimen) applications.

Telepathology is the practice of remote pathology using telecommunication links to enable the electronic transmission of digital pathology images. Telepathology can be used for remotely rendering primary diagnoses, second opinion consultations, quality assurance, education, and research purposes. The use of telepathology for clinical patient care has been limited mostly to large academic institutions. Barriers that have limited its widespread use include prohibitive costs, legal and regulatory issues, technologic drawbacks, resistance from pathologists, and above all a lack of universal standards. This article provides an overview of telepathology technology and applications.

Recent advances in hardware and computing power contained within mobile devices have made it possible to use these devices to improve and enhance pathologist workflow. This article discusses the possible uses ranging from basic functions to intermediate functions to advanced functions. Barriers to implementation are also discussed.

The single most important element to consider when evaluating clinical information systems for a practice is workflow. Workflow can be broadly defined as an orchestrated and repeatable pattern of business activity enabled by the systematic organization of resources into processes that transform materials, provide services, or process information.

This article provides surgical pathologists an overview of health information systems (HISs): what they are, what they do, and how such systems relate to the practice of surgical pathology. Much of this article is dedicated to the electronic medical record. Information, in how it is captured, transmitted, and conveyed, drives the effectiveness of such electronic medical record functionalities. So critical is information from pathology in integrated clinical care that surgical pathologists are becoming gatekeepers of not only tissue but also information. Better understanding of HISs can empower surgical pathologists to become stakeholders who have an impact on the future direction of quality integrated clinical care.

Translational bioinformatics and clinical research (biomedical) informatics are the primary domains related to informatics activities that support translational research. Translational bioinformatics focuses on computational techniques in genetics, molecular biology, and systems biology. Clinical research (biomedical) informatics involves the use of informatics in discovery and management of new knowledge relating to health and disease. This article details 3 projects that are hybrid applications of translational bioinformatics and clinical research (biomedical) informatics: The Cancer Genome Atlas, the cBioPortal for Cancer Genomics, and the Memorial Sloan Kettering Cancer Center clinical variants and results database, all designed to facilitate insights into cancer biology and clinical/therapeutic correlations.

This article presents an overview of the curriculum deemed essential for trainees in pathology, with mapping to the Milestones competency statements. The means by which these competencies desired for pathology graduates, and ultimately practitioners, can best be achieved is discussed. The value of case (problem)-based learning in this realm, in particular the kind of integrative experience associated with hands-on projects, to both cement knowledge gained in the lecture hall or online and to expand competency is emphasized.

Quality assurance encompasses monitoring daily processes for accurate, timely, and complete reports in surgical pathology. Quality assurance also includes implementation of policies and procedures that prevent or detect errors in a timely manner. This article presents uses of informatics in quality assurance. Three main foci are critical to the general improvement of diagnostic surgical pathology. First is the application of informatics to specimen identification with lean methods for real-time statistical control of specimen receipt and processing. Second is the development of case reviews before sign-out. Third is the development of information technology in communication of results to assure treatment in a timely manner.

SURGICAL PATHOLOGY CLINICS

RELATED INTEREST

Clinics in Laboratory Medicine
March 2015; Volume 35, Issue 1
Automated Hematology Analyzers: State of the Art
Carlo Brugnara and Alexander Kratz, *Editors*

THE CLINICS ARE AVAILABLE ONLINE!
Access your subscription at:
www.theclinics.com

Preface
Pathology Informatics

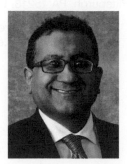

Anil V. Parwani, MD, PhD, MBA
Editor

Surgical pathology is a discipline that generates a spectrum of data, including text, images, and numbers, which contributes deeply to patient care either directly or via an interpretation from a pathologist who integrates the information to provide a diagnostic report. This is an exciting time in Pathology, particularly surgical pathology, as we are being confronted with a new frontier of knowledge base, which is impacting our diagnosis and even the morphologic assessment of surgical pathology entities.

Pathology informatics is a relatively new and emerging area of pathology focused on the acquisition, storage, analysis, and management of information. The data sources are multiple and may involve specialized technologies, nomenclature, and processes that are integral to the way information flows through pathology systems and into specialized output areas, such as the hospital information systems and other downstream systems. Tasks that a pathologist may perform, such as tissue examination and producing a pathology report, may rely on the processes crafted by an informatics-driven workflow. The art and science of surgical pathology is going through a transformation today as surgical pathologists are finding themselves integrating data from multiple sources and converting this into useful information, which in turn is contributing to knowledge that becomes instrumental in driving the care of a patient.

Pathology informatics is the first issue in the *Surgical Pathology Clinics* series that has been designed to provide an overview of specialized topics in pathology informatics that will be of interest to surgical pathologists either as an introduction to some key areas of this broad specialty, such as laboratory information systems, or as more in-depth review of some complex and newly emerging areas of pathology informatics, such as molecular pathology informatics. This is by no means a comprehensive textbook of pathology informatics but rather special topics to introduce the surgical pathologist to new technologies and information systems that impact or are going to impact the practice of surgical pathology. Each topic provides an overview of the topic with direct relevance to how this information may be used by the surgical pathologist. There are key illustrations with an emphasis on practical insights into the topic. Text is provided in a concise format for efficient use by the reader with a focus on pathology informatics as it relates to the practice of surgical pathology. References are collated at the end of the issue.

The vision for putting together the pathology informatics issue is that this text will serve both as an introduction to some emerging topics in the emerging and dynamic field of pathology informatics and as an up-to-date reference source for the practicing surgical pathologists as well as pathologists in training. The practice of surgical pathology is at this unique crossroads where

Surgical Pathology 8 (2015) xi–xii
http://dx.doi.org/10.1016/j.path.2015.04.001
1875-9181/15/$ – see front matter © 2015 Published by Elsevier Inc.

surgpath.theclinics.com

convergence of multiple knowledge domains is already occurring. A deep understanding of the information ecosystems and the workflow needed to accomplish the vital integration of various data points in compiling the next generation of surgical pathology report will be required for the surgical pathologist to remain in the forefront of the technology and information surge.

Anil V. Parwani, MD, PhD, MBA
Department of Pathology
University of Pittsburgh Medical Center
200 Lothrop Street
Pittsburgh, PA 15213, USA

E-mail address:
parwaniav@upmc.edu

Laboratory Information Systems

Walter H. Henricks, MD

KEYWORDS

- Laboratory information systems • Informatics • Laboratory operations • Laboratory management
- Computer systems • Pathology informatics • Workflow

ABSTRACT

Laboratory information systems (LISs) supply mission-critical capabilities for the vast array of information-processing needs of modern laboratories. LIS architectures include mainframe, client-server, and thin client configurations. The LIS database software manages a laboratory's data. LIS dictionaries are database tables that a laboratory uses to tailor an LIS to the unique needs of that laboratory. Anatomic pathology LIS (APLIS) functions play key roles throughout the pathology workflow, and laboratories rely on LIS management reports to monitor operations. This article describes the structure and functions of APLISs, with emphasis on their roles in laboratory operations and their relevance to pathologists.

OVERVIEW TO LABORATORY INFORMATION SYSTEMS

Pathologists and pathology laboratories depend on laboratory information systems (LISs) to support their operations and, ultimately, to carry out their patient care mission. Over the past few decades,[1,2] LISs have evolved from relatively narrow, often arcane, and/or home-grown systems into sophisticated systems that are more user-friendly and support a broader range of functions and integration with other technologies that laboratories deploy.

Modern LISs consist of complex, interrelated computer programs and infrastructure that support a vast array of information-processing needs of laboratories. LISs have functions in all phases of patient testing, including specimen and test order intake, specimen processing and tracking, support of analysis and interpretation, and report creation and distribution. In addition, LISs provide management reports and other data that laboratories need to run their operations and to support continuous improvement and quality initiatives.

This article describes the structure and functions of anatomic pathology LISs (APLISs), with emphasis on their roles in laboratory operations and their relevance to pathologists.

ELEMENTS OF LABORATORY INFORMATION SYSTEMS

LABORATORY INFORMATION SYSTEM INFRASTRUCTURE

LISs have a foundation of technical infrastructure. Such infrastructure consists in aggregate of hardware and related dedicated software that enable the LIS to carry out its functions (Box 1). Software is computer programming that consists of instructions for the components of the computer system to perform.

Servers are computers that house the main elements of the LIS software, including its main database (see later in this article). Servers provide, or "serve," LIS functions to system users and/or other processes (eg, printers) that request them. Servers can accommodate simultaneous access by multiple users in a networked system environment. An LIS may use one or more servers, and some servers may be dedicated to specific functions like managing communications with other systems (ie, interfaces).

LIS users (sometimes referred to as "end-users") in the laboratory gain access to the LIS through end-user devices, most commonly

---

The author has no competing financial interests to disclose.

Center for Pathology Informatics, Pathology and Laboratory Medicine Institute, Cleveland Clinic, L21, 9500 Euclid Avenue, Cleveland, OH 44195, USA

E-mail address: henricw@ccf.org

Surgical Pathology 8 (2015) 101–108

http://dx.doi.org/10.1016/j.path.2015.02.016

Box 1
Laboratory information system (LIS) infrastructure components

- Servers
- End-user devices: desktop PCs
- Monitors
- Printers: paper and label
- Scanners
- Networks

desktop computers (in this article generically referred to as PCs for personal computer). In a client-server environment (see later in this article), these devices are referred to as *client* devices. Use of LISs on other client devices, such as tablets and smartphones, is emerging as well.[3,4]

LISs require the use of networking technologies for connections among the LIS infrastructure components. Networks consist of physical media and related engineering software that together enable electronic data exchange. Networks in an LIS may include copper (Ethernet), fiber optics, wireless, and/or other media. The network to which an LIS is connected within an organization typically can gain access to the worldwide network of the Internet by way of an organization's gateway to external networks.

LISs also connect to various peripheral devices to execute certain functions. Computer display monitors are an obvious requirement at an end-user PC. The specification requirements for display monitors are getting increasing attention with the advent of whole slide imaging techniques and virtual microscopy, that bring with them need for higher-resolution displays.[5] Printers are necessary

for printing reports, and label printers of different form factors print labels for slides, specimen containers, and other assets. Digital scanners enable the capture of hard copy elements, such as paper requisitions or insurance information, into an LIS.

LABORATORY INFORMATION SYSTEM ARCHITECTURE

LIS architecture affects users' LIS experience. The *architecture* of an LIS refers to the model of how the hardware and software components function together to deliver LIS functions. LIS architecture defines the allocation of computing power among system components. LISs are commonly deployed as some variant of *client-server* architecture (**Fig. 1**). In client-server, end-users invoke LIS functions on their "client" devices. The functions go to servers as requests for services, for example editing a report, electronic sign out, data entry, or accessioning a case. Clients and servers work together to perform system functions, and computing resources and power are "distributed" in this manner.

Although older, the *mainframe*, or host-based, architecture exists in some LISs (**Fig. 2**). Mainframe set ups differ from client-server in that computing resources are centralized to a much greater degree on a single powerful computer ("mainframe"). The mainframe, or host, manages all LIS functions. Instead of using computing devices with software, end-users interact with the system using so-called "dumb" terminals that function only for data input and display functions.

Many laboratories now benefit from use of *thin client* LIS architecture (**Fig. 3**). In the thin client model, LIS client software is centralized onto a thin client-server, and end-users interact with the LIS by using client software that performs only

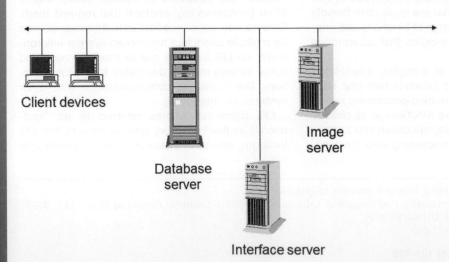

Fig. 1. Client-server LIS architecture.

Client devices

Database server

Interface server

Image server

Fig. **2.** Mainframe LIS architecture.

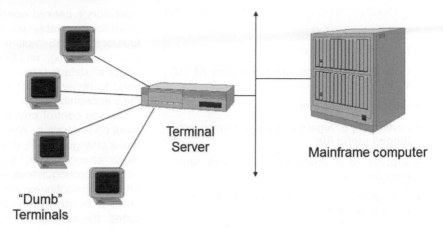

Terminal Server

Mainframe computer

"Dumb" Terminals

simple functions (= "thin" client) for communicating with the thin client-server. The benefits for laboratories of using thin client in an LIS are listed in **Box 2**. In short, thin client architecture greatly facilitates system administration by standardizing the client software available to users and because client software updates need only occur on the thin client-server(s) instead of on all individual PCs. Laboratories should be aware, however, that using thin client may incur additional license costs, and not all LIS functions may be available to users who access the LIS via thin client. For example, speech-to-text recognition or digital image capture into the LIS may not be possible using a thin client to access the system.

In what can be thought of as an extension of the thin client model, hospitals and laboratories are increasingly choosing to implement LISs based on software-as-a-service (SaaS) arrangement with an LIS vendor. These models are also referred to application service provider and "in the cloud." In these settings, a laboratory contracts with a vendor to provide an LIS application over secure network or Internet connections with the system that the vendor maintains at a remote location.

An SaaS arrangement offers laboratories benefits that include a lower cost of acquisition and the outsourcing of infrastructure and software maintenance and upgrades. On the other hand, the laboratory is reliant on the vendor to maintain high availability of the system, and the options for configuration or customization of LIS functions may be limited.

THE HEART OF AN LABORATORY INFORMATION SYSTEM: DICTIONARY TABLES AND DEFINITIONS

An LIS is at its core a database, and data are typically organized into tables or files that relate to one another based on system logic. Databases are described in detail in the article by Parwani elsewhere in this issue. Operating within the LIS, a database management system controls the access, organization, storage, management, retrieval, and integrity of data that reside in the LIS database. Broadly speaking, LIS tables are of 2 types: *record tables* and *maintenance tables*. Record tables consist of data generated during the

Fig. **3.** Thin client LIS architecture.

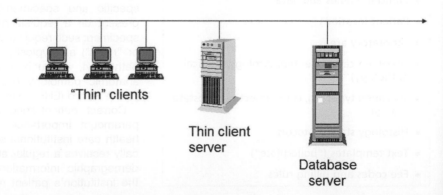

"Thin" clients

Thin client server

Database server

course of using the system for patient care activities, ranging from daily logs to long-term archive of pathology reports. Maintenance tables define and keep track of information about the system is configured, including data definitions and internal system operations.

LIS *dictionaries* are the maintenance tables in the LIS that determine and store the data definitions, terminology, naming conventions, report content and format, and other configurations for the laboratory. These definitions ultimately determine workflow and processes in the laboratory. The typical LIS contains dozens of dictionaries. Examples of important dictionaries in an APLIS are listed in **Box 3**.

LIS dictionary definitions tailor the LIS to the unique needs and expectations of an individual laboratory. Definition building requires planning, allocation of resources, and understanding of the

laboratory's desired operations. Careful attention to establishing table definitions in the LIS is crucial to successful LIS implementation and smooth operations. Although an LIS may have some "out-of-the-box" default table entries, the laboratory will need to review default entries carefully to determine acceptability.

Change control processes for LIS dictionaries merit consideration. When a laboratory desires to make changes to LIS definitions, even seemingly minor changes can lead to unintended and/or negative consequences. For example, when a laboratory discontinues use of a particular special stain, if dictionary entries are not properly updated, the stain code may remain embedded in some histology stain-ordering protocols and appear to be requested of the laboratory. This example also illustrates the important point that some dictionary entries are linked to entries in other tables or definitions and that knowledge of these relationships is important in managing changes.

FEATURES OF ANATOMIC PATHOLOGY LABORATORY INFORMATION SYSTEMS AND THEIR ROLES IN LABORATORY OPERATIONS

The APLIS has numerous "touch points" in pathology laboratory workflow throughout the specimen analysis and interpretation cycle. The following subsections describe roles of the LIS functions and data elements in preanalytic, analytical, and postanalytic phases of testing in the surgical pathology laboratory. Generally, these processes correspond to functional modules in the LIS that link to one another.

SPECIMEN INTAKE AND ACCESSIONING

On receipt of a specimen in the laboratory, the first step in processing is to register, or to "accession" the specimen into the LIS. This is the point at which the LIS first "learns" of the existence of the new specimen. Laboratory personnel enter patient-specific and specimen-specific data that are present on a requisition that accompanies the specimen; such requisitions (or test request forms, or "req's") are typically hard copy (in anatomic pathology), although electronic transmission of anatomic pathology orders from an electronic health record (EHR) to the LIS are possible.[6]

Correct patient-specimen identification is of paramount importance when accessioning. In health care institutional settings, the APLIS typically receives a regular electronic feed of patient demographic information via an interface with the institution's patient registration/management system. These "ADT" (admission-discharge-transfer) interfaces supply the LIS with data that (depending on the circumstances) include patient names, medical record numbers, gender, data of birth, location, physician, insurance, and others. An ADT feed enables laboratory users to select and to pull into the LIS all the necessary demographic data after entering only a name or medical record number. This process reduces the risk of patient misidentification or selection of the incorrect patient. In settings without an ADT feed to the LIS, new patient demographic records must be created in the LIS for patients not seen previously.

The other data elements entered during accessioning are typically a mixture of free-text entries and selection from dictionary entries defined for a particular data field. For example, the user will select a submitting physician from choices displayed from entries defined in the LIS Physician Dictionary. Other data elements that are commonly captured at accessioning are listed in **Box 4**. Additionally, dictionary elements, such as orders for histology protocols and default fee codes, can attach to the case (or part) automatically based on rules and linkages to specimen types that the laboratory defines in the LIS.

The outcome of the accessioning process is the LIS assigning a unique LIS accession number (case number) to the case. The LIS updates the

---

Box 4
Data elements entered into APLIS at time of case accessioning

- Patient identification number
- Patient name and other identifying information
- Specimen type[a] (eg, colon biopsy)
- Specimen description (eg, mass in gastric body)
- Submitting physician[a]
- "Copy to" physician(s)[a]
- Patient location[a] and/or client location[a]
- Date of procedure
- Date of receipt
- Pathologist assigned[a]
- Clinical history
- Histology protocols linked to specimen type[a]

[a] Indicates that entry is selected based on LIS dictionary entries.

---

specimen status to "accessioned" (or something analogous). Accession numbers are typically a combination of letters and numbers, and a laboratory may define various "number wheels" in the LIS to distinguish different categories of specimens (eg, by originating location, HS-15-123, CS-15-123). The LIS assigns a single accession number to cases that have multiple individual specimen parts (eg, multiple prostate needle biopsies). This capability keeps the case cohesive and enables a single report for multispecimen cases. By contrast, clinical laboratory LISs typically assign a unique number to each individual specimen container (eg, blood tubes), and a separate result is provided for multiple tests ordered on the specimen.

GROSS SPECIMEN PROCESSING AND SECTIONING ("GROSSING")

The gross processing phase begins with generation of a gross description of the specimen and ends with submission and designation of sections for histologic slide preparation. Users enter gross descriptions into the gross description field in the LIS. Defining specimen type-specific boilerplate, template text entries in LIS dictionaries can facilitate text entry. Many LISs also incorporate or accommodate speech-to-text ("voice recognition") entry, which can reduce reliance on transcription and speed processing.[7] Sections selected for histology designated in the gross description follow the laboratory-defined numbering scheme in the LIS for specimen parts and tissue blocks (eg, A1, A2, B1, B2). At the completion of sectioning, the prosector or other processor creates discrete entries in the designated tissue sections/blocks in the histology module (or similar), in preparation for the next steps. At the end of the grossing process and entries, the case status in the LIS can be updated to "Gross Complete," or something similar.

To optimize specimen identification and *specimen tracking*, a pathology laboratory may deploy an electronic interface between the LIS and cassette engravers that label the cassettes into which prosectors place tissue sections. Such interfaces establish a link between the asset (tissue cassette/block) and the LIS to improve specimen identification and tracking.[8] Data engraved on cassettes may include bar codes, particularly 2-dimensional bar codes, which increase data available to the LIS and other systems compatible with the bar code(s). Radiofrequency identification technologies hold promise as a future method for asset tracking once barriers of cost and system integration have been overcome.[9,10]

HISTOLOGY PROCESSING AND SLIDE CREATION

Histology laboratory processing begins with tissue fixation and preparation of tissue blocks and ends with creation of glass slides with stained tissue sections. Throughout this phase of processing, the LIS tracks and organizes the workflow in the laboratory, largely through the use of histology logs and histology protocols. The LIS logs are essentially lists of the specimens that a particular bench or area of the laboratory will process for an upcoming specified period of time (eg, work shift). The specimen data on the logs corresponds to data entered "upstream," for instance the tissue cassettes designated as submitted in the grossing phase. LIS histology logs often in use include embedding logs, routine histology logs, special stain request logs, and immunohistochemistry logs. A laboratory can configure the format of the logs and the data to be displayed, or may choose the system's default configurations. Data elements in histology logs typically include accession number, date/time stamp, patient and specimen data, histology protocol(s) ordered, other stains ordered, and comments about the specimen or the request.

Histology protocols are LIS dictionary entries that define the number of slides/levels, histologic stains, and other instructions for processing. For routine workflow (particularly for biopsies), these protocols often attach to the specimen part automatically during the accessioning process (see earlier in this article) and appear on logs that the LIS automatically prints at laboratory-defined intervals. For add-on stains, users order stains, protocols, or batteries of stains in the LIS by selecting from dictionary entries provided in the stain-ordering function. These protocol orders then appear on the corresponding log for the laboratory.

An LIS may support individual slide tracking.[8] At microtomy stations, a laboratory may deploy a combination of barcode scanners and slide labelers/engravers to enable histotechnologists to track each block and slide and to ensure concordance of identification between individual block and slide labels. These functions depend on connections with the LIS for data exchange and comparisons. LISs typically offer at least some capability for the laboratory to determine the format and content of its slide labels.

Pathologist Interpretation and Final Report Generation and Distribution

For each case, a "working draft" report in the LIS provides the pathologist with information about the case and processing up to the point that he or she has received the slides. The laboratory may choose to provide hard copies of working drafts, printed in batch mode and collated with the slides for each case, or pathologists may access working drafts paperlessly in the LIS. The laboratory can configure the format and content of working drafts in the LIS. Working drafts typically include gross description, including sections submitted, clinical information, frozen section results (as applicable), default fee codes, and data about the patient's previous pathology specimens available in the LIS.

Pathologists, or designees such as transcriptionists, enter pathologic diagnosis and, as applicable, descriptive comments and microscopic description, into the relevant data fields in the LIS. To facilitate entry of diagnosis text, an LIS may include capabilities such as speech-to-text conversion ("voice recognition")[7,11,12] and creation of predefined templates, checklists, and formats. Default codes for billing (Current Procedural Terminology) and/or diagnosis (International Classification of Diseases) codes linked to specimen type definitions may auto-populate into final reports.

Final diagnosis data fields in LISs are typically entered and stored as text "blobs" that are not further structured in the database. Even if a report template enables display of report content in a structured manner (eg, as a checklist or "synoptic" report), such display alone does not correspond to structure with discrete data elements in the underlying database. Some LISs and third-party solutions offer so-called true "synoptic" modules that enable report data entry and storage as discrete data elements,[13,14] which are then amenable to more effective criteria-based database query and analysis. Synoptic reporting is covered more extensively in the article by Parwani elsewhere in this issue.

Once a report is finalized, the LIS supports distribution of the reports, whether electronic or hard copy. A pathologist finalizes a report (ie, "signs out" a case) by entering an electronic signature (or by otherwise marking it as final if manual signatures are used), which locks the case in the database. For certain types of reports, or for certain physician groups, a laboratory may need to fax or to print remotely hard copies, and the LIS sends these reports based on rules and definitions (eg, recipient fax number). If there is an LIS-EHR interface for results, finalizing a report triggers transmission of the report to the EHR.

In EHRs, the screen design and formatting dictates the quality and readability of the display of interfaced pathology reports. Sometimes reports may appear quite different in the EHR compared with the LIS, with potential for misinterpretation.[15,16] An LIS may be able to provide interfaced electronic reports that preserve formatting (eg, portable document format, PDF), and if the receiving system can accommodate such reports, this may be a mechanism for improving readability.

Report Amendments and Addenda

LISs accommodate amended reports and report addenda through similar though not identical ways. Once an electronic signature is affixed to a report in the LIS, the report cannot be changed without creating an amendment, or amended report. If a report is changed or corrected, the LIS automatically marks the amended case as such in the database and automatically labels any new reports generated from the case as amended reports. An LIS may have the capability to categorize and to display the reasons for the amendment. An addendum report is created in the LIS in cases when new information, such as special stain results, is added to a previously finalized report. Addenda do not involve changing any information in the original report. Pathologists finalize amended and addended reports with a new electronic signature.

In the setting of an LIS-EHR interface, the amended report replaces and overlays the original report in the EHR. The same may be true for addenda, but depending on the setting, addenda may be appended to cases without completely overlaying the previous. Laboratories may have to ensure that amended or addended status is obvious in the format and display of reports in the LIS and the EHR. Audit trail functions ensure that original reports are accessible in the LIS and the EHR.

THE LABORATORY INFORMATION SYSTEM AND LABORATORY ADMINISTRATION

In addition to the capabilities necessary for daily operations and patient care in the laboratory, the LIS offers functions that support management and leadership activities in the laboratory. Laboratories rely on *management reports* from the LIS for data that reflect status of operations, laboratory performance, metrics, and maintenance. **Box 5** lists common categories of management reports in an APLIS. Laboratories will typically have options of using management reports that are predefined in the LIS, modifying predefined reports, or creating their own LIS management reports. LISs accommodate scheduling of management reports to fire off automatically at defined times or intervals (eg, every morning), and laboratory personnel can run reports on an ad hoc basis.

> **Box 5**
> **Categories of common management reports in an APLIS**
>
> - Turnaround time (TAT)
> - Cases not signed out (ie, pending case logs)
> - Volumes of specimens, blocks, slides
> - Utilization (eg, special stains)
> - Billing reports
> - Interface error logs

LISs provide for quality management activities beyond management reports. A laboratory may be able to configure its LIS to select cases automatically and randomly for secondary quality assurance review and assign to a second pathologist.[17] In residency training programs, LISs can track aspects of resident performance. Gynecologic cytopathology has multiple quality and regulatory requirements that LISs often have tools to facilitate.

LISs have tools for database queries. Although management reports are a type of database query, laboratories often need to conduct database searches based on criteria tailored to a specific question or need. Common examples are case finding for validation or development of stains in the laboratory, quality reviews, and investigative research. Efficacy of database searches in an LIS depends on the structure of underlying data (ie, discrete data elements vs unstructured text) and on the LIS tools available to define queries. More on database structures and data elements can be found in the articles by Parwani and Amin elsewhere in this issue.

ADVANCED FEATURES AND FUNCTIONS IN LABORATORY INFORMATION SYSTEMS

LISs now incorporate multiple features that were either unavailable or that not long ago required custom development.[18] Recently, the Association for Pathology Informatics created and published a detailed listing of basic and advanced LIS features as part of a toolkit to assess LIS capabilities.[19] Several such capabilities (speech-to-text conversion ["voice recognition"], barcoding, specimen/block/slide tracking, engraver interfaces) have been described in their context of laboratory operations in earlier sections of this article. LISs now routinely possess capabilities to store digital images linked to cases. With the increasing acceptance of whole slide imaging (WSI) for clinical purposes,[20,21] capabilities for interfaces or integration between WSI systems and LIS will likely increase. Various aspects of imaging in pathology are covered in other articles of this text.

With respect to further advances, future LISs are expected to have more sophisticated tools to support data mining and pathologists' analysis of pathology and clinical data sets.[22] Some experts believe that the LIS will evolve into multimodality pathologist "cockpits" that combine pathology imaging, access to clinical data (eg, EHR) and other data sources, LIS functions, and analytical tools.[23] As applications for molecular genetic pathology testing, including next generation sequencing, on pathology specimens continue to emerge, further innovation in LISs will be necessary to report and to correlate such data in concert with traditional pathologic findings in ways that are optimal for patient care.[24]

REFERENCES

1. Elevitch FR, Aller RD. The ABCs of LIS: computerizing your laboratory information system. Chicago: ASCP Press; 1989.
2. Carter AB, McKnight RM, Henricks WH, et al. Pathology informatics: an introduction. In: Pantanowitz L, Tuthill JM, Balis UJ, editors. Pathology informatics: theory and practice. Chicago: ASCP Press; 2012. p. 1–10.
3. Park S, Parwani A, Satyanarayanan M, et al. Handheld computing in pathology. J Pathol Inform 2012; 3:15.
4. Hartman DJ, Parwani AV, Cable B, et al. Pocket pathologist: a mobile application for rapid diagnostic surgical pathology consultation. J Pathol Inform 2014;5:10.
5. Krupinski EA. Virtual slide telepathology workstation of the future: lessons learned from teleradiology. Hum Pathol 2009;40(8):1100–11.
6. Georgiou A, Westbrook J, Braithwaite J. Computerized provider order entry systems: research imperatives and organizational challenges facing pathology services. J Pathol Inform 2010;1:11.
7. Henricks WH, Roumina K, Skilton BE, et al. The utility and cost effectiveness of voice recognition technology in surgical pathology. Mod Pathol 2002;15(5): 565–71.
8. Pantanowitz L, Mackinnon AC Jr, Sinard JH. Tracking in anatomic pathology. Arch Pathol Lab Med 2013;137(12):1798–810.
9. Leung AA, Lou JJ, Mareninov S, et al. Tolerance testing of passive radio frequency identification tags for solvent, temperature, and pressure conditions encountered in an anatomic pathology or biorepository setting. J Pathol Inform 2010;1:21.
10. Bostwick DG. Radiofrequency identification specimen tracking in anatomical pathology: pilot study of 1067 consecutive prostate biopsies. Ann Diagn Pathol 2013;17(5):391–402.
11. Kang HP, Sirintrapun SJ, Nestler RJ, et al. Experience with voice recognition in surgical pathology at a large academic multi-institutional center. Am J Clin Pathol 2010;133(1):156–9.
12. Singh M, Pal TR. Voice recognition technology implementation in surgical pathology: advantages and limitations. Arch Pathol Lab Med 2011;135(11):1476–81.
13. Kang HP, Devine LJ, Piccoli AL, et al. Usefulness of a synoptic data tool for reporting of head and neck neoplasms based on the College of American Pathologists cancer checklists. Am J Clin Pathol 2009;132(4):521–30.
14. Hassell LA, Parwani AV, Weiss L, et al. Challenges and opportunities in the adoption of College of American Pathologists checklists in electronic format: perspectives and experience of Reporting Pathology Protocols Project (RPP2) participant laboratories. Arch Pathol Lab Med 2010;134(8):1152–9.
15. Valenstein PN. Formatting pathology reports: applying four design principles to improve communication and patient safety. Arch Pathol Lab Med 2008;132(1):84–94.
16. Wilkerson ML, Henricks WH, Castellani WJ, et al. Management of laboratory information in the electronic health record. Arch Pathol Lab Med 2015; 139(3):319–27.
17. Owens SR, Dhir R, Yousem SA, et al. The development and testing of a laboratory information system-driven tool for pre-sign-out quality assurance of random surgical pathology reports. Am J Clin Pathol 2010;133(6):836–41.
18. Sinard JH, Gershkovich P. Custom software development for use in a clinical laboratory. J Pathol Inform 2012;3:44.
19. Tuthill JM, Friedman BA, Balis UJ, et al. The laboratory information system functionality assessment tool: ensuring optimal software support for your laboratory. J Pathol Inform 2014;5:7.
20. Pantanowitz L, Sinard JH, Henricks WH, et al, College of American Pathologists Pathology and Laboratory Quality Center. Validating whole slide imaging for diagnostic purposes in pathology: guideline from the College of American Pathologists Pathology and Laboratory Quality Center. Arch Pathol Lab Med 2013;137(12):1710–22.
21. Bauer TW, Schoenfield L, Slaw RJ, et al. Validation of whole slide imaging for primary diagnosis in surgical pathology. Arch Pathol Lab Med 2013;137(4):518–24.
22. Sepulveda JL, Young DS. The ideal laboratory information system. Arch Pathol Lab Med 2013;137(8): 1129–40.
23. Krupinski EA. Optimizing the pathology workstation "cockpit": challenges and solutions. J Pathol Inform 2010;1:19.
24. Gu J, Taylor CR. Practicing pathology in the era of big data and personalized medicine. Appl Immunohistochem Mol Morphol 2014;22(1):1–9.

Data Representation, Coding, and Communication Standards

Milon Amin, MD[a],*, Rajiv Dhir, MBBS, MBA[b]

KEYWORDS

• *ICD-10* • *CPT* • Standards • Pathology • Coding • Informatics

ABSTRACT

The immense volume of cases signed out by surgical pathologists on a daily basis gives little time to think about exactly how data are stored. An understanding of the basics of data representation has implications that affect a pathologist's daily practice. This article covers the basics of data representation and its importance in the design of electronic medical record systems. Coding in surgical pathology is also discussed. Finally, a summary of communication standards in surgical pathology is presented, including suggested resources that establish standards for select aspects of pathology reporting.

DATA REPRESENTATION: IT'S JUST A BUNCH OF WORDS, RIGHT?

The immense volume of cases signed out by surgical pathologists on a daily basis gives little time to think about exactly how these data are stored. Yet, an understanding of the basics of data representation has implications that affect a pathologist's daily practice.

DATA REPRESENTATION IN A PARAGRAPH: EVERYTHING COMES FROM BYTES

As reported by Sinard,[1] all data are stored in binary form; the fundamental unit of data is the byte, which can be "on" (1) or "off" (0). Eight bytes form a bit, and combinations of bytes that are on or off (ie, 00010001 or 10110010) are used to represent integers. Because each integer between 0 and 128 can represent letters and punctuation based on the American Standard Code for Information Exchange (ASCII), numerous possibilities emerge. Moreover, as bits are stacked (ie, 8-bit, 16-bit, and 32-bit), many combinations of off and on positions are possible, representing many possible forms of data (**Fig. 1**). Software, also created from these data, decodes these bits and bytes into something that pathologists can understand. While pathologists usually do not need to understand this decoding step in practice, the challenges in this step – a fundamental step – can generate frustration between pathologists and information technology (IT) departments, if IT members are not clear on what the pathologist needs to see and accomplish in his/her workflow.

DATA REPRESENTATION, VARIABLES, AND PATHOLOGY REPORTS: TOO IMPORTANT TO BE AN AFTERTHOUGHT

Variables are an important part of data representation and storage; they can be analogized as "containers" for information (**Fig. 2**). In pathology reports, there are variables for a patient's name, date of birth, paraffin blocks, gross description, final diagnosis, and so forth. A pathology report, however, is also a variable in itself, stored in a "database" of similar variables. Most importantly, how these variables are organized can optimize (or jeopardize) a physician's workflow. For example, Jackson describes[2] a case in which an abnormal pathology result was hidden in the

Disclosure statement: No disclosures.
[a] Affiliated Pathologists Medical Group, 19951 Mariner Avenue Suite 155, Torrance, CA 90503, USA;
[b] Department of Pathology, University of Pittsburgh Medical Center Shadyside Hospital, 5230 Centre Avenue, Room WG 02.6, Pittsburgh, PA 15232, USA
* Corresponding author.
E-mail address: milon.amin@outlook.com

surgpath.theclinics.com

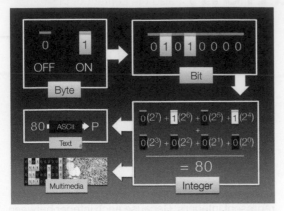

Fig. 1. The fundamental unit of data: the byte. Bytes are units of data with off (0) and on (1) positions; 8 bytes combine to form a bit. Combinations of bits are used to represent integers, text, and virtually limitless other types of data.

comments section of an electronic medical record (EMR) and initially missed by the clinician, who had to click around to finally locate the desired result. When revisiting the analogy of containers and variables, the abnormal result was likely accessible to pathologists in their laboratory information system (LIS); however, when transmitted to different EMRs for clinicians to access, it was sent to an inappropriately labeled (and less easily accessible) container. Sadly, such findings are not unexpected for EMRs catering to clinical services; developers of such records may think of pathology results as an afterthought, hence may not design organized

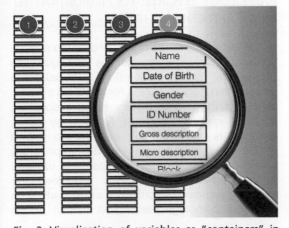

Fig. 2. Visualization of variables as "containers" in data storage. Pathology software may contain arrays of pathology reports. Each report, in turn, contains myriad variables to store information. When transferring reports to another information system, whether the other information system has "the same containers" must be considered. Information systems that follow standards, such as HL7, can transmit and accept these variables more easily.

and easily visible containers to hold such data (after they are transferred from pathologists' LIS). Thus, pathologists' input in the design of such EMRs, as well as interfaces between these EMRs, is crucial to ensure that data are properly represented.

Hernandez and Allen[3] emphasize the role of pathologists as leaders in transforming "raw data" into "meaningful information." This role prompts questions, such as, "Exactly how do I want to convey my points to the clinician?" "Do I just use words and numbers?" and "Do I want a table to show my immunohistochemical findings or a figure to depict prostate biopsy results?" Such questions prompted Sperberg-McQueen and Dubin's[4] review of 2 major types of data representation—analog and digital, which is different from the term *digital* most are accustomed to. In this case, they refer to *analog* data representation as a model that resembles physical properties as closely as possible, such as bar graphs/tables to represent numbers or colors to represent grading of dysplasia; conversely, *digital* data representation represents purely symbolic forms, such as actual numbers or text.[4] Examples are shown in **Fig. 3**. In particular, because standardized codes, such as ASCII, exist, it is much easier to transmit digital forms of data representation between EMRs, as opposed to analog forms. Given that clinicians are increasingly expecting laboratory results to interface with their currently available/implemented EMRs, the decision by a pathology laboratory to incorporate more analog forms of reports, although visually pleasing, may invoke more challenges in delivering information electronically to other EMR systems. Even seemingly simple items like a table of immunostains in Microsoft Word does not display properly in EMRs unless those EMRs are programmed to handle such elements. Such is one of many examples depicting the challenges of data representation in surgical pathology.

CODING IN SURGICAL PATHOLOGY: A DUTY TO DOCUMENT DUTIES

Regardless of the number of diagnoses made and cases signed out, medical coding is required to actually document pathology services in a way other departments understand. The use of codes, such as *Current Procedural Terminology* (*CPT*) and *International Classification of Diseases* (*ICD*), summarizes many services and diagnoses as simplified alphanumeric codes, which are interpreted by other parties (eg, researchers and billing departments). The use of such codes is mandated under the US Health Insurance Portability and Accountability Act.[5]

Summary of Findings

Carcinoma Biopsy Sites (containers A C D F): **right base lateral (1 of 2 cores); 58%; total 29%; CA length .7 cm); right apex lateral (1 of 2 cores; 45% 85%; total 67%; CA length 1.6 cm); right mid (1 core; 5%; CA length .07 cm); left mid lateral (2 of 2 cores; 25% 75%; total 45%; CA length .9 cm). No evidence of perineural or vascular invasion. The Gleason Score is 3+4=7.** Carcinoma confirmed with HMW cytokeratin.

Benign Biopsy Sites (no atypia, PIN or carcinoma; containers B E G H): right mid lateral; left base lateral; left apex lateral; left mid.

Clinical Information: stage by DRE is T1b; PSA is 8.
Indication for Biopsy: elevated PSA.

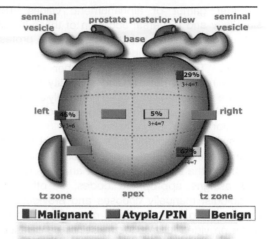

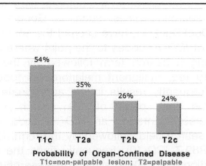

Partin Table: Organ Confined Disease

Probability of Organ-Confined Disease
T1c=non-palpable lesion; T2=palpable

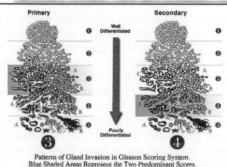

Gleason Score 3 + 4 = 7

Patterns of Gland Invasion in Gleason Scoring System.
Blue Shaded Areas Represent the Two Predominant Scores.

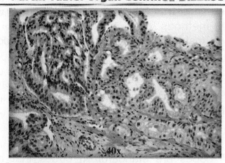

Low Power, Prostate
variably sized glands infiltrate the stroma

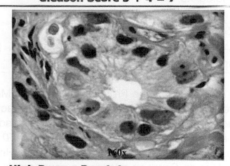

High Power, Prostate
Core biopsy, low power view; nuclei contain prominent nucleoli.

Fig. 3. Example of surgical pathology report with "analog" and "digital" data representation. ASCII characters (ie, numbers and text) represent digital data representation, whereas the prostate biopsy maps and bar graphs represent analog data representation. The decision to use either form (or both forms) of data representation may depend on what types of data a clinician's medical record system can accept and display properly without distortion. (Reproduced with permission from of Eric Glassy, MD, Pathology Inc, Torrance, CA.)

THE *INTERNATIONAL CLASSIFICATION OF DISEASES* AND ITS RELATION TO SURGICAL PATHOLOGY

According to the World Health Organization (WHO), *ICD* is the standard diagnostic tool for epidemiology, health management, and clinical purposes.[6] For any rendered diagnosis, the closest corresponding *ICD* code is also rendered. *ICD, Ninth Revision (ICD-9),* codes consist of numeric values; *International Classification of Diseases, Tenth Revision (ICD-10)* codes consist of a wider gamut of alphanumeric values. The simplicity and universal adoption of these codes allow global sharing between health care professionals, laboratories, insurance companies, and the like. They allow WHO member states to compile national mortality and morbidity statistics; they are also extensively used nationally and internationally to guide reimbursement and resource allocation.[6]

In surgical pathology, ICD codes must be provided with each final diagnosis report.[7] In some institutions, the billing department analyzes reports and assigns appropriate codes; in others, a pathologist manually chooses and provides ICD codes during final diagnosis entry. The pathologist's provided ICD codes must not be confused with the clinical ICD code, which may be listed on the surgical pathology requisition. Given that pathologists are physicians, a pathologist-assigned ICD code must be given on the basis of the pathologist's diagnosis.[8] Sometimes, this may not match the clinician-provided ICD code: an example is if a clinician submits an upper extremity skin lesion (ICD-10 code L98.9: disorder of skin, unspecified) and a pathologist diagnoses basal cell carcinoma (ICD-10 C44.61: basal cell carcinoma of skin of upper limb). Such situations necessitate knowledge of ICD codes by pathologists.

PASSING THE BATON: MANDATED TRANSITION FROM ICD-9 CODES TO ICD-10 CODES

On April 1, 2014, the Protecting Access to Medicare Act of 2014 (Pub L No. 113–93) was enacted, which delayed the originally scheduled deadline for all health care practices to adopt ICD-10 codes.[9] Accordingly, the US Department of Health and Human Services released a new compliance date (October 1, 2015) by which all clinical services should use ICD-10 codes. ICD-9 codes will remain for several years after this date, so knowledge of both ICD-9 and ICD-10 terminology is strongly encouraged.[10] Moreover, ICD, Eleventh Revision, codes have been developed for adoption at a future time.[6] This section focuses on ICD-10 codes.

THE INTERNATIONAL CLASSIFICATION OF DISEASE, TENTH REVISION, CODING SYSTEM: FINDING A WAY THROUGH

As discussed previously, ICD-10 codes consist of letters and numbers, whereas ICD-9 codes consist of only numbers and decimals. ICD-10 codes also cover approximately 10 times more medical conditions than ICD-9 codes. General categories of ICD-10 codes are summarized in **Table 1**. If a pathologist renders a descriptive diagnosis that may not be specific for a single entity, some ICD-10 codes may still be provided depending on the histologic context; examples of such instances are in **Table 2**. The entire list of ICD-9 and ICD-10 codes is detailed; it may be frustrating for a pathologist to search a coding manual for appropriate ICD-10 codes to match a final diagnosis. Fortunately, several ICD-10 code databases are available on-line and free of charge (at the time of this writing). Examples of such on-line databases, as well as mobile device applications, are listed in **Table 3**. Moreover, in the authors' experiences, Web search engines, such as Google, Bing, and DuckDuckGo, have cached the entire database of ICD-10 codes to the point where simply entering a search term followed by the term, ICD-10 (eg, malignant melanoma of foot ICD-10), frequently results in the appropriate code on the first page of the search results. Conversely, entering an ICD-10 code in the Web search field, followed by the term, ICD-10 (eg, R89.7 ICD-10), frequently finds the corresponding entity. One caveat is that search results may point to earlier revisions of ICD-10 databases (eg, from the year 2010); nonetheless, such methods can provide pathologists with nearly instant search results for ICD-10 codes and their entities.

CURRENT PROCEDURAL TERMINOLOGY: DOCUMENTATION OF PATHOLOGISTS' SERVICES

CPT codes are standardized codes that allow health care providers, including pathologist services, to request payment for procedures and services rendered to patients. The CPT coding manual is owned by the American Medical Association.[11] Essentially, CPT codes are 5-digit numeric codes representing all clinical procedures; a subset of these codes has modifiers that may increase the code to 7 digits. Most codes pertaining to surgical pathologists' services are between 88300 and 88399.

A comprehensive and regularly updated resource specifically for CPT coding in pathology is the American Pathology Foundation Service Coding Handbook (version 14.3 at the time of this writing; American Pathology Foundation, Laguna Hills, California); however, some consider the handbook too detailed to serve as

Table 1
General categories of *International Classification of Diseases, Tenth Revision*, codes

Chapter	Code Prefix	Title/Category
I	A00–B99	Certain infectious and parasitic diseases
II	C00–D48	Neoplasms
III	D50–D89	Diseases of the blood and blood-forming organs and certain disorders involving the immune mechanism
IV	E00–E90	Endocrine, nutritional, and metabolic diseases
V	F00–F99	Mental and behavioral disorders
VI	G00–G99	Diseases of the nervous system
VII	H00–H59	Diseases of the eye and adnexa
VIII	H60–H95	Diseases of the ear and mastoid process
IX	I00–I99	Diseases of the circulatory system
X	J00–J99	Diseases of the respiratory system
XI	K00–K93	Diseases of the digestive system
XII	L00–L99	Diseases of the skin and subcutaneous tissue
XIII	M00–M99	Diseases of the musculoskeletal system and connective tissue
XIV	N00–N99	Diseases of the genitourinary system
XV	O00–O99	Pregnancy, childbirth, and the puerperium
XVI	P00–P96	Certain conditions originating in the perinatal period
XVII	Q00–Q99	Congenital malformations, deformations, and chromosomal abnormalities
XVIII	R00–R99	Symptoms, signs, and abnormal clinical and laboratory findings, not elsewhere classified
XIX	S00–T98	Injury, poisoning, and certain other consequences of external causes
XX	V01–Y98	External causes of morbidity and mortality
XXI	Z00–Z99	Factors influencing health status and contact with health services
XXII	U00–U99	Codes for special purposes

a basic guide for surgical pathology staff. In 2010, Demenstein[12] published a set of basic principles and rules, accessible to not only pathologists but also all workers on the surgical pathology bench; this article is available on-line at the time of this writing. A basic primer of *CPT* codes is discussed, based on the authors' experiences.

Table 2
Select examples of *International Classification of Diseases, Tenth Revision*, codes in descriptive histopathologic findings

Histologic Situation with a Potentially Broad Differential Diagnosis	Possible *International Classification of Diseases, Tenth Revision*, Code
Nonspecific histologic findings or a generalized pattern on a skin biopsy (ie, superficial perivascular dermatitis) with multiple differential diagnoses	L98.9 (unspecified skin disorder) or L98.8 (other specified skin disorder)
Nonspecific abnormal findings on histology (eg, a minute focus of atypical cells in a uterine cervical biopsy; cannot exclude dysplasia)	R89.7 (nonspecific histologic findings in specimens from other organs and tissues)
Abnormal white blood cell population on histology, not diagnostic for lymphoma	D72.9 disorder of white blood cells, unspecified
Mildly active inflammation without specific features on a colon biopsy	K63.9 disease of intestine, unspecified

Table 3
Select examples of accessible *International Classification of Diseases, Tenth Revision*, code databases (on-line access and mobile device applications)

Name of Database/ Application	Location	Notes
ICD-10 (WHO)	http://apps.who.int/classifications/icd10/browse/2010/en	As of this writing, only 2010 and older editions of ICD-10 codes are covered by this database.
ICD10Data.com	http://www.icd10data.com/ICD10CM/Codes#	Continuously updated, searchable online database of ICD-10 codes. Also included are options to search and convert ICD-9 codes into ICD-10 codes.
ICD-10 (Centers for Disease Control and Prevention)	http://www.cdc.gov/nchs/icd/icd10cm.htm	CDC Database of ICD-10 codes. While newest revisions are typically found here, they are not searchable online; they are only available in portable document format (PDF) and Microsoft Excel format (XLS). Files are large with slower download times.
ICD-10 (Wikipedia)	http://en.wikipedia.org/wiki/ICD-10	Searchable database of ICD-10 codes; the year of revision is unspecified.
ICD 10 Lite 2012 (Google Play)	https://play.google.com/store/apps/details?id=com.ipremiumapps.icd10cm.lite&hl=en	Free mobile App for Android Devices. While the database is searchable and accessible offline, search results may not be refined as they are using online searching with a web browser.

THE ESSENTIAL *CURRENT PROCEDURAL TERMINOLOGY* NUMBERS—IN AN AVALANCHE OF NUMBERS

For a pathologist new to *CPT* codes in surgical pathology, the most commonly encountered codes are discussed for routine gross and/or microscopic examination, special histochemical stains, immunohistochemical stains, and select additional procedures (ie, frozen section diagnosis).

THE FIRST STEP: ASSIGNING A CODE BETWEEN 88300 AND 88309 FOR GROSS AND/OR MICROSCOPIC EVALUATION

When evaluating a specimen, the first *CPT* code assigned is for the gross and/or microscopic examination. This code typically is between 88300 and 88309 (or between G0416 and G0419), depending on the type of specimen (summarized

in **Table 4**). The code for microscopic examination supersedes that for the gross examination; thus, a gross examination code (ie, 88300) cannot be assigned if a code encompassing microscopic evaluation (ie, 88305) has already been applied. Each code is assigned per "specimen part" from the same patient. In most cases, this means that each code is assigned per separately labeled specimen, usually in the form of different containers. For instance, if a patient has 3 separately labeled skin biopsies, with each biopsy in a different container (ie, part 1: right arm; part 2: left arm; and part 3: left shin), each part in most cases is assigned a single *CPT* code (ie, part 1: 88305, part 2: 88305, and part 3: 88305). If a large specimen labeled as a single part is present in multiple containers, this does not give the pathologist the authority to assign multiple *CPT* codes to each container. Furthermore, if the specimen did not survive processing and no material is present on the slides for that specimen,

Table 4
Summary of surgical pathology *Current Procedural Terminology* codes 88300 to 88309 and G0416 to G0419, with examples of specimen types from the 2014 *Current Procedural Terminology*

Current Procedural Terminology Code	Level	Examples of Scenarios/Specimen Types
88300	Level I	Gross examination only specimens (ie, calculi, foreign body, hardware, intrauterine device)
88302	Level II	Confirmation of identification in the absence of disease (ie, confirm complete cross sections of vas deferens and fallopian tubes in sterilization procedures, incidental appendectomy, foreskin of newborn, hydrocele testis, hernia sac, plastic repair of skin, testicular castration)
88304	Level III	Induced abortion, skin tag, appendix for appendicitis, simple vascular specimens (ie, artery/vein for atheromatous plaque, varicosity, thrombus/embolus without neoplasia), simple cystic lesions (abscess, aneurysm, bartholin cyst, synovial cyst, ganglion cyst, epidermal inclusion cyst, cholesteatoma, mucocele, pilonidal cyst/sinus, spermatocele, variocele, single paratubal cyst, etc.), curettings/débridement of cartilage/bone (other than for pathologic fracture), carpal tunnel tissue, colostomy stoma, pterygium of conjunctiva, cornea, diverticulum of gastrointestinal tract, femoral head (other than fracture/fissure/fistula), foreskin of adult, gallbladder (ie, for stones, cholecystitis; not for tumor), intervertebral disc, loose body in joint, lipoma, meniscus, tonsils and/or adenoids, other vas deferens (ie, other than incidental/sterilization)
88305	Level IV	Vast majority of biopsies for assessment of disease (some exclusions apply, such as breast biopsies for which margins are assessed; see 88307 for clarifications), all skin excisions (even for large cutaneous neoplasms), exostosis of bone, spontaneous/missed abortion, heart valve, joint resection, placenta (other than third trimester), excision of spleen, orchiectomy (other than for neoplasia, castration), synovium, uterus for prolapse only (with or without adnexa)
88307	Level V	Excision of adrenal gland; bone fragments (for pathologic fracture), select biopsies (ie, brain, liver, testis), breast excision with assessment of margins (one 88307 code is assigned even if margins are in separate containers), most organ resections (includes non-neoplastic uterus without prolapse, uterus with fibroids, partial laryngectomy, partial nephrectomy, thyroid lobectomy, transurethral resection of urinary bladder lesion, etc.)
88309	Level VI	Predominantly total and subtotal organ resections for tumor, including extensive soft tissue resections for tumor, bone resection for tumor, mastectomy with regional lymph nodes extremity disarticulation (not disarticulation of digit); fetus, with dissection
G0416		Code used for reimbursement for governmental payers (ie, Medicare/Medicaid) only. Report a single G0416 code for an entire set of prostate biopsies with 10–20 parts from the same patient during the same procedure (for cases of <10 parts, each part is assigned 88305 instead).
G0417		Code used for reimbursement for governmental payers (ie, Medicare/Medicaid) only. Report a single G0417 code for an entire set of prostate biopsies with 21–40 parts from the same patient during the same procedure.
G0418		Code used for reimbursement for governmental payers (ie, Medicare/Medicaid) only. Report a single G0418 code for an entire set of prostate biopsies with 41–60 parts from the same patient during the same procedure.
G0419		Code used for reimbursement for governmental payers (ie, Medicare/Medicaid) only. Report a single G0419 code for an entire set of prostate biopsies with >60 parts from the same patient during the same procedure.

From Padget D. APF pathology service coding handbook: medical service, procedure, and diagnosis reporting policies and practices for the pathology profession. Laguna Beach (CA): American Pathology Foundation; 2014. p. 506–10; with permission. CPT codes copyright © 2013 American Medical Association. All Rights Reserved.

only the gross examination code 88300 can be assigned.

THE SECOND STEP: EXTRA STUDIES AND PROCEDURES, EXTRA *CURRENT PROCEDURAL TERMINOLOGY* CODES

Although a single *CPT* code per specimen part covers gross and/or microscopic examination, the interpretation of special stains imparts additional services by a pathologist—and hence—additional codes. Common examples of these codes (to include circumstances such as frozen section evaluation and select ancillary studies) are summarized in **Table 5**. If 2 special stains

are performed, that does not automatically imply that 2 *CPT* codes can be used. For instance, performing the same p63 immunostain on 2 different paraffin blocks from the same specimen part cannot generate two 88342 codes; only one 88342 code can be applied per different immunostain, per specimen part. Moreover, several new codes, including 88343; G0461; and G0462, emerged in 2013 for specific instances of immunohistochemical stains. These codes are also summarized in **Table 5**. Knowledge of when to use these codes may be of value, given that there has been considerable confusion in the pathology community on their proper usage.

Table 5
Quick reference of surgical pathology *Current Procedural Terminology* codes for select ancillary procedures

Current Procedural Terminology Code	Ancillary Procedure
88311	Decalcification on specimen

88312	Most histochemical (nonimmuno-) stains for evaluation of organisms:
	    periodic acid–Schiff (with or without diastase, include periodic acid–Schiff stains used to assess the basement membrane)
	    Grocott methenamine silver
	    Acid-fast bacilli
	    Giemsa
	    Gram

88313	Additional histochemical (nonimmuno-) stains:
	    Trichrome
	    Alcian blue
	    Colloidal iron
	    Iron
	    Fontana-Masson
	    Reticulin
	    Methenamine silver trichrome
	    Congo red

88342	Any single immunohistochemical stain (ie, pankeratin or Melan-A)
88343	Additional immunohistochemical stains performed on the same slide (example: for a p16/Ki-67 combination stain, the first stain counts as 88342 but the second stain counts as 88343)
G0461	Code used for reimbursement for governmental payers (ie, Medicare/Medicaid) only. Code G0461 is reported for the first stain per specimen. All subsequent stains are assigned G0462 each (see below).
G0462	Code used for reimbursement for governmental payers (ie, Medicare/Medicaid) only. Code G0462 is reported for each additional stain per specimen.
88321	Used for each specimen part where the block and/or slide originates from another institution (ie, codes such as 88305 should not be used for consultation cases)
88331	Intraoperative consultation involving a frozen section diagnosis on 1 block
88332	Intraoperative consultation involving a frozen section diagnosis on each additional block after the first block

From Padget D. APF pathology service coding handbook: medical service, procedure, and diagnosis reporting policies and practices for the pathology profession. Laguna Beach (CA): American Pathology Foundation; 2014. p. 506–10; with permission. CPT codes copyright © 2013 American Medical Association. All Rights Reserved.

CODING FOR SYSTEMATIZED NOMENCLATURE OF MEDICINE CLINICAL TERMS

Systematized Nomenclature of Medicine Clinical Terms (SNOMED CT) represents a merged library of 2 code sets created by the College of American Pathologists (CAP) and the National Health Service of the United Kingdom; SNOMED CT's development now continues via the International Health Terminology Standards Development Organisation.[13] More specifically, SNOMED CT covers more than 300,000 concepts in medicine and also more than a million descriptors (ie, synonyms and semantic relationships). Thus, although *ICD* and *CPT* codes cover medical conditions, the vast array of numeric SNOMED CT codes covers more-specific aspects of medical conditions on a multiaxial system, ranging from clinical findings, procedures/interventions, body structures (ie, anatomic site), and organisms to substances, pharmaceutical/biologic products, and even social contexts. **Fig. 4** demonstrates an example of this scope. The translation of so many medical terms and relationships into these numeric codes enables information systems that recognize SNOMED CT codes to store and share sizable amounts of medical information. At the time of this writing, a searchable on-line SNOMED CT database (v17.0.0, April 2014; National Pathology Exchange, Brighouse, United Kingdom) available at http://www.snomedbrowser.com.

The vast range of this information is not, however, without challenges. Although some LISs incorporate computer-assisted coding, where SNOMED CT codes are submitted based on final diagnosis templates chosen by a pathologist,

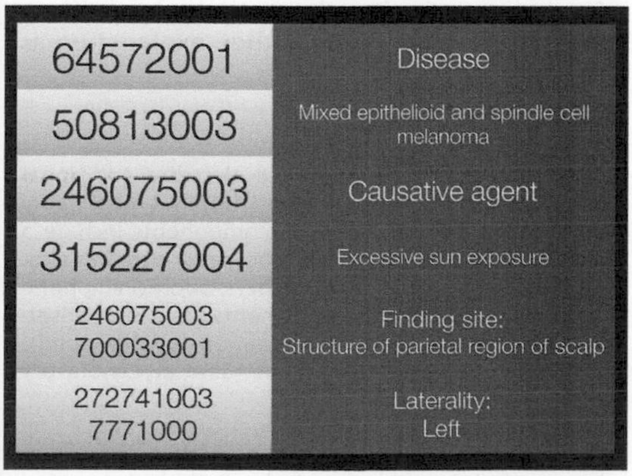

caution when designing such systems—to include input from pathologists—is needed. For instance, if a pathologist includes the term, "granuloma," in the report, how does the system know if the pathologist is describing a granuloma of inflammatory bowel disease, a peripheral granuloma of the oral cavity, an isolated nonspecific finding in a background of inflammation, a foreign body reaction, or some other form of inflammation? Although SNOMED CT codes offer generous flexibility to provide codes for a variety of languages used by pathologists, care must be taken such that codes cover the proper histologic context. Some studies have expressed concern that histopathologic findings may not be properly represented for patient information exchange and research unless further modifications to SNOMED CT concept models are developed.[14–16]

COMMUNICATION STANDARDS IN PATHOLOGY: EFFORTS TO SPEAK THE SAME LANGUAGE

Standards—set levels of expected quality or attainment—are all around and are abided by daily for safety and quality assurance. How many citizens would board an airplane if there were no air traffic rules, with no set method of flying aircraft (and likely a higher number of fatal airplane crashes)? How many would drive cars if each suburb had different sets of colors and signs for their traffic lights? The same can be said for pathology—how many clinicians would trust pathologists if pathologists did not share a common language of terms in surgical pathology reports? This is where standards are helpful. Yet, even if all pathologists spoke exactly the same language, this language can be broken if different medical record systems used by pathologists and clinicians cannot understand each other. Communication standards are crucial in this regard.

WHO SETS THE COMMUNICATION STANDARDS FOR PATHOLOGY?

Most standards are established by standards organizations. Examples of such organizations are listed in **Table 1.** Existing standards range from familiar units of measurement (ie, the micron) adopted by the International System of Units (SI), to entities, such as Health Level Seven International (HL7), a standards organization for hospital information systems accredited by the American National Standards Institute. HL7 allows for messaging protocols that simplify the interface between health care software applications and vendors. If 2 completely

64572001	Disease
50813003	Mixed epithelioid and spindle cell melanoma
246075003	Causative agent
315227004	Excessive sun exposure
246075003 700033001	Finding site: Structure of parietal region of scalp
272741003 7771000	Laterality: Left

Fig. 4. Examples of related SNOMED CT codes. Note the coverage of not only a medical condition but also the relationship of this condition with other terminologies, including anatomic site and causative factors.

different information systems follow HL7, they can transmit patient demographics, clinical notes, and diagnoses between each other without loss or misinterpretation of information.

Available standards do not cover the full realm of reporting entities encountered in surgical pathology. Some standards have emerged, particularly for malignant neoplasms; examples include the American Joint Committee on Cancer staging guidelines, the CAP cancer templates synoptic reporting, and the CAP biomarker reporting templates. Nonetheless, for lesions other than malignancies, standards in surgical pathology reporting are not widely addressed, to the authors' knowledge. Although pathology textbooks provide a wealth of information about pathologic lesions (and all their variants), they typically leave it to pathologists to decide how (and now much) to report these findings. For instance, what margins should be reported for benign neoplasms? To which benign neoplasms does this apply? How should reports with minimal tissue be addressed? What pertinent negatives might be suggested to report for cases with mild or benign findings? Although answers to these questions are not concrete, they may contribute to the establishment of standards of pathology reporting. The authors acknowledge that it is impossible to fully address each and every situation in this section; instead, a general set of experience and evidence-based perspectives is presented as a guide, with emphasis on the final diagnosis and comment sections of the surgical pathology report.

HOW DOES A PATHOLOGY PRACTICE MEET "THE STANDARDS" OF PATIENT CARE?

The most common means of meeting pathology standards is to be accredited by a supporting organization such as the CAP. Checklists for criteria to meet these standards as well as applications for CAP accreditation can be requested from the Laboratory Accreditation and Program Accreditation section of the CAP Web site (see References for full Web address).[17]

STANDARDS OF BASIC COMPONENTS OF THE SURGICAL PATHOLOGY REPORT

An in-depth description of standards for surgical pathology report components has been published by Goldsmith and colleagues[18] and is accessible on-line (as of this writing). A brief summary of mandatory elements in surgical pathology reports, as recommended by Goldsmith and colleagues, is presented in **Box 1**.

Box 1
Required elements for surgical pathology diagnosis reports, as described by Goldsmith and colleagues

Name of laboratory

Phone number of laboratory

Service performed by laboratory (eg, histology, immunohistochemistry)

Patient name

Patient date of birth

Other patient identification (such as a medical record number)

Patient history/clinical information, including preoperative and postoperative diagnoses if applicable

Full name of ordering/submitting physician

Full names of all physicians to receive copies of report

Date of specimen collection

Date specimen was received in laboratory

Case accession number (specimen identification number)

Report title (ie, surgical pathology report)

Report status (ie, preliminary, amended)

Report page number, including total number of pages in the report

Date and time the original report was completed

Gross description of specimen, including container, container labels (and fixative with length of time of fixation, if applicable)

Final diagnosis lines by pathologist (with a diagnosis comment if further explanation is needed)

Pathologist signature

Goldsmith and colleagues also describe additional components that are preferred but not necessarily mandatory; examples of such components include a graphic/logo of the laboratory (ie, service/trademark), laboratory fax and billing numbers, additional phone numbers of laboratory departments (ie, customer service), additional contact information for the submitting physician (ie, pager), and Clinical Laboratory Improvements of 1988 number.

Data from Goldsmith JD, Siegal GP, Suster S, et al. Reporting guidelines for clinical pathology reports in surgical pathology. Arch Pathol Lab Med 2008;132:1608–16.

STANDARDS FOR PATHOLOGY REPORTING/FINAL DIAGNOSIS LINES IN SURGICAL PATHOLOGY REPORTS

The availability of standards for the reporting of final diagnosis lines depends on the pathologic entity identified. Although standards for the reporting of some entities (ie, primary malignancies) have been established, standards for the reporting of most other lesions (in particular, benign/low-grade neoplasia) have not been established. It is impossible to cover each and every scenario in

the scope of this article (or, perhaps, in the scope of this entire issue); rather, available resources for pathologists to use are presented.

STANDARDS FOR PATHOLOGY REPORTING: PRIMARY MALIGNANCIES

Standards for the reporting of several primary malignancies (including features, such as size, margins, specific histologic features, TNM pathologic staging, and recommended ancillary testing) are listed in the CAP cancer protocols and

---

Table 6
Example styles of diagnosis lines for select benign lesions

Scenario	Sample Diagnosis/Comment Lines	Additional Comments
A shave biopsy of a compound melanocytic nevus broadly involves the inked biopsy margins.	Compound melanocytic nevus of the skin, incompletely excised, negative for dysplasia and malignancy.	
A shave biopsy of a junctional melanocytic nevus focally involves an inked peripheral biopsy margin.	Junctional melanocytic nevus of the skin, negative for dysplasia and malignancy (see note). NOTE: The nevus focally extends to a peripheral edge of the biopsy, but neither architectural disorder nor atypia is seen.	To avoid confusion with clinicians, the authors prefer to use the term "peripheral and deep" instead of "lateral and deep" to describe the inked slide section margins for unoriented skin biopsies.
A shave biopsy of a vulvar hemangioma extends to the deep margin of the biopsy.	Hemangioma, incompletely excised, negative for malignancy.	The authors prefer not to use phrases, such as "transected at base." In the authors' experiences, clinicians have preferred terms that more directly assess the completeness of an excision.
A local excision of a poroma involves the deep and peripheral biopsy margins.	Poroma, extending to the deep and peripheral margins (see note). NOTE: Re-excision of this lesional site with therapeutic margins is recommended to prevent lesional recurrence and/or progression.	Some benign neoplasia, such as poroma, can progress to porocarcinoma; this is one of several examples in which reporting of margins for benign lesions is necessary.
A 5-cm lipoma is excised. Adipocytes broadly involve the resection margins.	Lipoma (5 cm). Negative for malignancy.	The authors do not report margins for benign lipomas and their variants. If a call is received, the pathologist explains that margin assessment is precluded by the identical appearance of lesional cells and non-neoplastic adipocytes.

Important note: This table is not intended to provide mandatory rules for pathologists to follow; rather, it represents a few samples from the authors' perspectives that are less likely to be followed by questions for clarification after the pathology reports are signed out.

checklists (see References for Web address). These checklists, available in Portable Document Format (PDF) and Microsoft Word format (DOC), are organized by organ system. The American College of Surgeons has mandated that at least 90% of reported primary malignancies from a laboratory (not including squamous cell and basal cell carcinomas of the skin <2 cm in greatest dimension) be accompanied by synoptic reports.[19] Reporting primary malignancies in the formats provided by these checklists satisfies this mandate as long as the information is presented in a list, similar to the way each checklist is written. Further details on synoptic reporting are presented in the article by Anil Parwani, elsewhere in this issue. The authors acknowledge that different institutions may have minor variations in ways these synoptics are filled out. Some institutions use an Extensible Markup Language (XML) graphical user interface (GUI) for the user to mark checkboxes for each of the data parameters. Other institutions elect to simply list the diagnosis followed by copying and pasting the synoptic text from the checklist directly into a basic text editor to remove text formatting, followed by copying and pasting into the surgical pathology report. Some institutions report the diagnosis in their own format, followed by a separate synoptic summary; however, some pathologists may not favor this method because it essentially forces pathologists to report all information twice, increasing the possibility of errors.

STANDARDS FOR PATHOLOGY REPORTING: BENIGN LESIONS AND THE QUESTION OF MARGINS

To the authors' knowledge, although several lesions are considered benign and, based on outcomes, typically do not require continued follow-up, definite standards do not exist for reporting these lesions in a surgical pathology report (ie, not to the same degree that exists for malignant neoplasia). In addition, some lesions are considered premalignant and require closer surveillance, yet the margin status may not necessarily affect the interval of follow-up. In other lesions, margin status may predict the risk of recurrence and prompt further treatment, such as conservative re-excision. Through training in pathology, pathologists typically acquire a mental list of such lesions for which margins or additional information do (or do not) bear clinical significance. In other cases, pathologists may report limited additional data, such as the size of a lesion or a histologic subtype, to correlate with the clinical impression (ie, seborrheic keratosis, pigmented, in a patient clinically suspected of having a melanocytic nevus). At some institutions, pathologists and clinicians have agreed on a subset of cases in which pertinent negatives are listed with the diagnosis ("negative for dysplasia and malignancy" for nevi that are not dysplastic, "negative for hyperplasia and malignancy" for endometrial curettings to rule out endometrial hyperplasia, "negative for dysplasia and malignancy" and the presence/absence of muscularis propria [detrusor muscle] for urinary bladder biopsies, "negative for neovascularization and malignancy" for corneal grafts, and so forth). Such pertinent negatives have been integrated into quick texts and templates designed by pathologists in anatomic pathology software. Examples of such cases from the authors' practices are listed in **Table 6**.

SUMMARY

Data representation, coding, and communication standards in pathology are important concepts that facilitate communications from pathologists to others, such that a communicated message remains unambiguous and easily understood. As the involvement of IT in pathology grows in tandem with pathologists' case volumes, so will the importance of such concepts in pathology practices.

REFERENCES

1. Sinard JH. Practical pathology informatics: demystifying informatics for the practicing anatomic pathologist. New York: Springer Science + Business Media; 2006. p. 65–76.
2. Jackson, BR. PI 13–16 (PI-10). ASCP Case Reports in Pathology Informatics (formerly ASCP CheckSample). 2013; 2(6): 1–13.
3. Hernandez JS, Allen TC. Transformation of pathologists responding in a volatile, uncertain, complex, and ambiguous environment. Arch Pathol Lab Med 2013;137:603–5.
4. Sperberg-McQueen CM, Dubin D. Data representation. DH curation guide: a community resource guide to data curation in the digital humanities. University of Illinois; 2012. Available at: http://guide.dhcuration.org/representation. Accessed July 12, 2014.
5. U.S. Department of Health and Human Services. NPRM: standards for electronic transactions. Office of the Assistant Secretary for Planning and Evaluation Website; 2013. Available at: http://aspe.hhs.gov/admnsimp/nprm/tx04.htm. Accessed July 8, 2014.

6. World Health Organization. International classification of diseases (ICD). World Health Organization Website; 2015. Available at: http://apps.who.int/classifications/icd10/browse/2015/en. Accessed March 5, 2015.

7. Castillo LA, Dettwyler WK, Dunston G, et al. Pathology lab coding alert. Coding Institute 2001;2(6):41–8.

8. Department of Health and Human Services. Centers for medicare and medicaid services. Program memorandum intermediaries/carriers, transmittal AB-01–144. ICD-9-CM coding for diagnostic tests. Washington, DC: Department of Health and Human Services; 2001.

9. Centers for Medicare and Medicaid Services (CMS). Medicare – ICD-10. Centers for Medicare and Medicaid Services (CMS); 2014. Available at: http://www.cms.gov/Medicare/Coding/ICD10/index.html?redirect=/icd10. Accessed July 6, 2014.

10. American Academy of Professional Coders. ICD-10 delay: frequently asked questions. American Academy of Professional Coders Website; 2013. Available at: http://www.aapc.com/icd-10-2014-delay/faq.aspx. Accessed July 14, 2014.

11. American Medical Association (AMA). CPT – current procedural terminology. American Medical Association (AMA); 2014. Available at: http://www.ama-assn.org/ama/pub/physician-resources/solutions-managing-your-practice/coding-billing-insurance/cpt.page. Accessed July 18, 2014.

12. Dimenstein IB. Principles and controversies in CPT coding in surgical pathology. Lab Med 2011;42(4): 242–9.

13. Benson T, editor. Principles of health interoperability HL7 and SNOMED. London: Springer; 2012. p. 233–6.

14. Campbell WS, Campbell JR, West WW, et al. Semantic analysis of SNOMED CT for a post-coordinated database of histopathology findings. J Am Med Inform Assoc 2014;21:885–92.

15. Nachimuthu SK, Lau LM. Practical issues in using SNOMED CT as a reference terminology. Stud Health Technol Inform 2007;129(1):640–4.

16. Rector A, Iannone L. Lexically suggest, logically define: quality assurance of the use of qualifiers and expected results of post-coordination in SNOMED CT. J Biomed Inform 2012;45(2):199–209.

17. College of American Pathologists (CAP). Laboratory accreditation checklists. College of American Pathologists (CAP); 2014. Available at: http://www.cap.org/apps/cap.portal?_nfpb=true&cntvwrPtlt_actionOverride=%2Fportlets%2FcontentViewer%2Fshow&_windowLabel=cntvwrPtlt&cntvwrPtlt%7BactionForm.contentReference%7D=laboratory_accreditation%2Fchecklists%2Fchecklist.html&_state=maximized&_pageLabel=cntvwr. Accessed July 4, 2014.

18. Goldsmith JD, Siegal GP, Suster S, et al. Reporting guidelines for clinical pathology reports in surgical pathology. Arch Pathol Lab Med 2008;132:1608–16.

19. Kang HP, Devine LJ, Piccoli AL, et al. Usefulness of a synoptic data tool for reporting of head and neck neoplasms based on the college of American pathologists cancer checklists. Am J Clin Pathol 2009;132:521–30.

Bar Coding and Tracking in Pathology

Matthew G. Hanna, MD[a,*], Liron Pantanowitz, MD[b]

KEYWORDS

- Bar codes • Tracking • Pathology informatics • RFID

ABSTRACT

Bar coding and specimen tracking are intricately linked to pathology workflow and efficiency. In the pathology laboratory, bar coding facilitates many laboratory practices, including specimen tracking, automation, and quality management. Data obtained from bar coding can be used to identify, locate, standardize, and audit specimens to achieve maximal laboratory efficiency and patient safety. Variables that need to be considered when implementing and maintaining a bar coding and tracking system include assets to be labeled, bar code symbologies, hardware, software, workflow, and laboratory and information technology infrastructure as well as interoperability with the laboratory information system. This article addresses these issues, primarily focusing on surgical pathology.

OVERVIEW

Bar codes are standardized identification tools that allow for asset tracking. They have widespread use in point of sale purchases, delivery companies, automobile industry, and health care. With advances in technology over the past few decades, there have been tremendous improvements in bar code and scanner performance. Some of the main purposes of implementing a bar coding and tracking system are to reduce errors and increase efficiency. Instead of manual logging entries, bar coding has reduced human errors by automating identification and tracking. Regarding health care, bar coding is a hospital-wide operation. From patient wristbands to hospital beds, different bar codes or RFID tags are used to identify, locate, and audit labeled assets.

The clinical laboratory has demonstrated positive effects of implementing bar coding and tracking systems.[1–6] Similar use of this technology, however, has only recently been introduced in anatomic pathology. Ever-increasing specimen volumes, complex testing, and a desire for decreased turnaround times without increasing costs and errors provide a pressing impetus for pathology laboratories to implement tracking solutions. There are myriad pathology assets that can be identified and tracked, including order requisitions, specimen containers, tissue cassettes/blocks, glass slides, and reagents. Interfacing bar codes or RFID tags with the LIS have become essential for contemporary pathology laboratories to reap the benefits of asset tracking, such as driving workflow, automation, error reduction, digital pathology, and improved patient safety.

HISTORY

Bar codes, which are ubiquitous today, made their debut approximately 80 years ago (Table 1). The first mention of bar coding was US patent 1985035A, published on December 18, 1934, by John Kermode, Douglass Young, and Harry Sparkes. Their patent included "sorting machines which employ photo-electric cells or other light-responsive means for sorting cards, records or the like in response to a code or designation marked thereon, or for tabulating, recording or effecting other controls in accordance with the marks on the cards or records." In October 1949, Norman Woodland and Silver Bernard filed a patent (US patent 2612994A), which delineated the first bar code process, entitled "Classifying apparatus and method." Bernard and Woodland were devising a method to automatically scan products at grocery stores to

Disclosure Statement: The authors have no disclosures.

[a] Department of Pathology, The Mount Sinai Hospital, 1 Gustave L Levy Place, New York, NY 10029, USA;
[b] Department of Pathology, University of Pittsburgh Medical Center, 5150 Centre Avenue, Pittsburgh, PA 15232, USA
* Corresponding author.
E-mail address: matthew.hanna@mountsinai.org

Surgical Pathology 8 (2015) 123–135
http://dx.doi.org/10.1016/j.path.2015.02.017

surgpath.theclinics.com

Table 1
Historical events of bar codes

Date	Event
December 18, 1934	US patent 1985035A is the first mention of bar code technology
October 20, 1949	US Patent 2612994A filed, describes the first bar code process
1961	Color bar codes first used on railroad cars
June 23, 1973	Announcement of the first UPC point of sale system
June 26, 1974	First product bar code scanned in a supermarket (Wrigley gum)
September 21, 1981	US Department of Defense adopts Code 39 bar code
September 1982	US Postal Service use POSTNET bar code to represent zip codes
1987	ISO 9000 quality management standards first created
February 2004	US Food and Drug Administration requires medications use bar codes
October 12, 2005	AABB requires ISBT 128 bar code for accreditation

Abbreviations: AABB, American Association of Blood Banks; POSTNET, Postal Numeric Encoding Technique.
Adapted from UPC History. ID History Museum.[7]

minimize time in checkout lines. Woodland eventually continued developing bar codes at IBM. The earliest bar coding system was used in a railroad company to identify railroad cars, called KarTrak automatic car identification. This color bar code system has many similarities to bar codes in use today. KarTrak used 13 horizontal labels of different width and spacing, a start and stop line, and a line checker. Due to high human reading error rates, however, their system was abandoned in the 1970s. The supermarket industry started using candidate bar code formats for automated checkout systems in the mid-1960s. In 1973, after many ad hoc committee meetings, the uniform product code (UPC) was designated the national standard by the National Association of Food Chains for grocery product identification. The International Organization for

Standardization (ISO) 9000 quality-management standards, first created in 1987, have pushed companies to ensure compliance with bar coding systems.[7–9] Because of these advancements, bar codes have a global presence. Health care subsequently also widely adopted bar code technology.

TYPES OF BAR CODES

A bar code is defined as an optical machine-readable symbol representing a set of data. Bar codes use light reflection on different-sized white and black bars or dots to encode a binary (1s and 0s) string of data. There are hundreds of different bar code varieties that can be created, most of which are grouped into categories of a linear (1-D) or 2-D bar code symbology (**Fig. 1**).

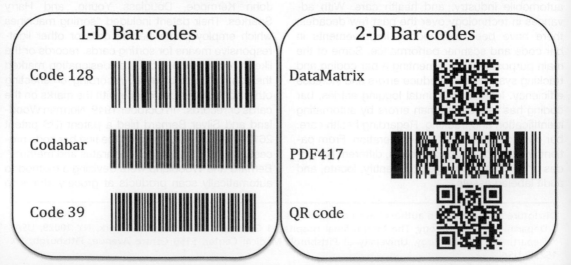

1-D Bar codes

Code 128

Codabar

Code 39

2-D Bar codes

DataMatrix

PDF417

QR code

Fig. 1. Linear (1-D) and 2-D bar code symbology examples. 1-D bar codes with data encoded only on the horizontal axis are represented by differentially spaced and sized line bars. 2-D symbologies are represented as black and white dots with data encoded along the vertical and horizontal axis.

The mapping between the bar code and message is called a symbology. Bar code symbology defines the technical details of a particular type of bar code (eg, encodable character set, bar spacing and width, and checksum specifications). 1-D symbologies include numeric or alphanumeric data. 2-D symbologies can include a much greater character count (higher data density), require a smaller footprint, and have fewer scan and printer failures compared with 1-D symbologies.[10–12] There is no single bar code that encompasses all uses and needs of a laboratory; consequently, using a combination of symbologies is commonplace and recommended based on a particular laboratory's needs. In efforts to standardize bar coding in laboratories, the Clinical and Laboratory Standards Institute (CLSI) published AUTO02-A2 (Laboratory Automation: Bar Codes for Specimen Container Identification) and AUTO12-A (Specimen Labels: Content and Location, Fonts, and Label Orientation).[13,14] These guidelines established an April 29, 2014, deadline for laboratories to comply with bar code standardization on specimen labels. Compliance will likely affect laboratory accreditation in future years by The Joint Commission and College of American Pathologists.

1-D SYMBOLOGY

Still regarded as the standard by many, 1-D symbologies eventually may be replaced by 2-D. 1-D bar codes, however, are still used frequently in most laboratories. These symbologies require a larger space on labels, have higher error detection rates (even minor bar code defacement can cause scan errors), and have fewer data density capabilities. The most prevalent and standard 1-D symbology used in laboratories is Code 128; due to its 3 subtypes (A, B, and C) that can encode all 128 characters of American Standard Code for Information Interchange (ASCII) (all alphanumeric characters, upper and lowercase, 0–99). Each Code 128 bar code can shift between its 3 subtypes, which allows for a high character density to be encoded and reduces errors with a checksum. Code 128 is used by the International Society of Blood Transfusion (ISBT) for the ISBT 128 standard and has largely replaced the older blood bank Codabar bar code. Codabar was one of the first symbologies to incorporate error detection schema, thereby reducing the need for a discrete check digit.[12]

2-D SYMBOLOGY

In the 1990s, with the mass production of charge-coupled devices (CCDs), scanner manufacturers were able to depend on 2-D scanning. These scanners use complex image analysis algorithms to decode 2-D symbologies, with better detection rates. In recent years, 2-D bar codes have seen increasing use in laboratories. They are scalable, require less label space, can encode much higher character densities, and have significantly decreased error detection rates; a 30% defacement of a 2-D bar code surface area can still be read. The 2-D symbology that has shown the most rapid adoption in laboratories is DataMatrix (**Fig. 2**). Depending on the matrix size and coding schema, DataMatrix can code up to 3116 numeric characters, 2335 alphanumeric characters, or 1555 bytes of binary data. This delivers more

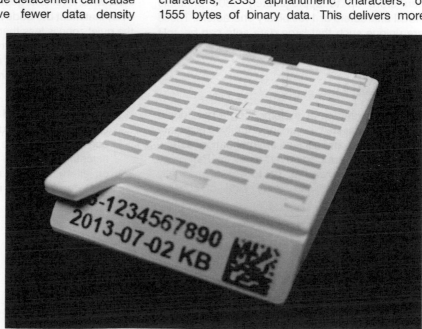

Fig. 2. Sample 2-D Data-Matrix symbology printed on a white cassette. Bar code placement on the opposite side of the upper cassette lip enables easier access for scanners.

efficient encoding of ASCII characters into a fixed set of data. The ASCII string and error correction system are encoded into the bar code based on a specific algorithm that places all data into particular positions of the matrix. The initial installments of DataMatrix codes used convolutional error correction (referenced as ECC-000 to ECC-140). A more recent second subset of DataMatrix codes (recommended standard ECC-200), however, uses Reed-Solomon (RS) error correction techniques (allowing for correct reading even when a portion of the bar code is defaced), which has error detection rates in the Six Sigma confidence interval range. To further lower error detection rates, check digits have been incorporated in the encoded character sequence used concurrently with DataMatrix's RS error correction, diminishing error rates to as low as 1 in 10^{15} scan events.[12,15,16]

Another 2-D symbology, quick response (QR) code, has seen widespread adoption in all areas of the world. QR codes can encode up to 7089 numeric characters or 4296 alphanumeric characters. Similar to DataMatrix codes, they have high data density capabilities and RS error reduction techniques. QR codes have different versions, related to physical size, and 4 error correction levels (L, M, Q, and H). The variables that regulate the amount of data stored in a QR code include data type, version (smallest, 1; largest, 40), and error correction level. PDF417 is another 2-D symbology that is used in hazardous material labeling, storing technical specifications and calibration data on electronic instruments, and encoding civilian data on drivers' licenses. These codes can store up to approximately 1800 printable ASCII characters or 1100 binary characters. These are unique such that large data sets can be split into multiple organized PDF417 codes.[10,15]

ERROR RATES

A major advantage of implementing a bar coding and tracking system is the opportunity to eliminate labeling errors and achieve optimal patient safety, consequently reducing adverse events. Pathology studies have shown that up to 1% of manually labeled specimens and up to 72% of adverse events have problems related to specimen identification.[17-20] Other pathology studies identified that the greatest percentage of misidentification occurred at grossing.[21-23] Implementing barcoding and tracking solutions in anatomic pathology laboratories can help minimize such errors (Fig. 3).[24,25] Bar code error tolerance rates are high, which makes their use many fold more dependable than manual logging. Bar codes are robust tools that have created vast efficiency in identification and traceability of assets. With proper implementation of a bar code and tracking system, virtually all errors can be avoided. Data from the Henry Ford Hospital reported a 62% decrease of overall misidentification case rate, 92% decrease in slide misidentification defects, and 125% increased technical throughput at their microtomy workstations after bar codes were introduced.[26]

BAR CODE FAILURES

Bar codes are not without fault (see Fig. 2).[27] Using pattern recognition, bar code scanners can identify code. Position finders can be found at the start/stop patterns of the opening and closing bars in a 1-D code or 3 bull's-eye corners of a QR code (or outer L shape of DataMatrix). The most common reason for bar code read failures is quiet zone violations. The quiet zone is the blank margin directly at the sides or around the periphery of the bar code; it is used to isolate the code of interest and ensure transfer of information of only the code being scanned. Bar code standards require a quiet zone of 10 times the smallest bar width, or 0.1 inch, whichever is largest. It has been shown, however, that most bar code readers do not work well if the quiet zone is less than 0.25 inches.[10,15]

Although bar codes are robust, there are a few reasons for why a bar code may fail (Table 2). Bar codes should be read accurately, quickly, and consistently.

- An intermittent read failure may result when a bar code scanner does not readily detect a code and continues to use signal processing algorithms to have a delayed correct read or, alternatively, may have a misread. Reasons for potential intermittent read failures

AMP Grossing Station Warning   ✕

STOP! The cassette you scanned does not match with case number S-15-1234567. Please set aside block for use with case number S-15-7654321. Press OK to continue.

[OK]

Fig. 3. Warning for improperly scanned cassette. The cassette for case S-15-7654321 was scanned while the specimen S-15-1234567 was previously scanned and opened.

Table 2
Types of bar code reader failures

Bar Code Failures	Description	Potential Harm
Intermittent read failure	Delayed scanner read	May lead to misread or delayed correct read
Nonread failure	Bar code not read	Least harm because bar code is not read
Misread failure	Inaccurate read	Most harm if not detected

are maximum print head dot density, typically measured in lines per inch or dots per inch, maximum printed media reproduction fidelity, and maximum spatial density of a scanning image.

- A misread failure occurs when a bar code is inappropriately read, where a new encoded string represents a valid bar code sequence but not the intended sequence of the scanned bar code. These errors can be produced via bar code defacement or other defects while printing, from inadequate error detection methods, or from optical-mechanical scanner defects. Misread failures, if not prevented, may lead to serious adverse effects due to the difficulty in detecting this error.
- Nonread failures occur when a bar code is effectively defaced to the point of nonrecognition by a scanner and can no longer be decoded. These failures are readily identified because no data are decoded from an illegible bar code.

Bar code defacement is likely to occur in a histology laboratory, where bar codes are exposed to blades, heat, harsh chemicals, and microwaves. As discussed previously, this may lead to nonread or misread failures. To thwart these failures, bar codes have an intrinsic design to allow for redundancy. These redundancy factors exist in both 1-D and 2-D symbologies. The greater the height of a 1-D bar code, the greater is its redundancy factor. For instance, if a 1-D bar code has a hole punched in it, scanning at a different level where the code is complete likely still ensures accurate scanning. 2-D symbologies have more sophisticated redundancy factors, where the data are placed in several areas of the code, such that localized defacement unlikely prevents an accurate scan of the bar code.[10]

Another error correction technology that bar codes implement is a checksum. This uses an algorithm to calculate all numeric values of each character in the bar code string to a final summation value. The check digit is usually the last number on the 1-D symbologies and it must correlate with the checksum. Bar code scanning hardware and software must utilize this feature to corroborate that the checksum and check digit are correct to ensure successful decoding of the code; and safeguard against a potential misread. Checksums are largely represented, however, on 1-D and older symbologies. Newer and more robust error detection strategies, such as redundancy checking, have since been developed.

MEDIA AND LABELS

Other factors that may affect bar code readability stem from incompatible scanners, printing defects, or the media used to print the bar code/label itself. For instance, when a printer head malfunctions, due to wear and tear, it may not properly transfer heat to the printing media. Lengthy archival times may also have an impact on the durability of labels. Clinical Laboratory Improvement Amendments mandates that laboratories retain paraffin blocks for a minimum of 2 years, cytology slides for a minimum of 5 years, and histopathology slides for a minimum of 10 years.[28] It is, therefore, suggested that the selected media be tested to sustain at least 10 times the allotted storage time to account for thermal changes or other media transfer failures. It is important to select reliable media marker technologies that ideally endure many years. Because bar codes must remain on their assets somewhat indefinitely, their indelibility or impossibility of being removed or washed away is of prime importance. During the life cycle of histology slides and blocks, they experience significant time with abrasive chemical solvents and high temperatures. High temperatures may darken direct thermal labels or cause label adhesive to detach. Darkened labels may render bar code symbology illegible.[10] Hence, before investing in labels it is recommended to run several trials of printed labels through a rigorous histology workflow (eg, 72-hour xylene test or 1 week in a 65°C slide dryer) to demonstrate label fidelity.

STANDARDIZATION

Due to advancements in technology and the variety of bar code formats and systems available, complete standardization remains a challenge. For example, legacy bar code symbologies may still be used in older blood banks that need to deal with both Codabar and ISBT 128. A not-for-profit organization, GS1, has provided comprehensive standards for bar code numbers on a global scale. European, Asian, and Australian countries now use a European Article Number bar code (13 digits) whereas the United States and Canada use UPC bar codes (12 digits). CLSI has developed laboratory standards for bar codes and labeling, which are available in their publications, AUTO02-A2, AUTO04-A (Laboratory Automation: Systems Operational Requirements, Characteristics, and Information Elements), and AUTO12-A (Fig. 4).[13,14,29] Hitherto, there were no set regulations to direct laboratory personnel when designing specimen labels, bar coding assets, or tracking specimens. AUTO12-A explains the required human-readable elements, locations, fonts, and font sizes needed on specimen labels. This standard also offers details about label size and layout and identifies Code 128 as the symbology to be used.[14] Continued focus on standardizing bar coding and specimen labels in anatomic pathology is still required. Lack of interoperability hinders sharing of assets between institutions and possibly locks laboratories in, preventing them from using existing bar codes on newer devices, such as automated immunostainers or whole-slide imaging scanners.

Bar coding reduces slide mislabeling.[30] Interinstitutional consultations remain problematic because laboratories are usually unable to read foreign bar codes (eg, bar codes generated by another laboratory). Solutions to address this problem, however, are starting to emerge. Certain LISs support foreign bar codes. This capability is available mainly for clinical laboratories. Hence, when an outside client sends samples with bar-coded identifiers already affixed, if the foreign bar code can be read, this prevents the need to relabel the specimen. In anatomic pathology, the traditional practice of handling consult materials (slides, blocks, specimen containers, and accompanying paperwork) involves manually staff relabeling these assets on arrival, which may lead to clerical errors. One solution is to apply temporary slide and/or cassette labels that are easily removed without defacing the consulting laboratory's underlying label (Fig. 5). These labels can be easily removed when materials are returned to the primary facility.

HARDWARE

As technology advanced, newer models of barcode readers, printers, and computers became available. With the advent of CCD sensors, barcode readers were able to utilize 2-D bar coding on a large, economical scale. 2-D bar codes are smaller, encode higher data density, and include better error correction methodologies, which make them ideal for labels that require less space on assets. Each bar code reader in an anatomic pathology laboratory is typically connected to an individual computer. Depending on the workflow, therefore, wherever bar codes need to be scanned, a computer system needs to be in place (eg, accessioning, grossing stations, tissue processors, microtomy, staining, slide assembly, slide distribution, and pathologist workstations). Adequate computers and network bandwidth to sustain these laboratory operations are necessary for smooth workflow.

Bar code readers by default are enabled to detect a wide array of symbologies; hence, configuration of these readers may be needed to recognize certain bar codes or to negate symbologies not used in the laboratory. Different bar code readers are available, including contact wands, laser bar code scanners, and image-based (camera) bar code readers. Scanners can be wired, wireless, or fixed/mounted. Omnidirectional scanners are preferred to single-line laser scanners because they can read symbologies in any orientation.[10]

Name, Patient
123456789

1/1/1987 28y M

MH287-123789123-98B

Attending Physician   Collection Date/Time

Fig. 4. AUTO12-A compliant label layout. Instead of the bar code as the most superior data element, the patient name is situated in the upper left corner in landscape format.

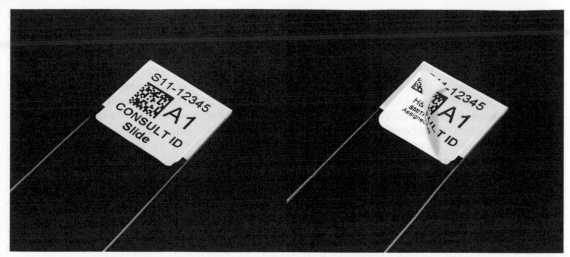

Fig. 5. Piggyback labeling of a glass slide for a consultation case. New labels that are easily removable are placed over existing labels and avoid the need to stick them on the opposite glass surface. (*Courtesy of* General Data Healthcare; with permission).

Bar code printers are essential for labeling specimen containers, cassettes, and slides. Labels usually need to include bar codes as well as other patient identification information (case accession number, patient name, slide number, and so forth). Printing can be performed on an adhesive label or directly onto the cassette or slide. Bar code printing technology includes impact (dot matrix) and nonimpact (ink-jet, laser, and thermal) printing **(Table 3)**.[15]

- Dot matrix printers print bar codes as a construct of numerous dots. These printers are the least expensive but have the lowest scanner readability.
- Ink-jet printers have high output capabilities but suffer from inconsistent print quality and readability on different materials. Certain materials may cause the media to diffuse and render a bar code illegible.
- Laser printers create electrostatic energy to attract ions in the ink to the necessary areas of bar codes and are bonded together by heat and pressure. These printers have high quality and readability but often cannot be used with chemical resistant labels.
- Thermal printers use a series of chemical reactions to form rows of dots as the media passes through the heating printhead. Thermal transfer has improved using specialized inked ribbon. These bar code printers have excellent long-lasting print quality and scanner readability but are more costly than other printers.

SOFTWARE

Software is an integral piece of bar coding and tracking systems. Solutions currently exist as either a component the LIS, third-party vendor middleware, or custom-built tracking solutions.[31] The key to success is to properly interface the software with the LIS and all laboratory instruments to be used. Software systems may have most, but not all, desired asset tracking attributes. Laboratories may use software as is, contract with their vendor for additional support, obtain third-party software, or custom develop sought-after tools in-house. This may be hampered by proprietary systems that do not integrate seamlessly with existing LISs or other tracking solutions. Some laboratories have implemented a dual bar code system for this purpose. The ideal tracking software should be user friendly, be easily configurable with diverse options, and have the ability to be used on multiple computer platforms (eg, desktop, tablet, and touch-screen devices).

Table 3
Comparison of bar code printer technology

Printer	Cost	Print Quality	Scanner Readability
Dot matrix	$	Good	Good
Ink-jet	$$$	Better	Good
Laser	$$	Better	Better
Thermal	$$	Best	Best

Testing software compatibility should be trialed extensively to identify workflow amity.

WORKFLOW

Workflow should be analyzed to create a streamlined set of operations that produce the highest yield in the fewest steps. When implementing a new tracking system, it may be necessary to adjust workflow as needed. Specimen tracking should ideally start when a specimen is obtained from a patient (eg, in a doctor's office or operating room). This requires, however, bedside, operating room, and/or outreach remote printers and in-depth integration of the electronic medical record (in which orders accompanying the specimen are placed) and the LIS. Such labels could be placed on specimen containers and be preaccessioned in an LIS long before reaching a pathology laboratory. Tracking of patient assets for most anatomic pathology laboratories usually begins at the accessioning stage, using manual logs as the traceable record of custody during specimen procurement. At the time of accessioning, labels are printed when the case gets activated. It is at this time that some laboratories may also choose to print a predetermined number of cassettes, depending on the specimen type. Accessioners should be made aware of preprinting, sorting, and distribution errors. Otherwise, just-in-time printing should be deferred until the time of grossing.[12]

All patient specimen labels must be accurate and coincide with each asset (eg, container, cassette, or slide) for that patient. Bar coding can be used to audit and track each step in an anatomic pathology laboratory (Fig. 6), creating soft stops that require an asset bar code to be scanned before proceeding with each successive step (eg, microtomy, staining, slide distribution, sign-out, and transcription). When scanning a bar code at microtomy, the system should be able to automatically identify the case and display ordered instructions (cut on edge, cross section, and so forth) and any other special orders to help drive workflow (use charged slides, send slides to immunohistochemistry, and so forth). This requires training laboratory personnel to use the system and how/when to scan bar codes. Although

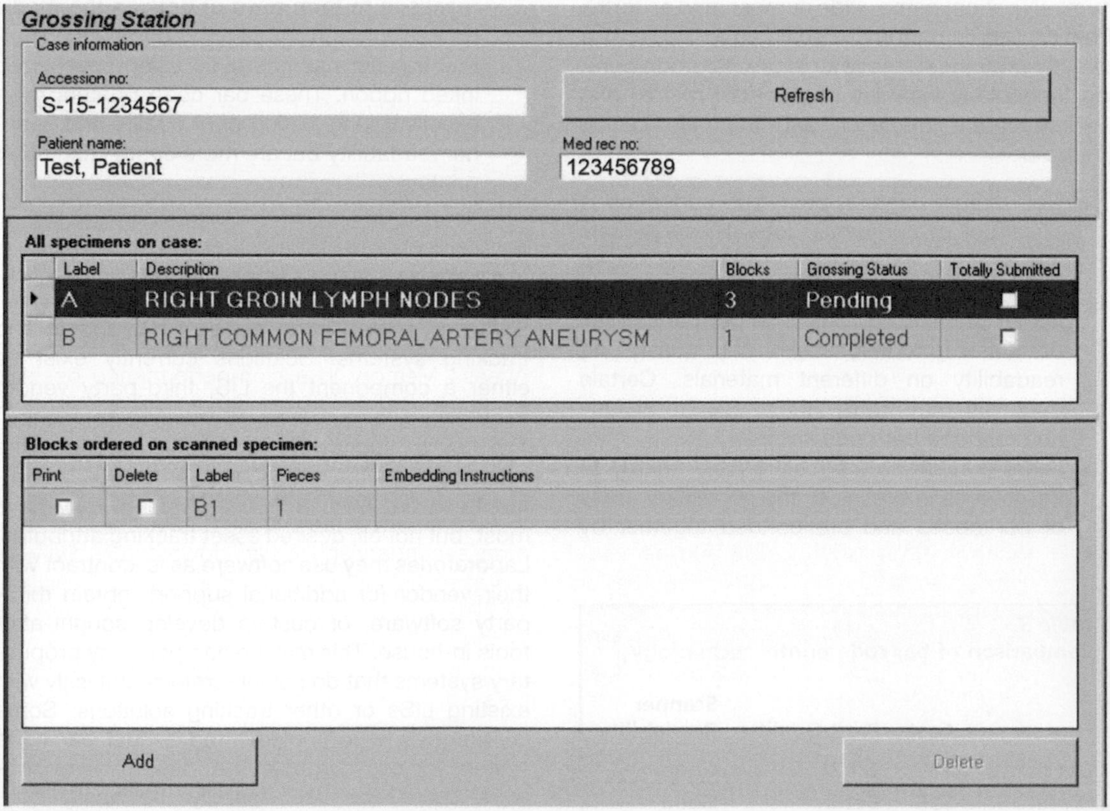

Grossing Station

Case information

Accession no:
S-15-1234567   Refresh

Patient name: Med rec no:
Test, Patient   123456789

All specimens on case:

	Label	Description	Blocks	Grossing Status	Totally Submitted
▶	A	RIGHT GROIN LYMPH NODES	3	Pending	■
	B	RIGHT COMMON FEMORAL ARTERY ANEURYSM	1	Completed	□

Blocks ordered on scanned specimen:

Print	Delete	Label	Pieces	Embedding Instructions
□	□	B1	1	

Add   Delete

Fig. 6. Grossing station phase of the test cycle. In this example, the grosser has scanned specimen B's container label; specimen B is hence highlighted green. One cassette has been ordered and scanned (B1). Specimen A has not yet been scanned; however, 3 cassettes have been preordered.

this may create additional steps when scanning these assets, overall it saves back-end time and energy when tracking a particular asset, if needed. Each scanned entry can record the time and workstation location where the asset was scanned and who was logged into the LIS at the time for this case, which is documented in the software for easy retrieval. Ongoing success depends on laboratory staff compliance and the capability of the tracking system to permit exceptions to be handled to avoid workarounds.

Workflow can be facilitated by using color-coding of stat specimens and/or specimens assigned to various subspecialties. There are numerous color cassettes available. For example, some laboratories choose to use red cassettes to indicate priority processing or designate tan to identify resident grossed specimens. Color-coding labels offers another option. It is recommended that all bar-code readers and labels be tested beforehand for machine-readable legibility to identify bar code readers that may have difficulty reading bar codes on select colors. Bar codes are often hard to read on dark red- or aqua-colored cassettes.

DASHBOARDS/STATUS MONITORS

Dashboards, or status monitors, are visual, tabular representations of scanned assets in the tracking system. They can be used to analyze workflow to identify areas of improvement or to check on the status of assets. For instance, with a quick glance at a dashboard, users can check to easily determine what time a specimen was accessioned, grossed, processed, embedded, cut, or stained or if the completed slides of a given case are assembled and ready for distribution. Users can

audit case distribution and workload volume (**Fig. 7**). Each tracked step can display the length of time needed dealing with an asset. Each workstation with a bar code reader can be used as a soft stop. The more stops involved, the more granular the data on the dashboard (**Fig. 8**). Priority assignments can be segregated by flags or colors, or colors can be used to display delayed cases. Distribution of information on a dashboard can be sent out as quality measures via spreadsheets in an e-mail on the Web or publicly displayed on large monitors in a histology laboratory. These monitors can display up-to-date information, which promotes real-time tracking.[12,32]

IMPLEMENTATION

Until recently, many anatomic pathology laboratories traditionally used manual logging systems to track their cases. In such laboratories, implementing a tracking system usually involves radical changes. Planning should begin long before any particular solution is pursued. The exact how, where, and when specimen assets are tracked and what the data will be used for must be carefully planned. More specifically, it is important to perform an analysis of existing versus desired workflow, select labels, determine space availability for devices, and develop a downtime strategy as well as garner what degree of IT support and finances is needed.[12] After the preliminary assessment is made, choosing a vendor tracking solution is the next step, keeping in mind the goal of maintaining interoperability with what already exists in a laboratory (eg, LIS, instruments, and computers). Although several solutions have been developed, each laboratory likely needs individual configuration of its tracking solution.

Event Time	Accession No	Material Description		Event Description	Event Location
07/23/2014 10:12:22 AM	S-14-321	Specimen A	MEDIAL MARGIN OF THE RIGHT LEG MASS	Scanned by HANNA, MATTHEW.	Peds-grossing
07/23/2014 10:12:40 AM	S-14-321	Block A1	PROCESS AND EMBED A PARAFFIN BLOCK	Block verified by HANNA, MATTHEW.	Peds-grossing
07/23/2014 10:13:00 AM	S-14-321	Specimen B	DISTAL MARGIN OF THE RIGHT LEG MASS	Scanned by HANNA, MATTHEW.	Peds-grossing
07/23/2014 10:13:18 AM	S-14-321	Block B1	PROCESS AND EMBED A PARAFFIN BLOCK	Block verified by HANNA, MATTHEW.	Peds-grossing
07/23/2014 10:13:37 AM	S-14-321	Specimen C	DEEP MARGIN OF THE RIGHT LEG MASS	Scanned by HANNA, MATTHEW.	Peds-grossing
07/23/2014 10:13:57 AM	S-14-321	Block C1	PROCESS AND EMBED A PARAFFIN BLOCK	Block verified by HANNA, MATTHEW.	Peds-grossing
07/23/2014 10:14:20 AM	S-14-321	Specimen D	PROXIMAL MARGIN OF THE RIGHT LEG MASS	Scanned by HANNA, MATTHEW.	Peds-grossing
07/23/2014 10:14:43 AM	S-14-321	Block D1	PROCESS AND EMBED A PARAFFIN BLOCK	Block verified by HANNA, MATTHEW.	Peds-grossing
07/23/2014 10:15:04 AM	S-14-321	Specimen E	LATERAL MARGIN OF THE RIGHT LEG MASS	Scanned by HANNA, MATTHEW.	Peds-grossing
07/23/2014 10:15:23 AM	S-14-321	Block E1	PROCESS AND EMBED A PARAFFIN BLOCK	Block verified by HANNA, MATTHEW.	Peds-grossing
07/23/2014 10:15:46 AM	S-14-321	Specimen F	SUPERFICIAL MARGIN OF THE RIGHT LEG M...	Scanned by HANNA, MATTHEW.	Peds-grossing
07/23/2014 10:16:04 AM	S-14-321	Block F1	PROCESS AND EMBED A PARAFFIN BLOCK	Block verified by HANNA, MATTHEW.	Peds-grossing
07/25/2014 3:47:30 PM	A-14-123	Specimen B	PLACENTA	Scanned by HANNA, MATTHEW.	Grossing-GI Station
07/25/2014 3:47:40 PM	A-14-123	Block B1	Resident Block	Block verified by HANNA, MATTHEW.	Grossing-GI Station
07/25/2014 3:47:44 PM	A-14-123	Block B2	Resident Block	Block verified by HANNA, MATTHEW.	Grossing-GI Station
07/25/2014 3:47:49 PM	A-14-123	Block B3	Resident Block	Block verified by HANNA, MATTHEW.	Grossing-GI Station
07/25/2014 3:47:53 PM	A-14-123	Block B4	Resident Block	Block verified by HANNA, MATTHEW.	Grossing-GI Station
07/25/2014 3:47:58 PM	A-14-123	Block B5	Resident Block	Block verified by HANNA, MATTHEW.	Grossing-GI Station
07/25/2014 3:48:03 PM	A-14-123	Block B6	Resident Block	Block verified by HANNA, MATTHEW.	Grossing-GI Station
07/25/2014 3:48:07 PM	A-14-123	Block B7	Resident Block	Block verified by HANNA, MATTHEW.	Grossing-GI Station
01/19/2015 8:40:15 PM	S-15-282	Specimen C	LEFT PELVIC LYMPH NODE	Scanned by HANNA, MATTHEW.	Grossing-GYN

Fig. 7. Workstation user audit. This inquiry allows all scan events by a user to be identified in real time, displaying the event time, case (accession) number, specimen, user, and location.

Processing History

Performed On	Action Name	Material ID	Action D&T	Employee	Site	Workst
Specimen	Specimen Collected		3/5/2015 11:23 AM	HANNA, MATTHEW	m	HACC1
Specimen	Specimen Collected		3/5/2015 11:23 AM	HANNA, MATTHEW	m	HACC1
Material	Material Received	MS-15-204-A	3/5/2015 11:23 AM	HANNA, MATTHEW	m	HACC1
Specimen	Specimen Received		3/5/2015 11:23 AM	HANNA, MATTHEW	m	HACC1
Order	Order Inserted		3/5/2015 11:23 AM	HANNA, MATTHEW	m	HACC1
Material	PRINT CASSETTES	MS-15-204-A	3/5/2015 11:27 AM	HANNA, MATTHEW	m	HACC1
Specimen	Gross Description Modified		3/5/2015 11:29 AM	HANNA, MATTHEW	m	GROS1
Material	Grossing	MS-15-204-A	3/5/2015 11:29 AM	HANNA, MATTHEW	m	GROS1
Material	Grossing Complete- Scan block	MS-15-204-A1	3/5/2015 11:29 AM	HANNA, MATTHEW	m	GROS1
Material	RBS - Store Material in Storage	MS-15-204-A	3/5/2015 11:29 AM	HANNA, MATTHEW	m	HACC1
Material	ASSIGN AND LOAD CASSETTES IN TISSUE PROC	MS-15-204-A1	3/5/2015 11:29 AM	HANNA, MATTHEW	m	TISPR1
Material	SEND SPECIMEN TO STORAGE	MS-15-204-A	3/5/2015 11:29 AM	HANNA, MATTHEW	m	HACC1
Material	Specimen Storage Check In	MS-15-204-A	3/5/2015 11:29 AM	HANNA, MATTHEW	m	HACC1
Material	ASSIGN TISSUE PROCESSOR	MS-15-204-A1	3/5/2015 11:29 AM	HANNA, MATTHEW	m	TISPR1
Material	BLOCK EMBEDDING	MS-15-204-A1	3/5/2015 11:29 AM	HANNA, MATTHEW	m	EMBD1
Material	Microtomy	MS-15-204-A1	3/5/2015 11:40 AM	HANNA, MATTHEW	m	MCR1
Panel Slide S1	Microtomy	MS-15-204-A1	3/5/2015 11:40 AM	HANNA, MATTHEW	m	MCR1
Material	BLOCKS TO FILE	MS-15-204-A1	3/5/2015 11:40 AM	HANNA, MATTHEW	m	HACC1
Panel Slide S1	Slide Stain	MS-15-204-A1	3/5/2015 11:41 AM	HANNA, MATTHEW	m	STA1
Panel Slide S1	CASE DISTRIBUTION	MS-15-204-A1	3/5/2015 11:41 AM	HANNA, MATTHEW	m	DIST1
Final Interpret...	Order Interpreted		3/5/2015 4:17 PM	HERZFELD, EMILY	m	PATH2
Interpretation	N - RBS - Assign interpretation for Proreview		3/5/2015 4:27 PM	HERZFELD, EMILY	m	PATH2
Final Interpret...	Final Report Signed Out		3/5/2015 4:31 PM	HERZFELD, EMILY	m	PATH2

Fig. 8. Case processing history. Audit trail of different workstations, tracking a single case through the laboratory workflow (specimen collection to final case interpretation).

Field-testing of instruments, labels, various bar-code symbologies, and hardware is useful to demonstrate suitability and forecast potential integration difficulties. Frequent discussions with vendors or hired consultants hopefully address any issues that arise. Implementation from the time of deployment to training requires support from informatics and IT staff, personnel (end users) in the laboratory, pathologists, and senior administration.[33]

INVENTORY MANAGEMENT SYSTEMS

Inventory of a pathology laboratory may include a plethora of items. To control the supply and demand of such supplies, inventory management systems have been developed, either as a stand-alone product or as part of an LIS. The focus of these systems is to assimilate product identification, asset tracking, and order management. Manually logging items in a pathology laboratory is a tremendous burden and importantly more prone to errors. These systems help ensure appropriate availability of reagents, cassettes, glass slides, personal protective equipment, and so forth. Important directives to establish include

product lists, monthly usage, frequency of ordering, storage, expiration dates, and cost. Systems have been developed to alert or automatically order new supplies when inventory runs low. Having a constant supply of supplies in a pathology laboratory is vital for an efficient operation. Shared resource facilities (eg, tissue biorepository) may greatly benefit from such inventory management systems.[34]

FUTURE DIRECTIONS

RFID is an emerging but recently introduced technology in pathology (**Table 4**).[35,36] RFID is a method of uniquely identifying items using radio wave signals emitted from an RFID tag that are detected by a reader with an antenna. These tags can encode data about an asset but do not always necessitate user action to physically scan the tag. Where bar codes fall short of only allowing individual static data to be encoded, RFID tags have the ability to allow multiple dynamic data updates, with rapid read rates and batch readability. Radio frequencies can penetrate nonmetallic objects. In laboratories, RFID tags can be placed

Table 4
Comparison of bar code and radiofrequency identification technologies

| | Bar Code | | Radiofrequency Identification | | |
	1-D	2-D	Passive	Active	Near-field Communication
Data density	Low	Intermediate	High	High	High
Line of site	Required	Required	None	None	None
Manual or automated	Manual	Manual	Automated	Automated	Automated
Batch capability	No	No	Yes	Yes	Yes
Frequency interferences	None	None	More sensitive	Less sensitive	Less sensitive
Battery requirement	None	None	None	Yes	None
Read vs read-write	Read	Read	Read-write	Read-write	Read-write

on each specimen/asset to be traced. RFID tags exist in passive or active forms, where passive tags draw electromagnetic energy from the radio waves of a reader, and active tags have their own power source. Active tags are battery powered, enabling longer read ranges (up to 100 m); however, this limits their longevity for assets being archived or for use in tissue repository laboratories. Passive tags have shorter read ranges (less than 25 m) and a reported life span of approximately 20 years. Active tags are also larger and cost more. Tags can be preserialized, programmable, or both. Preserialized tags are proprogrammed at the time of manufacturing and are assigned a unique sequential character sequence. Programmable tags are encoded at the time of use by the user. RFID technology is currently more expensive than bar codes. Also, few vendors offer them as a part of their tracking solution.[10,37] RFID tags have been shown to be resilient in anatomic pathology laboratories.[38] It is likely that RFID technology will be increasingly used in laboratories in the near future.

NFC has been recently popularized in smartphone technology related to contactless payment systems. NFC is a specialized subset of RFID technology. RFID frequencies exist as low (<0.3 MHz), high (3–30 MHz), ultrahigh (860–950 MHz), and microwave (2450–5800 MHz) ranges.[37] NFC technology operates at the same high frequency range (predominantly 13.56 MHz) as other RFID tags; however, its distinguishing factor is that an NFC-labeled item can serve as a reader and a tag simultaneously. Depending on the frequency, RFID tags can be read at far or near distances, NFC technology is built to have secure reads at only a few centimeters. It is anticipated that similar technology will likely be used to improve tracking in health care, including pathology.[39–42]

SUMMARY

Anatomic pathology laboratories have a responsibility to modernize and sustain increasing efficiency, leverage automation, and foster patient safety. Misidentification errors in laboratories have the capability to cause devastating events. The use of bar coding and tracking systems for anatomic pathology laboratories has, therefore, become common. Although workflow changes may incorporate dramatic reforms, this technology has the ability to decrease laboratory blunders while proportionately increasing efficiency. As technology has advanced, more robust products and innovative solutions have been witnessed. As with the introduction of 2-D high data density bar codes in laboratories, RFID technology offers similar promising benefits.

REFERENCES

1. Becich MJ, Gilbertson JR, Gupta D, et al. Pathology and patient safety: the critical role of pathology informatics in error reduction and quality initiatives. Clin Lab Med 2004;24(4):913–43.

2. Sharma G, Parwani AV, Raval JS, et al. Contemporary issues in transfusion medicine informatics. J Pathol Inform 2011;2:3.

3. Richmond L. Barcoding in the lab: achieving error-free efficiencies. Healthc Inform 1994;11:26–30.

4. Snyder SR, Favoretto AM, Derzon JH, et al. Effectiveness of barcoding for reducing patient specimen and laboratory testing identification errors: a Laboratory Medicine Best Practices systematic review and meta-analysis. Clin Biochem 2012;45(13–14):988–98.

5. Pagliaro P, Turdo R, Capuzzo E. Patients' positive identification systems. Blood Transfus 2009;7:313–8.

6. Morrison AP, Tanasijevic MJ, Goonan EM, et al. Reduction in specimen labeling errors after

implementation of a positive patient identification system in phlebotomy. Am J Clin Pathol 2010;133: 870–7.

7. ID History. Progression of proposed product ID symbols. ID History Museum. 2013. Available at: http://www.idhistory.com/. Accessed January 17, 2015.

8. Ashford P, Distler P, Gee A, et al. ISBT 128 implementation plan for cellular therapy products. J Clin Apher 2007;22(5):258–64.

9. Butch S, Distler P, Georgsen J, et al. ISBT 128: an introduction. 3rd edition. 2006. Available at: http://www.transfusionmedicine.ca/sites/transfusionmedicine/files/articles/ISBT%20128_Attachments/ISBT%20an%20Introduction.pdf. Accessed January 18, 2015.

10. Balis UJ, Pantanowitz L. Specimen tracking and identification systems. In: Pantanowitz L, Balis UJ, Tuthill JM, editors. Pathology informatics: theory & practice. Chicago: ASCP Press; 2012. p. 283–304.

11. Specification for bar code symbols, vol. MH10.8M-1983. ANSI; 1983.

12. Pantanowitz L, Mackinnon AC Jr, Sinard JH. Tracking in anatomic pathology. Arch Pathol Lab Med 2013;137:1798–810.

13. Mountain PJ, Callaghan JV, Chou D, et al. Laboratory automation: bar codes for specimen container identification; approved standard. In: CLSI document AUTO02-A2, vol. 25, 2nd edition. Wayne (PA): CLSI; 2005. p. 25.

14. Hawker CD, Agrawal Y, Balis UJ, et al. Specimen labels: content and location, fonts, and label orientation; approved standard. In: CLSI document AUTO12-A, vol. 31, 1st edition. Wayne (PA): CLSI; 2011. p. 48.

15. Palmer RC. The bar code book: a comprehensive guide to reading, printing, specifying, evaluating, and using bar code and other machine readable symbols. 5th edition. Victoria, BC, Canada: Trafford Publishing; 2007.

16. Cowan DF. Bar coding in the laboratory. In: Cowan DF, editor. Informatics for the clinical laboratory: a practical guide for the pathologist. New York: Springer; 2005. p. 156–68.

17. Lippi G, Blanckaert N, Bonini P, et al. Causes, consequences, detection, and prevention of identification errors in laboratory diagnostics. Clin Chem Lab Med 2009;47:143–53.

18. Nakhleh RE, Zarbo RJ. Surgical pathology specimen identification and accessioning: a College of American Pathologists Q-Probes Study of 1 004 115 cases from 417 institutions. Arch Pathol Lab Med 1996;120(3):227–33.

19. Dunn EJ, Moga PJ. Patient misidentification in laboratory medicine: a qualitative analysis of 227 root cause analysis reports in the Veterans Health Administration. Arch Pathol Lab Med 2010;134:244–55.

20. Valenstein PN, Sirota RL. Identification errors in pathology and laboratory medicine. Clin Lab Med 2004;24(4):979–96.

21. Nakhleh RE, Idowu MO, Souers RJ, et al. Mislabeling of cases, specimens, blocks, and slides: a College of American Pathologists study of 136 institutions. Arch Pathol Lab Med 2011;135(8):969–74.

22. Layfield LJ, Anderson GM. Specimen labeling errors in surgical pathology: an 18-month experience. Am J Clin Pathol 2010;134:466–70.

23. Nakhleh RE. Patient safety and error reduction in surgical pathology. Arch Pathol Lab Med 2008;132: 181–5.

24. Simpson NJ, Kleinberg KA. Implementation guide to barcoding and auto-id in healthcare: improving quality and patient safety. Chicago: HIMSS; 2009.

25. Informatics for the Clinical Laboratory. A practical guide for the pathologist. New York: Springer; 2002. p. 156–68.

26. Zarbo RJ, Tuthill JM, D'Angelo R, et al. The henry ford production system: reduction of surgical pathology in-process misidentification defects by bar code- specified work process standardization. Am J Clin Pathol 2009;131(4):468–77.

27. Snyder ML, Carter A, Jenkins K, et al. Patient misidentifications caused by errors in standard barcode technology. Clin Chem 2010;56:1–7.

28. Eiseman E, Haga SB. Handbook of human tissue sources. Chapter 6 Pathology specimens, 1999. Available at: http://www.rand.org/content/dam/rand/pubs/monograph_reports/MR954/MR954.chap6.pdf Accessed January 11, 2015.

29. Tomar RH, Aller RD, Arkin CF, et al. Laboratory automation: systems operational requirements, characteristics, and information elements; approved standard. In: CLSI document AUTO04-A, vol. 21, 1st edition. Wayne (PA): CLSI; 2001. p. 40.

30. Sharma G, Piccoli A, Kelly SM, et al. Reduction of anatomical pathology slide mislabel rate due to implementation of barcoding at two tertiary care hospitals. Mod Pathol 2011;24(Suppl 1):342A.

31. Sinard JH, Gershkovich P. Custom software development for use in a clinical laboratory. J Pathol Inform 2012;3:44.

32. Sinard JH, Mutnick N, Gershkovich P. Histology asset tracking dashboard: real-time monitoring and dynamic work lists. J Pathol Inform 2010;1:18.

33. Force HB. Implementation guide for the use of bar code technology in healthcare. Chicago: Healthcare Information and Management Systems Society; 2003.

34. Dash RC, Robb JA, Booker DL, et al. Biospecimens and biorepositories for the community pathologist. Arch Pathol Lab Med 2012;136(6):668–78.

35. Briggs L, Davis R, Gutierrez A, et al. RFID in the blood supply chain: increasing productivity, quality

and patient safety. J Healthc Inf Manag 2009;23: 54–63.

36. Knels R, Ashford P, Bidet F, et al. Guidelines for the use of RFID technology in transfusion medicine. Vox Sang 2010;98:1–24.

37. Lou JJ, Andrechak GA, Riben M, et al. A review of radio frequency identification technology for the anatomic pathology or biorepository laboratory: much promise, some progress, and more work needed. J Pathol Inform 2011;2:34.

38. Leung AA, Lou JJ, Mareninov S, et al. Tolerance testing of passive radio frequency identification tags for solvent, temperature, and pressure conditions encountered in an anatomic pathology or biorepository setting. J Pathol Inform 2010;1:21.

39. Swedberg C. Brigham and Women's Hospital Tests NFC RFID for patient bedsides. RFID Journal 2013. Available at: http://www.rfidjournal.com/articles/view?10511/. Accessed January 7, 2015.

40. Agrawal A. Medication errors: prevention using information technology systems. Br J Clin Pharmacol 2009;67:681–6.

41. Section of Pharmacy Informatics and Technology, American Society of Health-System Pharmacists. ASHP statement on bar-code-enabled medication administration technology. Am J Health Syst Pharm 2009;66:588–90.

42. Poon EG, Keohane CA, Yoon CS, et al. Effect of barcode technology on the safety of medication administration. N Engl J Med 2010;362:1698–707.

Enhancing and Customizing Laboratory Information Systems to Improve/Enhance Pathologist Workflow

Douglas J. Hartman, MD

KEYWORDS

- Image-embedded reports • Voice recognition • Pre–sign-out quality assurance
- Computerized provider order entry

ABSTRACT

Optimizing pathologist workflow can be difficult because it is affected by many variables. Surgical pathologists must complete many tasks that culminate in a final pathology report. Several software systems can be used to enhance/improve pathologist workflow. These include voice recognition software, pre–sign-out quality assurance, image utilization, and computerized provider order entry. Recent changes in the diagnostic coding and the more prominent role of centralized electronic health records represent potential areas for increased ways to enhance/improve the workflow for surgical pathologists. Additional unforeseen changes to the pathologist workflow may accompany the introduction of whole-slide imaging technology to the routine diagnostic work.

OVERVIEW

The workflow for pathologists constitutes a broad category due to the many roles that surgical pathologists must engage in during a workday. These roles include interpreting histopathologic findings, generating a diagnostic report to clearly convey pathologic findings, communicating critical results when appropriate, ensuring quality of the pathology system, educating future pathologists (residents and fellows), and, when appropriate, having quality assurance performed on the diagnostic findings. To understand various ways that a pathologist's workflow can be enhanced, understanding the practice workflow for pathologists is critical.

Many academic practices and some community pathology practices have converted into a subspecialized sign-out service.[1-3] Several factors are contributing to this trend: (1) increased pressure for consolidation or concentration of hospital services into a centralized center, (2) increasing complexity of the knowledge base, and (3) requests from clinical colleagues for subspecialty expertise. There is variability among how the subspecialization works by practice, with most academic practices having pathologists dedicated to a single subspecialty whereas community practices may rely on subspecialty expertise in a consultative role for specific or difficult cases. A mixture of subspecialty-only pathologists with general pathologists is appealing from a management standpoint because caseload balancing can be readily performed when adjustable pathologist labor is possible, depending on the volume of a particular organ specimen type. With the ongoing health care changes, subspecialty expertise demand is likely to increase in order to deliver higher-quality, outcome-driven health care. Just as pathologists are becoming subspecialized, the clients that pathologists serve have been changing as well.

Disclosure Statement: author for one up-to-date on topic - Clinical Pathological Cases in Gastroenterology, otherwise no disclosures.
Department of Anatomic Pathology, University of Pittsburgh Medical Center, 200 Lothrop Street, A-607, Pittsburgh, PA 15213, USA
E-mail address: hartmandj@upmc.edu

Surgical Pathology 8 (2015) 137–143
http://dx.doi.org/10.1016/j.path.2015.02.006
1875-9181/15/$ – see front matter © 2015 Elsevier Inc. All rights reserved.

Clinical teams have become a mixture of attending physicians who themselves are becoming more and more subspecialized, house staff (fellows and residents), nurse practitioners or physician assistants, nurse coordinators, nurses, and so forth. The secondary team members are sometimes interacting with the pathology department more than the attending physician due to time constraints. Additionally, pathology reports have many different intended audiences—for instance, a surgical resection report is completed predominantly for the operating surgeon, but a primary care physician/oncologist/radiation oncologist (and so forth) may be interested in report content that differs from the surgeon. Additionally, greater transparency of records is demanded by the public, which is leading to surgical pathology reports going directly to the patients themselves. These challenges present an opportunity for pathology to demonstrate its contribution to the clinical team but the solutions often involve balancing various competing needs.

It is within this setting that pathologists must complete the many diverse tasks that are requested of them. Within this article, I discuss several possible ways to enhance/customize surgical pathology workflow. Many of these may be more helpful depending on the clinical practice setup.

VOICE RECOGNITION TECHNOLOGY

Several studies have explored the use of voice recognition technology in pathology with mixed interpretation of the results. One component to consider when looking at voice recognition is the current practice environment. If there is a delay between dictation and completion of reports, voice recognition technology is an attractive alternative. In a system where transcription completes reports quickly, however, the altered workflow associated with voice recognition is not welcomed because there is little gain compared with the prior system. Voice recognition technology is particularly suited to filling in template forms rather than generating a final (free text–based) diagnosis.[4] Henricks and colleagues[4] demonstrated that targeted deployment of voice recognition was cost effective (reduced 2 full-time equivalent positions and payback period was less than 2 years). Kang and colleagues[5] also found that voice recognition technology was amenable to use predominantly for gross description. The use of preprogrammed templates facilitated less text editing of the reports and allowed for greater acceptance.[5] Kang and colleagues[5] discussed several barriers to adoption of voice recognition technology for final diagnosis. These barriers boil down to a lack of standardization in pathology reporting.[5] The

pathology department at State University of New York at Stony Brook adopted voice recognition for the complete surgical pathology workflow (from gross description to final diagnosis sign-out).[6] Although not explicitly stated in their study, this group seems to have experienced long turnaround time with their transcription service, and some pathologists submitted handwritten copies of reports to be transcribed.[6] Within this background, the investigators found voice recognition technology a marked improvement, but, despite its improvements over the prior system, some pathologists still used the prior system for report generation.[6]

WORK PROCESSING

Many articles have been written in recent years describing implementation of lean principles based on the Toyota Production System.[7] Other articles also describe efficient processing as the Henry Ford Production System.[8] These systems are largely taken from the manufacturing world. The systems describe changes to the workflow of a specimen of pathology into a continuous flow system. Although continuous flow systems reduce errors and are efficient, some steps in the processing of pathology specimens require batch processing. The biggest batch process for pathology specimen workflow is the specimen processors. Numerous articles have described implementation of continuous process flow to gross processing or continuous flow to slide generation but few if any studies have described a 100% continuous flow specimen processing system.[7–12] This may be because this physically cannot be done. Therefore, the processing of specimen has been turned into a mix of batch and continuous flow processes. Therefore, for a sign-out pathologist, considering an optimal workflow depends on the method for receiving the slide—continuous flow or batch processes. Theoretically, if a pathologist is receiving 1 slide every 10 minutes, then the pathologist can advance that case within a 10-minute window before the next slide comes out. Most departments, however, deliver slides in batches, leading to the pathologist working within a batch processing workflow. This process can include house staff also within the process, which can add another step in batch processing. In the future, with the introduction of whole-slide imaging into the workflow process, continuous flow may be more of a reality than can be achieved in practical terms now. A sample diagram of the workflow from slides leaving histology to report delivery to downstream end users within a pathology department is described in **Fig. 1**. Although continuous flow

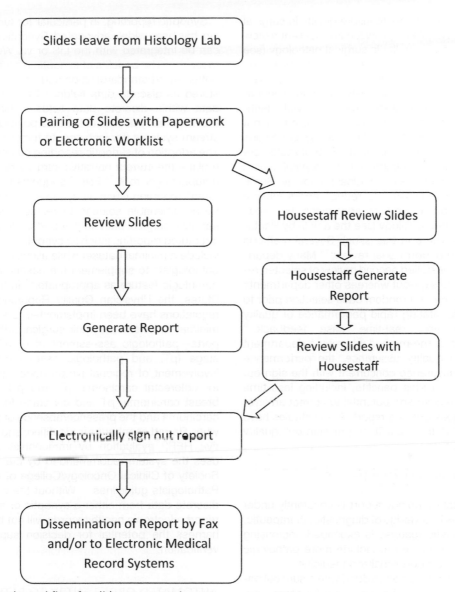

Fig. 1. Sample workflow for slides to report signout.

systems seem the most efficient method, batch processing is currently an integral component of the health care system.

To this end, new iterations of laboratory information systems (LIS) software have tested providing case status updates to sign-out pathologists, for instance, the cases accessioned, the cases of gross complete, and the cases of final diagnosis. Although it is difficult to know how this functionality will work from a practical standpoint, this functionality suggests that the dynamic process of specimen processing can be interactive. Some institutions have instituted specimen tracking through their LIS systems (see the article by Pantanowitz elsewhere in this issue).[13] This specimen tracking may also interact with the clinical systems from which specimens are received. The current workflow is less granular, but perhaps as bar coding expands, this functionality will become more granular. This type of system may also be helpful when whole-slide imaging is implemented (notification of scanning status for slides and so forth).

QUALITY ASSURANCE

Since the release of the Institute of Medicine 1999 report, "To Err is Human: Building a Safer Health System,"[14] several articles have been published describing quality assurance measures and proposing novel ways to insure quality in surgical pathology. Nakhleh[15] provided an excellent review of all aspects of quality in surgical pathology (see also the article by Nakhleh elsewhere in this issue). A simple representation of errors breaks them down into preanalytical, analytical, and postanalytical errors.[15] Pathologists can assist with identifying preanalytical and postanalytical errors but these errors are often influenced by conditions outside pathology's control. Pathologists are able to monitor and improve the analytical aspect of quality assurance for surgical pathology. Some proposed mechanisms to reduce errors include bar code processing of specimens by gross room staff and histology (see the article by Pantanowitz elsewhere in this issue). Several methods are used to perform peer review.[15] Many departments have installed second review of selected reports prior to sign-out whereas other departments have implemented random case selection prior to sign-out, facilitating rapid performance of quality assurance and real-time case feedback.[16] Regardless of the method whereby a department determines quality assurance, the performance of quality assurance concurrent with the sign-out of a case provides benefits, including less time locating the case and potential to correct an error before it goes out in a report. A few studies have documented the benefit of pre–sign-out quality assurance.[16,17]

SURGICAL PATHOLOGY REPORT

The surgical pathology report is constantly under evolution as knowledge of diagnostic, therapeutic, and prognostic features is expanded. Increasing demands are placed to include more pathologic data in an era of personalized medicine.[18]

Histologic images embedded within surgical pathology reports have been possible for some time. This system of surgical pathology reporting has been provided predominantly by commercial pathology groups.[18] In my opinion, the lack of widespread adoption of whole-slide imaging systems and the difficulty of representing the pertinent pathologic findings in a single image have impeded more widespread adoption of image embedded surgical pathology reports. Additionally, the lack of transmission of images across interfaces within the electronic medical record and the lack of widespread color printing delivery of pathology reports (many reports are still delivered via fax) also impede the adoption of this method for reporting. Besides the increased use of images in reports, commercial laboratories also use templates with graphics and synoptics to enhance and market their pathology reports.[19,20]

Synoptic reporting, in particular for tumor staging, has been widely advocated. Synoptic reporting can be integrated with the LIS or via Web-based tools.[21–23] The benefits of synoptic reports include better report standardization and allow data to be stored as discrete data fields.[23] Storing synoptic data within discrete data fields within an LIS provides ready access to the data points for downstream systems (for instance, to tumor registries). The adoption of synoptic reporting can be used to replace the current narrative surgical report or as a supplement to it.[24] Ellis[24] suggests that "structured" reporting (such as synoptic reporting) may be an amenable solution to replace the current narrative surgical pathology reports. Ellis envisions structured reporting (such as synoptic reporting) to include a minimal dataset while allowing individual pathologists to supplement the description of the pathologic feature as appropriate.[24] In the United States, the Physician Quality Reporting System regulations have been implemented to encourage minimal data elements within surgical pathology reports—pathologic assessment of primary tumor stage (pT) and pathologic assessment of the involvement of regional lymph nodes (pN) stage for colorectal carcinoma, pT and pN stage for breast carcinoma, pT and pN stage for prostate carcinoma and the presence/absence of dysplasia when Barrett esophagus is identified; and quantitative HER2 evaluation by immunohistochemistry uses the system recommended by the American Society of Clinical Oncology/College of American Pathologists guidelines.[25] Without the creation of discrete data from either a synoptic or structured report, electronic health records will not be able to harness the potential for decision support and verification.

AUTOMATED ORDER ENTRY TO PATHOLOGY LABORATORY INFORMATION SYSTEMS

The introduction of computerized physician order entry (CPOE) has been driven largely to reduce medication-related errors.[26] The use of CPOE for laboratory test order entry provides an opportunity to improve laboratory test ordering efficiency, laboratory utilization, and patient care.[27] The benefits of CPOE in clinical pathology laboratory testing include reduced risk for mislabeled specimens, incorrect container types, lost requisitions, and incorrect testing.[27] CPOE is being introduced, however, into the surgical pathology system. This offers the ability to increase efficiency within the health care system; however, it leads to nonpathology workers entering information into the pathology LIS. Some of the benefits (such as incorrect testing and incorrect container types) associated with CPOE for clinical pathology laboratory testing do not apply to anatomic pathology. This change in the delivery of order to anatomic pathology will require pathology departments to educate the clinical administrative staff about the type of information needed to perform an appropriate pathologic examination. In the past, this task has been accomplished by requiring the completion of a requisition form, although the requirement of a requisition does not always mean all of the clinical information is provided.[28] One study of dermatopathology requisitions found no difference between hand-written requisitions (3.0%) and electronic requisitions (3.9%).[29] With the implementation of a CPOE system, the possibility of clinical decision support can be introduced[27]; however, it is unclear how clinical decision support systems would affect the performance of anatomic pathology services. Although clinical pathology laboratory is more advanced than the surgical pathology laboratory when it comes to electronic order entry, the current order entry systems do not support add-on testing (additional studies and so forth).[27]

USE OF IMAGES IN SURGICAL PATHOLOGY

It is said, "a picture can say a thousand words."[30] The possible uses of images within surgical pathology extend from scanning of documents (either outside reports or requisitions) to gross images to and microscopic images.

In recent years the advent of high throughput document scanning has created an opportunity to scan specimen requisitions into an LIS. One of the drawbacks of this ability is that it encourages hand-written orders that may be illegible (discussed previously regarding order entry as an alternative system). Even in an electronic order system, there may be a role for document scanning ability within the LIS, particularly for downtime procedures, additional/follow-up orders on specimens, or documentation of extradepartmental consultations. The image file type can be customized to contain specific properties related to the file extension—for instance, at the University of Pittsburgh Medical center, we have created a specific file type for requisitions, which allows for printing of the surgical pathology working draft along with the requisition. In this example, the need to match a requisition with the printed working draft (printed after the gross complete status was made) was eliminated because the file type from the case was matched when the case was ready to print the working draft. Some potential future directions might be to automate notification

of the sign-out pathologist when additional tests have been requested or an extradepartmental consultation has been received. Within our department, as part of quality assurance, it is policy to issue an addendum statement when an outside consultation on a pathology report is received. Reduction of manual entry of documents via document scanning is ideal but unlikely to be completely eliminated in the current system.

Image documentation of gross abnormalities of surgical specimens may represent an alternative documentation of the type of specimen/gross findings received. It is our departmental policy to obtain gross images of surgical specimens. Given the expanded use of pathologist assistants for most grossing responsibilities, the images obtained sometimes may not be of optimal quality. One possible solution to encourage more optimal gross images is to integrate the image capture work into the gross description work. Currently, the acquisition of the image is one more task assigned to a pathologist assistant on top of other responsibilities. Integrating this into the workflow would encourage appropriate gross documentation and potentially reduce a pathologist assistant's time per case. If the gross measurements could be derived from the image, it might be possible to store these measurements as discrete values for later use within the LIS, for instance, in the generation of the final report or the completion of a synoptic report. This workflow is currently not possible and our pathologist assistants mostly generate narrative gross descriptions based on grossing manual or institutional guidelines on top of acquiring gross images of the surgical specimens.

The use of microscopic images within surgical pathology reports is discussed previously. With the lack of widespread whole-slide imaging devices, the acquisition of microscopic images is tedious. At the University of Pittsburgh Medical Center, using the same LIS software for microscopic image integration into the surgical pathology report, we have experimented with placing a 2-D bar code on surgical pathology reports. The 2-D bar code linked to a Web site with content related to the final diagnosis of the surgical pathology report (no diagnostic information was present within the link). The intent of this code would be to provide information to the end-user information above and beyond the diagnostic aspect of the surgical pathology report. At the University of Pittsburgh Medical Center, we have yet to assess the end-user viewpoint of this strategy but no feedback was directed after instituting this experiment. Several conclusions could be suggested by this small experiment: (1) paper reports are no longer the primary method by which end users access their surgical pathology reports, (2) end users focus only on the diagnostic part of the reports, or (3) there was no to limited novelty of having a 2-D bar code on the report. Within the past 10 years, there has been an expansion of electronic records from departments other than radiology or pathology. This change may reflect why a paper surgical pathology report no longer is used by end users. A recent article described a delayed identification of errors in dates associated with laboratory test reporting with the implementation of a new order entry system.[31] This likely reflects overworked clinical colleagues and a lack of awareness to pathology quality issues from clinical colleagues. One of the fundamentally most important functions for our surgical pathology reports is to communicate results to the end users.[32] To the extent that it is possible, this effort could represent a further method to communicate with clinical colleagues pertinent information to their practice or a given medical condition. Future directions for adding supplemental data will require coordination between the downstream clinical systems and the pathology LIS. This function might pair well with efforts to electronically order additional studies/tests on a surgical pathology specimen. Coded diagnostic information (such as the implementation of *International Classification of Diseases, Tenth Revision*) represents an increased granularity of medical coding and the potential to use this by pathology to supplement clinical decision support systems is vast.[33]

Pathologist workflow is affected by many different variables, predominantly related to the setup of the practice that they work for. Surgical pathologists are tasked with many different roles that culminate in the final pathology report. Several software systems can be used to enhance/improve pathologist workflow. These systems include voice recognition software, pre–sign-out quality assurance, microscopic image embedding within surgical pathology reports, and computerized provider order entry. Recent changes in diagnostic coding and centralized electronic health records represent potential areas for increased ways to enhance/improve the workflow for surgical pathologists. Additional unforeseen changes to pathologist workflow may accompany the introduction of whole-slide imaging technology to the routine diagnostic work.

REFERENCES

1. Sarewitz SJ. Subspecialization in community pathology practice. Arch Pathol Lab Med 2014;138(7): 871–2.

2. Black-Shaffer WS, Young RH, Harris NL. Subspecialization of surgical pathology at the Massachusetts General Hospital. Am J Clin Pathol 1996;106(4 Suppl 1):S33–42.

3. Groppi DE, Alexis CE, Sugrue CF, et al. Consolidation of the North Shore-LIJ Health System Anatomic Pathology Services: the challenge of subspecialization, operations, quality management, staffing and education. Am J Clin Pathol 2013;140(1):20–30.

4. Henricks WH, Roumina K, Skilton BE, et al. The utility and cost effectiveness of voice recognition technology in surgical pathology. Mod Pathol 2002;15(5):565–71.

5. Kang HP, Sirintrapun J, Nestler RJ, et al. Experience with voice recognition in surgical pathology at a Large Academic Multi-Institutional Center. Am J Clin Pathol 2010;133:156–9.

6. Singh M, Pal TR. Voice recognition technology implementation in surgical pathology. Arch Pathol Lab Med 2011;135:1476–81.

7. Serrano L, Hegge P, Sato B, et al. Using LEAN principles to improve quality, patient safety, and workflow in histology and anatomic pathology. Adv Anat Pathol 2010;17:215–21.

8. Zarbo RJ, Tuthill JM, D'Angelo R, et al. The Henry Ford Production System: reduction of surgical pathology in-process misidentification defects by bar code-specified work process standardization. Am J Clin Pathol 2009;131:468–77.

9. D'Angelo R, Zarbo RJ. The Henry Ford Production System: measures of process defects and waste in surgical pathology as a basis for quality improvement initiatives. Am J Clin Pathol 2007;128(3):423–9.

10. Zarbo RJ, D'Angelo R. The Henry Ford Production System: effective reduction of process defects and waste in surgical pathology. Am J Clin Pathol 2007;128(6):1015–22.

11. Persoon TJ, Zaleski S, Frerichs J. Improving preanalytic processes using the principles of lean production (Toyota Production System). Am J Clin Pathol 2006;125(1):16–25.

12. Jimmerson C, Weber D, Sobek DK 2nd. Reducing waste and errors: piloting lean principles at Intermountain Healthcare. Jt Comm J Qual Patient Saf 2005;31(5):249–57.

13. Grimm EE, Schmidt RA. Reengineered workflow in the anatomic pathology laboratory: costs and benefits. Arch Pathol Lab Med 2009;133:601–4.

14. Kohn LT, Corrigan JM, Donaldson MS, editors. To err is human: building a safer health system. Washington, DC: National Academy Press; 1999.

15. Nakhleh RE. What is quality in surgical pathology? J Clin Pathol 2006;59:669–72.

16. Owens SR, Dhir R, Yousem SA, et al. The development and testing of a laboratory information system-driven tool for pre-sign-out quality assurance of random surgical pathology reports. Am J Clin Pathol 2010;133:836–41.

17. Owens SR, Wiehagen LT, Kelly SM, et al. Initial experience with a novel pre-sign-out quality assurance tool for review of random surgical pathology diagnoses in a subspecialty-based University practice. Am J Surg Pathol 2010;34:1319–23.

18. Parwani AV, Mohanty SK, Becich MJ. Pathology reporting in the 21st century: the impact of synoptic reports and digital imaging. Lab Med 2008;39(10):582–6.

19. Leong AS. Synoptic/Checklist reporting of breast biopsies: has the time come? Breast J 2001;7:271–4.

20. Leong FJ, Leong AS. Digital imaging in pathology: theoretical and practical considerations, and applications. Pathology 2004;36:234–41.

21. Qu Z, Ninan S, Almosa A, et al. Synoptic reporting in tumor pathology: advantages of a web-based system. Am J Clin Pathol 2007;127:898–903.

22. Baskovich BW, Allan RW. Web-based synoptic reporting for cancer checklists. J Pathol Inform 2011; 2:16.

23. Lankshear S, Srigley J, McGowan T, et al. Standardized synoptic cancer pathology reports – so what and who cares? A population-based satisfaction survey of 970 pathologists, surgeons, and oncologists. Arch Pathol Lab Med 2013;137(11):1599–602.

24. Ellis DW. Surgical pathology reporting at the crossroads: beyond synoptic reporting. Pathology 2011; 43(5):404–9.

25. Available at: http://www.ascp.org/PDF/Advocacy/Performance-Measures.pdf. Accessed August 29, 2014.

26. Devine EB, Hansen RN, Wilson-Norton JL, et al. The impact of computerized provider order entry on medication errors in a multispecialty group practice. J Am Med Inform Assoc 2010;17(1):78–84.

27. Baron JM, Dighe AS. Computerized provider order entry in the clinical laboratory. J Pathol Inform 2011;2:35.

28. Nakhleh RE, Gephardt G, Zarbo RJ. Necessity of clinical information in surgical pathology: a College of American Pathologists q-probes study of 771475 surgical pathology cases from 341 institutions. Arch Pathol Lab Med 1999;123:615–9.

29. Kinonen CL, Watkin WG, Gleason BC, et al. An audit of dermatopathology requisitions: hand written vs. electronic medical record data entry accuracy. J Cutan Pathol 2012;39:850–2.

30. Available at: http://en.wikipedia.org/wiki/A_picture_is_worth_a_thousand_words. Accessed August 30, 2014.

31. Appleton A, Sadek K, Dawson IG, et al. Clinicians were oblivious to incorrect logging of test dates and the associated risks in an online pathology application: a case study. Inform Prim Care 2012; 20(4).241–7.

32. Nakhleh RE. Quality in surgical pathology communication and reporting. Arch Pathol Lab Med 2011; 135:1394–7.

33. Available at: http://www.cms.gov/Medicare/Coding/ICD10/index.html?redirect=/icd10. Accessed August 30, 2014.

Specialized Laboratory Information Systems

Bryan Dangott, MD

KEYWORDS

- Specialty LIS • Report integration • Niche LIS • Multimodality LIS • Streamlined LIS • Custom-build
- Efficient LIS

ABSTRACT

Some laboratories or laboratory sections have unique needs that traditional anatomic and clinical pathology systems may not address. A specialized laboratory information system (LIS), which is designed to perform a limited number of functions, may perform well in areas where a traditional LIS falls short. Opportunities for specialized LISs continue to evolve with the introduction of new testing methodologies. These systems may take many forms, including stand-alone architecture, a module integrated with an existing LIS, a separate vendor-supplied module, and customized software. This article addresses the concepts underlying specialized LISs, their characteristics, and in what settings they are found.

OVERVIEW: WHAT IS A SPECIALIZED LABORATORY INFORMATION SYSTEM?

Broadly speaking, a specialized LIS is designed to perform a limited number of functions extremely well rather than trying to serve the needs of an entire laboratory. Because specialty systems are more customized than general LISs, they can take many forms. For example, a specialty LIS may exist as a stand-alone commercial application that is installed alongside an existing LIS architecture. Alternatively, they may consist of a markedly enhanced or customized spin-off or module of an existing LIS. Additionally, in practice settings where subspecialty sign-out is the norm, a specialty-specific LIS or LISs may fulfill all the needs of the organization. In rare instances, a specialty LIS may be developed entirely in-house to serve as the backbone of a laboratory. Some

examples and characteristics of specialized LISs are listed in **Box 1**.

IDENTIFYING SHORTCOMINGS

POTENTIAL SHORTCOMINGS OF AN EXISTING LABORATORY INFORMATION SYSTEM

Some laboratories or laboratory sections have unique needs that traditional anatomic and clinical pathology systems may not address. Settings where a specialized LIS may thrive are listed in **Box 2**. The factors contributing to perceived or real shortcomings in a given laboratory with a given LIS are usually complicated and multifactorial. In most instances, laboratory sections do not have the luxury of choosing an LIS up front. More often than not, a laboratory with an existing LIS adapts its functions to the changing or growing role of the laboratory or laboratory subsections. Unfortunately, these adaptations may sometimes fall short of the desired outcome. Challenges for traditional LISs are listed in **Box 3**.

POTENTIAL SHORTCOMING OF A NEW LABORATORY INFORMATION SYSTEM

When a laboratory is in the rare position of choosing a new LIS, the needs of the laboratory as a whole need to be considered in comparison to the needs of individual laboratory subsections. LIS purchase decisions are major financial investments with long-term contracts and significant organizational impact. The scale and complexity of these decisions may cause some unique or lower-priority requests to be outweighed by the operational needs of the laboratory or organization as a whole. The needs of every section in the laboratory often cannot be met by a single product.

East Carolina University, 600 Moye Blvd, Greenville, NC 27834, USA
E-mail address: dangottb@ecu.edu

Surgical Pathology 8 (2015) 145–152
http://dx.doi.org/10.1016/j.path.2015.02.003
1875-9181/15/$ – see front matter © 2015 Elsevier Inc. All rights reserved.

surgpath.theclinics.com

Box 1
General characteristics of a specialized laboratory information system

Performs a critical function

Example: interfaces with equipment that a traditional LIS does not support, allows future scalability

Enhances operations

Example: improved turnaround time, specimen tracking, enhanced reports, diagnostic data representation, correlation with previous results, etc.

Fills a major gap in existing systems

Example: allows meaningful and efficient storage and use of genomic or molecular testing, allows laboratories to adopt new testing methodologies

Tailored to specific practice environment

Example: subspecialty sign-out, molecular diagnostics, pharmaceutical industry

---

Box 2
Settings where a specialized laboratory information system may thrive

High-volume subspecialty sign-out

Example: dedicated sign-out of gastrointestinal, genitourinary, hematopathology, dermatopathology, etc.

Limited practice sign-out

Example: pharmaceutical or research setting, flow cytometry laboratory, molecular laboratory

Pathology practices trying to gain competitive advantage with enhanced functions

Example: customer relationship management, Web-based reports, integration of whole-slide images, molecular testing data, or photomicrographs with reports

Esoteric or cutting-edge testing

Example: transplant pathology, immunophenotyping, donor matching, flow cytometry, molecular testing, and proprietary testing methodologies, such as multigene tumor profiles, whole-slide imaging

High-throughput laboratories

Example: large commercial laboratory systems with LIS dashboards designed to track business and operational metrics and to streamline high-volume workflows

---

Box 3
Challenges for traditional laboratory information systems

Rapid growth of a laboratory section

Example: a previously considered low-priority feature may become critically important with laboratory growth

Evolving or proprietary test methodologies

Example: in-house developed test

New markets

Example: gene expression tumor profiling

New data types

Example: genomic sequencing

Integrated reports

Example: integration of histology, clinical laboratory data, flow cytometry, and molecular and cytogenetic testing methodologies as may be found in a hematopathology case

---

This may leave some laboratory sections with unmet needs. Furthermore, strong consideration should be given to the challenges of switching an LIS. Although technical barriers are in themselves difficult, an LIS conversion can be challenging from the perspectives of personnel and managing change within an organizational culture. The larger the organization, the greater the challenge in replacing a major component of an operational infrastructure.

SHORTCOMINGS DUE TO EVOLVING TECHNOLOGY

Some clinical laboratory analyzers were originally designed for a research setting. These instruments may include their own software, which was designed to interact with the instrument. However, the software may not have well-developed options for interfacing with the traditional LIS or electronic medical (EMR) systems. These stand-alone systems may themselves be considered a specialty LIS. This is more common when a vendor focuses heavily on hardware, and, as a result, the software that accompanies the equipment may be underdeveloped. These systems can be harder to maintain and may require on-site experts to handle customization and technical support issues.

SHORTCOMINGS DUE TO NONTRADITIONAL DATA SETS

Laboratory testing is a rapidly evolving field with a significant number of new tests and techniques introduced every year. Gene sequencing and molecular testing can create massive data sets, which require customized storage and data processing solutions. A traditional LIS is not designed to handle these data sets. Even technologies, such as whole-slide imaging, can create a need for a specialty LIS. Most whole-slide imaging systems come with their own software, which in many cases fits the definition of a specialty LIS. In well-established laboratories, some modalities of testing may not even have existed when the original LIS was chosen, which can leave gaps in function for the LIS as other technologies mature.[1]

MEETING UNIQUE NEEDS

As discussed previously, there are many settings where a laboratory may have unique needs that are not addressed by the current LIS. If the needs for a laboratory are too unique, the market for software to address these needs may be small. Another laboratory that has similar needs may also have just enough differences in its requirements to make the design of a broadly marketable solution difficult. From a software design point of view, these site-to-site differences lead to market fragmentation. Large LIS vendors may avoid small niche markets for these exact reasons. Common features of a niche market are listed in **Box 4**. A specialty LIS vendor needs to generate enough revenue from a small customer base to overcome the high development costs. If demand or profitability is strong enough, a few vendors may be willing to take the risk of developing custom software.

OPTIONS FOR FILLING GAPS

Option 1: Buying from an Existing Vendor

In many cases, LIS vendors offer add-on modules to augment their flagship systems. If an add-on exists that addresses an application gap, it should be strongly considered. Usually, a vendor-offered add-on can seamlessly integrate with existing infrastructure. The costs of implementing a vendor solution, however, can be too high if the specialty testing volume is low or if there are unknown/uncertain reimbursement streams. Rapidly evolving laboratory technologies are especially challenging because they may lack LIS vendor support initially. If the existing LIS vendor does not address the needs of a particular subsection, the laboratory could consider adding a specialty LIS to fill the gaps.

Option 2: Buying from a Separate Vendor

Some specialized LIS products comprise a self-contained LIS that exists in concert with an existing LIS. Adding infrastructure from a separate vendor raises considerable organizational costs in terms of licensing, personnel, and maintenance of multiple disparate systems. Balancing the complexity, efficiency, cost, technical support, and operational needs for these decisions is a challenge that is unique to every individual setting. For a laboratory purchasing a stand-alone LIS, this may translate to high up-front and long-term support costs. Some specialty LISs are hosted and supported off-site through cloud technologies that allow Web-based access and management. Off-site hosting may work well for some purposes, but there have to be clear Health Insurance Portability and Accountability Act protections in place and clear methods for archiving or exporting data if a vendor ever goes out of business. A special section is dedicated to discussing Web-based LIS reporting and off-site LISs later in this article.

Option 3: Bridging or Building

In some cases, buying a market ready product meets the needs of a laboratory. In other cases, alternative approaches to address the shortcomings are needed. For laboratories that are not satisfied with the existing market options, there are essentially 2 other approaches: bridge or build. These options can only be considered realistic if advanced technical skills are readily available within the organization. Building requires more technical expertise than bridging, but both approaches need an experienced information technology (IT) team.

Bridging

Some vendors or in-house LIS teams are able to add functions to existing systems to enhance the performance of an LIS. For example, several anatomic LISs have macro or scripting languages or are built around word processing solutions,

---

Box 4
Features of a niche market

1. Current products do not offer an adequate solution.

2. There is a motivated customer base with unmet needs.

3. Product development and marketing are tailored to a particular market segment.

4. Niche product offers better performance or unique attributes in comparison to other solutions.

which have this capacity. Using these programming tools, menus and forms can be built to fill gaps in functionality. An advantage of this method is these changes can be made without major alteration in the LIS. The difficulty with this technique is maintaining consistency throughout all workstations because macro code is frequently deployed locally. Other solutions may be developed within an existing middleware product. However, as volumes increase, parent LISs are updated, or when new technologies are adopted, these bridge solutions may be overwhelmed or become outdated.

Building

Some laboratories take greater ownership of the design and support of their LISs by designing their own modules or code where needed. Designing and implementing software to act as a specialized LIS requires significant planning, preparation, and training. Organizations that are considering this option usually undergo extensive evaluation of the initial and long-term economic implications of building their own systems.

Large-scale commercial laboratory

Large-scale laboratories may think that available LIS products do not adequately meet all of their needs. In some exceptional settings, the right mix of technical staff, organizational need, and capital backing may exist to produce an entirely custom-built LIS product. A software system designed specifically for the needs of a laboratory not only can address shortcomings of other products but also can provide strategic advantages by addressing the specific needs of the organization, its workforce, and its customers. The up-front financial and time investments can be substantial, but the rewards come in the form of gained efficiencies and application flexibility. Considerations for building an in-house LIS are listed in **Box 5**. The long-term support of these products is usually performed in-house. In the right setting, the up-front costs may also be offset by lower long-term support and licensing fees.

Box 5
Considerations for building an in-house laboratory information system

1. Scalability

2. Building a design team

3. Support costs

4. Total cost of ownership versus long-term benefit

CONSIDERATIONS FOR BUILDING AN IN-HOUSE LABORATORY INFORMATION SYSTEM MODULE

SCALABILITY AND TIMELINESS

Initially, an in-house LIS module may be developed to optimize a specific workflow. If a laboratory later decides to add additional testing modalities or workflows, a separate module may need to be built. This can be a slow development process and may delay a laboratory's entry into some testing markets. Many commercial LISs already have modules that may fit the general needs of the added modality. The implementation time for these new modules can, therefore, generally be done more quickly with a commercial product if one exists. If there is no acceptable product, then developing in house may be faster than waiting for a vendor solution.

EXPERIENCE OF THE DESIGN TEAM

The LIS is more than just a software product. It is a home to diagnostic patient information that has a critical function to the organizational mission. In addition, it is subject to extensive regulatory oversight by Clinical Laboratory Improvement Amendments and other accrediting agencies. The design team must be familiar with those constraints and also be able to work in concert with them. The design team needs to be staffed in such a way that the organization is protected from loss of one or several key personnel. A custom-built solution may be well understood by a few individuals. Retiring or departing staff who possess this intellectual capital can leave a knowledge gap that can be hard to fill. Extensive documentation and use of common coding languages and common backend architectures can be helpful in avoiding major knowledge gaps.

SUPPORT COSTS

An in-house product has to factor in long-term maintenance costs before a project starts. An off-the-shelf LIS product usually comes with predictable maintenance costs. For sizable laboratories, the annual maintenance fees for a commercial LIS can exceed several hundred thousand dollars annually. Staff needs for developing a new system may far exceed the staff necessary to support the system. How to reallocate personnel on completion of the development phase of the project becomes a challenging question.

COST VERSUS BENEFIT

The costs of implementation and support must be weighed in each setting to determine the best course of action. Some key questions to answer are

1. Will the system deliver strategic advantages to the laboratory?
2. Will the workflow be more efficient or allow more automation?
3. Will the in-house system allow customized reports that are strategically valuable to the client base?
4. Can integration with other systems and instrumentation be easily achieved?
5. Are Web-based reports a priority?
6. Are dollars that would be invested in LIS development better spent elsewhere?
7. What is the long-term impact of the LIS on the organization?
8. Does the in-house product allow better-quality management and improve operational efficiency?

NEWER TECHNOLOGIES AND REPORTING OPTIONS

THE OFF-SITE LIS

Web-based LISs are relatively new and not widely implemented. The workflow of a Web-based LIS is well suited for integrated or enhanced result reporting. Several of the larger commercial laboratories have already implemented Web-based LISs for at least some of their workflow. In some respects, large commercial laboratories with Web portals act as specialized LISs for their clients. This is well suited for flow cytometry reporting, molecular reporting, cytogenetics, and esoteric testing. Web-based reporting may take on several forms depending on market conditions and client types. In a reference laboratory setting, the clientele may consist of hospitals, medical groups, individual physicians, or even individual patients. Web-based resulting offers the ability to download a fully graphical PDF report.[1,2] Clients may then use these graphical reports to show to patients.

There are some technical challenges of incorporating Web-based results with an existing LIS. First, a Web-based report may create a separate data stream which can present challenges for tracking the status of pending tests. Second, the results may be delivered in a format that is less conducive to integration with current systems. Many modern anatomic LISs have the capacity to archive an external document by attaching it to an existing accession number. This has big advantages for integrating various results and data sources with a case. Some LISs and EMRs allow importation of graphical elements via scanning, attaching an electronic file

such as a PDF, or using Health Level Seven Clinical Document Architecture (CDA).[3]

REPORTING RESULTS TO CLIENTS

For Web-based resulting, the design of reporting groups is an important consideration. This is understood more clearly by considering that many individual users of a Web-based system may belong to the same client. Individual users may also share responsibility for patient results. Groups are created by allowing individual users to see results of other members in that group. Various levels of reporting groups are listed in **Box 6**. In general, more members in a reporting group may yield gains in convenience at the possible expense of security. No matter how the reporting groups are assigned, each user should always have a unique user name and password.

Example 1—Client Level Access

Consider that physicians 1, 2, 3, and 4 all work for Hospital ABC. A reference laboratory may wish to consider all the pathologists from Hospital ABC as a group. The individual users that are granted group level access may see results from all specimens sent in by any other user of that group. This setup helps with cross-coverage so that results for a case can be seen and acted on without delay if the original ordering pathologist is on vacation when the ancillary test results are delivered.

Example 2—Client Subgroups

In some settings, small groups of pathologists handle subspecialty sign-out for the practice. In

---

Box 6
Reporting groups

Client level

Users in this group have access to all results for the client ID.

Group level

Users in this group only have access to a specific reporting group. Individual users may belong to more than one group.

Individual level

Individual users can only log in to see results from tests they are designated as responsible for. Individual level access may be for a physician or even a patient.

Result level

Result level reporting means that each result is in its own group and the login only allows viewing of that specific test result.

sub-specialty diagnostic settings, physicians 1 and 2 may handle hematopathology results whereas physicians 3 and 4 handle dermatopathology testing. In this setting, it may be more beneficial to create client subgroups. This way the hematopathologists only have access to hematopathology testing data whereas the dermatopathologists only have access to dermatopathology data.

Example 3—Individual Access

Physician or individual level login is more limited and only allows given users to see results they have responsibility for on a given patient. Some direct-to-consumer laboratories use similar user level reporting so that patients may log in to see their own results through a portal.

Example 4—Result Level Reporting

Result level reporting means a unique login is created for each result. This is the most restrictive form of Web-based reporting. In this scenario, a unique login has to be delivered to the user for each result. If the credentials for viewing a Web-based result are delivered via reporting to a remote LIS, then the ability to track who has viewed the result is also lost because several users may view the log-in credentials, but it is not possible to track who actually logs in. When a user logs in, only the results from that specific test are viewable.[4]

EXAMPLE: HEMATOPATHOLOGY, THE SPECIALTY THAT CHALLENGES THE SPECIALIZED LABORATORY INFORMATION SYSTEM

SPECIALIZED LABORATORIES

Highly specialized laboratories that deal exclusively with specific specimen types occasionally have needs that can be better addressed by specialized LISs. Benefits may be gained in workflow solutions that are specifically tailored for the specimens and environment of the laboratory. Examples where this may occur include flow cytometry, hematopathology, gastrointestinal pathology, dermatopathology, and molecular testing. Of these, a hematopathology bone marrow specimen is a complex workflow that is good for illustrative purposes due to the amount of ancillary testing that may accompany a given specimen. Potential complexities of subspecialty testing are listed in **Box 7**.

COMPLEX WORKFLOW

Complex workflows may not be well addressed by traditional anatomic pathology LISs. Traditional anatomic pathology practice involves examining

> **Box 7**
> **Complexities of subspecialty testing**
>
> 1. Complex workflow
> 2. Multimodality testing and data types
> 3. Varied reporting timeline
> 4. Integration of various data types and tests which may have their own reporting paradigm or be signed out at an off-site facility
> 5. Integration of various IT systems/varied control/ownership of testing modalities
> 6. Evolving technologies

histologic sections in conjunction with appropriate use of immunohistochemical stains, special stains, in situ hybridization studies, and/or immunofluorescence studies. In general, these testing methods are available for interpretation within 1 day of being requested. A complete histologic interpretation for most surgical specimens is usually completed within a few days but same-day turnaround services exist.[5,6] The testing modalities of most surgical specimens are readily handled by a traditional anatomic LIS. Using the hematopathology bone marrow example (proposed previously), the complexity of data integration increases and reports can deviate significantly from traditional histopathology workflows.[7] With a bone marrow sample, the peripheral blood and bone marrow aspirate specimens may be morphologically evaluated on 1 day with a bone marrow core examined on day 2 after decalcification and paraffin embedding. Another day may pass while waiting for immunohistochemistry evaluation of the bone marrow core. If these specimens are triaged and dictated by a pathologist, this can involve multiple sessions of dictation, review, and editing before the slides are completely evaluated and a diagnostic report can be issued.

MULTIMODALITY TESTING AND DATA TYPES

Common testing methods that may challenge anatomic LISs include flow cytometry, diagnostic molecular studies, clonality studies, and cytogenetic studies. The usual turnaround times for some of the more complex ancillary testing methodologies can take days or weeks. This can present a problem for reporting these ancillary results when a diagnostic report has already been issued. The example bone marrow specimen frequently includes flow cytometry testing, fluorescence in situ hybridization (FISH) testing, cytogenetic testing, and/or various forms of molecular testing. The challenge for pathologists and LISs in general is integrating these varied testing methodologies and data types into a concise report. Flow cytometric, cytogenetic, and FISH reports may include images in addition to textual reports. Molecular testing may include graphs of historical values of transcript levels to show how a patient is responding to targeted agents.

TIMELINE

The third challenge in the hematopathology multimodality testing example is incorporating testing results into the diagnostic workflow with a timeline that is extended and unpredictable. Flow cytometry results are usually available in sync with the timeline of a primary bone marrow report. Cytogenetic results are usually not available before the bone marrow is ready for sign-out and must be added as an addendum. FISH and molecular testing have varied timelines but are generally available post–sign-out. Molecular clonality studies and esoteric gene profiling tests can take several weeks to perform. For pathologists, it may be difficult to keep track of where all specimens are in the testing timeline. A system that tracks pending tests and laboratory contact information can be helpful for updating the diagnostic report, for updating clinicians with findings of the ancillary studies, and for following up on "overdue" results. Most practices deal with these timeline incongruencies by adding addendums/amendments to the original histologic report to include ancillary testing results with a comment on the impact on the final diagnosis.

DATA INTEGRATION FROM MULTIPLE LABORATORIES

Another major challenge of specialty sign-out is that some testing may be performed off-site.[7] Off-site testing can get even more complex if a commercial laboratory triaged the specimen to multiple separate facilities. This adds complexity to both the uncertain timeline and interfacing issues (discussed previously). An ideal solution alerts a pathologist when a new result is available or automatically injects the data into a field on a pending amendment for later review. Automatic injection is only realistic for ancillary testing that is performed in the parent institution where contextual fields can be predefined and controlled. The structure of an ideal integrated report would approximately follow a synoptic template[8] to let clinicians know that some tests are still pending or that some tests were not performed. Design consistency helps clinicians find information quickly and provides a standardized structure where specific test results

are expected to be found.[9] Using a well-structured report, the data from a particular testing methodology consistently fall in a specific location or under a specific header.

MULTISYSTEM

The fifth challenge of integration is crossing data between clinical pathology and anatomic pathology systems. If a laboratory has in-house testing, the results for FISH and molecular testing may be reported into the clinical pathology system. If testing is performed off-site, the results may or may not be interfaced to an existing clinical pathology system. If the systems are interfaced at all, they are most likely only transmitting textual data. Although technically possible, the probability of receiving graphical data over an interface at the present time is low. At the present time, integrating results from disparate systems into a single anatomic pathology report is generally done manually.

EVOLVING TECHNOLOGIES

As discussed previously, instrumentation and testing methodologies are rapidly evolving, which presents challenges to a traditional LIS. Hematopathology has a high adoption rate of new testing methodologies. Few LISs are designed to meet the data storage, integration, and reporting needs across anatomic pathology, flow cytometry, molecular, and cytogenetic modalities.

SUMMARY

This article examines the concepts underlying specialized LISs, their characteristics, and in what settings they may perform well. Opportunities for specialized LISs continue to evolve as whole-slide imaging, genetic testing, and personalized medicine efforts continue to grow.

REFERENCES

1. Park S, Pantanowitz L, Sharma G, et al. Anatomic pathology laboratory information systems: a reivew. Adv Anat Pathol 2012;19(2):81–96.
2. Winsten D. The Web-enabled LIS. Advance for the Laboratory 2005;14:9 38.
3. Dolin R, Alschuler L, Boyer S, et al. HL7 clinical document architecture, release 2. J Am Med Inform Assoc 2006;13:30–9.
4. Shirts B, Larsen N, Jackson B. Utilization and utility of clinical laboratory reports with graphical elements. J Pathol Inform 2012;3:26.
5. López A, Graham A, Barker G, et al. Virtual slide telepathology enables an innovative telehealth rapid breast care clinic. Hum Pathol 2009;40:1082–91.

6. Barentsz M, Wessels H, van Diest P, et al. Same-day diagnosis based on histology for women suspected of breast cancer: high diagnostic accuracy and favorable impact on the patient. PLoS One 2014; 9(7):1–6.

7. Hess J. What hematopathology tells us about the future of pathology informatics. Arch Pathol Lab Med 2009;133:908–11.

8. Mohanty S, Piccoli A, Devine L, et al. Synoptic tool for reporting of hematological and lymphoid neoplasms based on World Health Organization classification and College of American Pathologists checklist. BMC Cancer 2007;7:144.

9. Valenstein P. Formatting pathology reports: applying four design principles to improve communication and patient safety. Arch Pathol Lab Med 2008;132:84–94.

Laboratory Information Systems Management and Operations

Ioan C. Cucoranu, MD

KEYWORDS

- LIS management • LIS operations • Change control • End-user training • Quality control reports
- Help desk

ABSTRACT

The main mission of a laboratory information system (LIS) is to manage workflow and deliver accurate results for clinical management. Successful selection and implementation of an anatomic pathology LIS is not complete unless it is complemented by specialized information technology support and maintenance. LIS is required to remain continuously operational with minimal or no downtime and the LIS team has to ensure that all operations are compliant with the mandated rules and regulations.

OVERVIEW

The main mission of an LIS is to manage a laboratory's workflow (both specimens and patient data) and to deliver accurate results for clinical management, in a timely manner. A modern LIS should have built-in functionality for other required activities, such as regulations, billing, or quality assurance. Currently, in the United States, pathology laboratories are under continuous pressure to improve workflows by using lean initiatives. Technologies, such as tracking systems and automation, have been used successfully for decades in clinical laboratories; they are finally becoming the norm in pathology laboratories as well. Other useful LIS functions, particularly when used in an academic environment, are support for pathology education and research.

The successful selection and implementation of an anatomic pathology LIS is not complete unless it is complemented by long-term specialized information technology (IT) support. This should be

provided by both in-house informatics and IT resources as well as by an LIS vendor. Nevertheless, optimal LIS operations depend on the availability of adequate, dedicated, and skilled informatics and IT personnel. For large health care systems, collaboration and communication between a laboratory's LIS staff and the hospital-wide IT personnel play a key role in the successful LIS maintenance.[1]

A LIS is required to remain continuously operational with minimal or no downtime. At the same time, an LIS team has to ensure that all operations are compliant with the mandated rules and regulations. As is the case for any health information system (HIS), close attention should also be shown to a system's development life cycle to further improve its functionality and usability. **Box 1** lists key operations that any LIS team needs to handle post–system implementation.

SYSTEM VALIDATION

Although a tedious and costly process, LIS validation must be performed to prove that an implemented system is fit for its intended use and that the system manages information well, with the expected accuracy, reliability, and file integrity, both initially and over time.[2] During the validation process, various LIS functions are performed while data are collected, maintained, and independently reviewed to demonstrate that the system performs consistently according to specifications. Pathology laboratories must establish protocols and standards for the validation process. All the validation steps and results must be well documented.

Department of Pathology and Laboratory Medicine, University of Florida College of Medicine - Jacksonville, 655 West 8th Street, Room 1-078, Jacksonville, FL 32209-6596, USA
E-mail address: ioan.cucoranu@jax.ufl.edu

Surgical Pathology 8 (2015) 153–157
http://dx.doi.org/10.1016/j.path.2015.02.002
1875-9181/15/$ – see front matter © 2015 Elsevier Inc. All rights reserved.

Box 1
Key operations that laboratory information system teams need to handle post–system implementation

- Training
- Help desk support
- Change control
- System security
- System data backup
- Interface monitoring and maintenance
- Downtime management (unscheduled vs scheduled)
- Database maintenance
- Upgrades (software and hardware)
- Administrative and management reporting
- Budgeting and cost analysis
- System validation
- Documentation
- New product evaluation
- Quality assurance and quality improvement initiatives

LIS vendors perform initial, internal system validations; however, any system must be revalidated whenever end users, vendors, or third parties add modifications or customizations. The Clinical and Laboratory Standards Institute published important factors that should be considered when developing validation protocols for LISs, including recommendations for preparation of validation protocols, to assess the accuracy and dependability of LISs in storing, retrieving, and transmitting data.[3]

INTERFACE MAINTENANCE AND MONITORING

Electronic interfaces are critical components of any HIS, having a significant impact on the overall performance of information exchange and health care delivery. They allow transmission of data and information between LISs and other clinical information systems (eg, electronic medical records and billing systems) or between LISs and laboratory equipment (eg, automated immunohistochemistry slide stainers). Although electronic interfaces have been in use for years and attempts have been made to standardize their implementation, the whole process is still a time- and resource-consuming process. Interface customization depends significantly on the laboratory and clinical systems being connected and on how those systems have been implemented.

Once implemented, additional activities are necessary to monitor and maintain interfaces, especially whenever changes are performed on any of the systems involved. Pathology laboratories are responsible for identifying interface problems (eg, laboratory orders not being processed or report formatting issues). Laboratory directors must ensure the outcomes of critical LIS functionality.[4] These include

- Accurate and complete flow of information between LISs and electronic health records
- Logical and human-readable report formatting on the receiving end and maintaining the essential elements of reports, as they were entered into the LIS
- Appropriate transmission of any coded information used to correctly identify results, such as LOINC
- Appropriate handling of report versioning, comments, or abnormality flags

Software packages to automate interface testing and validation are currently available. Keystrokes or data entry can be simulated and screen output reading can be performed electronically, to verify achievement of the desired outcomes. There are several advantages when using validation software tools, including the following:

- Scenarios can be checked multiple times.
- Outputs may be rigorously compared against intended outcomes.

- All interactions can be audited.
- A complete set of testing can be easily run whenever an adjustment is made to any system.

Key points to consider when maintaining and validating interfaces:

- Design a standardized process for recurrent interface validation.
- Perform the test on the entire chain of interfaces.
- Ensure that interface error logs work as expected and that there is a monitoring procedure in place.
- Use a test environment whenever possible.
- Use test patients when working in a live environment.
- Consider automated testing software to make the testing process faster, more accurate, more complete, reproducible, and better documented.
- Have a written agreement with the management of any receiving system, acknowledging the responsibility to inform the laboratory of any significant changes (eg, upgrades) so that timely revalidation can be performed.

TRAINING

End-user training is a critical component for a successful HIS implementation. Training components include

- Initial trainin—training administered to all users immediately before implementation of a brand-new LIS as well as training administered to newly hired staff
- Additional training—sessions provided to end users as their role and activities performed are changed or as additional features are added to the LIS.

For an effective training program development, it is important to assess end users' training needs by using techniques that reveal end users' cognitive processes. Usability testing methods have the ability to gather data related to human computer interaction.[5] These methods can be combined with traditional methods, such as interviews and questionnaire surveys.

HELP DESK SUPPORT

It is essential to implement well-planned support processes and procedures to minimize end-user frustration. The support system outcome could ultimately have a direct impact on LIS functionality. Help desk is a resource made available to end

users when they encounter problems with their LIS services. Usually, the LIS help desk support specialists provide technical assistance with personal computers, operating systems, and LIS-related applications (eg, password log-ins and word processors) and sometimes with peripheral devices (eg, digital cameras) or add-on software (eg, voice recognition software) used in the laboratory. Help desk personnel may provide ad hoc end-user training on the proper use of all these components. Based on laboratory size and the help desk request volume, software applications can be implemented to support this process.

Implementation of best practices for help desk support include

- Knowledge management—system that improves operational efficiencies by reducing the time spent to rediscover previous incidents or problems
- Problem management—system that gathers information during incident management to help identify problems. Thus, the root cause of frequent recurring incidents can be identified by capturing information in a knowledge database.
- Access management—maintains end-user accounts along with password resets to ensure quick response time

CHANGE CONTROL AND DOCUMENTATION

Once an LIS is implemented, additional changes may be required by the vendor, IT services, or laboratory (eg, fine-tune, add functionality or add additional tests and protocols). Change control is a systematic approach used to manage all the changes made to an LIS. This approach ensures that no unnecessary or unauthorized changes are made, that all changes are documented and monitored in a controlled and coordinated fashion, that LIS services are not unnecessarily disrupted, and that laboratory IT and informatics resources are used efficiently. Planning, policies, and standard operation procedures (SOPs) as well as adherence to change control processes can potentially prevent a laboratory from costly mistakes (eg, system crashes, security breaches, or data corruption). Change control applies to any changes (eg, revisions, alterations, additions, enhancements, or upgrades) performed on both hardware and software. Furthermore, regulatory bodies, such as the College of American Pathologists, mandate documentation of all changes. LIS managers are responsible for change control documentation. **Table 1** lists recommended items to be documented as part of change control.

Table 1
Change control documentation

Documentation Items	Explanation of Change
Description of change	Detailed explanation of the change performed
Reason for change	Needs and benefits of the performed change
Persons responsible for change implementation	Allow for identification of personnel that actually performed the change
Change category	Hardware, software, process, or procedural
Degree of change	Minor vs major—based on overall impact on the LIS, health care IT system, and laboratory, including cost
Change sign off	Identifies the person responsible for the overall change
Risk assessment	Allows for problems that may occur as result of the change to be assessed and planning for resolution if such problems occur
Evaluation and monitoring of the implemented changes	Evaluate outcome and determine the success of change implementation

Adapted from Cucoranu I, Parwani A, Pantanowitz L. Laboratory information system operations and regulations. In: Pantanowitz L, Parwani AV, editors. Practical informatics for cytopathology, vol. 14. New York: Springer; 2014. p. 64; with permission.

MANAGEMENT REPORTING AND QUALITY ASSURANCE/QUALITY IMPROVEMENT INITIATIVES

A modern LIS should be capable of generating automated or on-demand management reports, such as documentation for regulatory compliance, quality assurance, or monitoring performance and productivity (eg, turnaround time, abnormal results, reimbursement, or frozen section correlations). The LIS team should work closely with laboratory administration and the quality assurance team to create and generate the reports needed. If deemed necessary and cost effective, additional tolls could be developed and/or implemented either in

collaboration with an LIS vendor (vendor-assisted software modifications) or by using third-party middleware software packages.[6] A further detailed description of the informatics role in patient safety and quality assurance is provided in the article elsewhere in this issue.

DATABASE MAINTENANCE

Accurate and reliable data are integral to all the pathology laboratory processes that involve the use of LISs. Increased data processing and electronic data exchange heavily rely on accurate, reliable, controllable, and verifiable data recorded in databases. Data dictionaries are used to ensure data accuracy and standardization. LIS database dictionaries are dynamic documents that must be updated as data collection requirements change. Procedures should be in place to standardize database dictionaries maintenance.

NEW PRODUCT EVALUATION

Modern LISs in pathology laboratories provide an opportunity for implementation of data automation. Therefore, it is desirable when selecting, purchasing, and implementing new equipment in a laboratory to have the LIS team actively involved in evaluating the possibility and cost-effectiveness of data transfer via electronic interfaces. Similarly, when implementing digital imaging equipment, the LIS team should be involved in assessing digital imaging format compatibility with the current LIS.

Other LIS operations include LIS data security, reliability, and privacy of patient health information. These are important functions for any pathology laboratory; therefore, they are discussed in detail in a separate article.

REFERENCES

1. Cucoranu I, Parwani A, Pantanowitz L. Laboratory information system operations and regulations. In: Pantanowitz L, Parwani AV, editors. Practical informatics for cytopathology, vol. 14. New York: Springer; 2014. p. 61–70.
2. Cowan DF, Gray RZ, Campbell B. Validation of the laboratory information system. Arch Pathol Lab Med 1998;122:239–44.
3. Pearson S, Fuller J, Kowalski B, et al. Managing and validating laboratory information systems; Approved Guideline AUT08-A. 2007. 26. Available at: http://www.clsi.org/source/orders/free/AUTO8-A.pdf. Accessed August 31, 2014.
4. Beckwith BA, Brassel JH, Brodsky VB, et al. Laboratory interoperability best practices: ten mistakes to

avoid. College of American Pathologists; 2013. Available at: http://www.cap.org/apps/docs/committees/informatics/cap_dihit_lab_interop_final_march_2013.pdf. Accessed August 31, 2014.

5. Qiu Y, Yu P, Hyland P. A multi-method approach to assessing health information systems end users' training needs. Stud Health Technol Inform 2007; 129:1352–6.

6. Kamat S, Parwani AV, Khalbuss WE, et al. Use of a laboratory information system driven tool for pre-signout quality assurance of random cytopathology reports. J Pathol Inform 2011;2:42.

Informatics and Autopsy Pathology

Bruce Levy, MD, CPE

KEYWORDS

- Autopsy • Pathology • Forensic • Informatics • Synoptic • Virtopsy • Images

ABSTRACT

Many health care providers believe that the autopsy is no longer relevant in high-technology medicine era. This has fueled a decline in the hospital autopsy rate. Although it seems that advanced diagnostic tests answer all clinical questions, studies repeatedly demonstrate that an autopsy uncovers as many undiagnosed conditions today as in the past. The forensic autopsy rate has also declined, although not as precipitously. Pathologists are still performing a nineteenth century autopsy procedure that remains essentially unchanged. Informatics offers several potential answers that will evolve the low-tech autopsy into the high-tech autopsy.

OVERVIEW—WHAT IS AN AUTOPSY?

An autopsy is a systematic examination of a deceased human body to document the cause of death and document the extent of disease or injury. The word autopsy originally comes from the Greek roots *autos* (self) and *optos* (sight). In combination they have been expressed as "to see for oneself" or "eyewitness." The history of the autopsy stretches back for 5000 years, but the autopsy as currently conceived has its origins during the Renaissance, with physicians such as Andreas Vesalius and Giovanni Morgagni. In the nineteenth century, Carl von Rokitansky performed thousands of autopsies using a method of in situ examination of the organs, although many investigators have erroneously ascribed the en bloc removal method of Maurice Letulle to Rokitansky. Rudolf Virchow is credited with incorporating the widespread use of the microscope with autopsies in addition to the organ-by-organ evisceration technique.[1]

The autopsy procedure begins with an examination of the exterior of the body, which includes a description of the body, basic measurements such as height and weight, and documentation of significant external findings. The body is then opened with a Y-shaped incision of the anterior torso and a bitemporal incision of the scalp. The internal organs are removed, weighed, measured, and examined. Sample tissues from the organs are typically submitted for microscopic examination. In many instances, more typically in forensic examinations, blood and other body fluids are examined for the presence of drugs or poisons. Occasionally microbiology cultures are obtained or other ancillary testing is performed. The autopsy procedure practiced today has changed little from the procedure performed in the second half of the nineteenth century by Rokitansky and Virchow.

The medical autopsy performed in hospitals is to be distinguished from forensic autopsies performed in medical examiner and coroner offices. Autopsies in a hospital setting are typically requested by a clinician or family member and require the informed consent of legal next of kin. Clinicians frequently have general and specific questions to be answered by the pathologist performing the autopsy. Families, besides wanting to know why their loved one died, are increasingly interested in identifying any inheritable risk that might have an impact on the health of surviving family members.[2] A medical autopsy may identify disease that had not been diagnosed or even suspected by the clinical team.[3–5] It is also an excellent tool for the investigation of the utility and potential complications of new diagnostic tests, treatments, or procedures.

In contrast, forensic autopsies are ordered by a medical examiner or coroner in deaths involving injury, chemical intoxication, or unexpected natural deaths and do not require the permission of the next of kin. The goals of forensic autopsies are focused on detailed documentation of injuries

Department of Pathology, University of Illinois at Chicago, MC847, 840 South Wood Street 130 CSN, Chicago, IL 60612, USA

E-mail address: bplevy@uic.edu

Surgical Pathology 8 (2015) 159–174

http://dx.doi.org/10.1016/j.path.2015.02.010

in trauma cases, quantization and interpretation of substances found within the body in poisonings or intoxications, and determination of the medical cause(s) of death for sudden unexpected natural deaths. A forensic pathologist anticipates the questions that the criminal justice or public health systems might have regarding these deaths and attempts to answer these questions through their examination. These examinations are typically more focused compared with hospital autopsies, although they may involve more extensive dissection in certain instances.

DECREASE IN THE AUTOPSY RATE

In the early years of the twentieth century, the autopsy rate in American hospitals hovered at approximately 10% of all hospital deaths. After the issuing of the Flexner Report in 1910, there was a steep rise in the autopsy rate into the middle of the century, with approximately half of all hospital deaths receiving an autopsy in 1950. Then began a gradual decline in the autopsy rate to approximately 45% in the middle 1960s and approximately 30% in 1970. In 1971, the Joint Commission on Accreditation of Hospitals eliminated the minimum autopsy requirement for hospital accreditation. The autopsy rate continued its decline and a century after the Flexner Report has come full circle, once again at less than 10%. Academic teaching hospitals have variable rates generally higher than 10%, but many community hospitals perform no autopsies at all (**Fig. 1**).[6–8]

Not only have the autopsy rates changed over time but also the distribution of the types of deaths and ages of those autopsied have changed over time. Although the autopsy rate for deaths from disease decreased from 16.9% to 4.3% between the years 1972 and 2007, the autopsy rate for deaths due to external causes increased from 43.6% to 55.4%. Of the 10 most common causes of death autopsied in 2007, only 1 (pregnancy, childbirth, and puerperium) was related to disease. Over the same years, the age distribution of those autopsies has also changed, with fewer autopsies performed with increasing age (**Figs. 2 and 3**).[9]

This decrease in the autopsy rate led George Lundberg, in an editorial in 1998, to state, "The autopsy is not dead, but it slumbers deeply, apparently the victim of a vast cultural delusion of denial."[10]

REASONS FOR AUTOPSY RATE DECLINE

Dr Lundberg goes on in his editorial to opine, "In fact, there is still a giant gap between what high-tech diagnostic medicine can do in theory in ideal circumstances and what high-tech diagnostic medicine does do in practice in real life circumstances."[10] Approximately 20 years after this editorial many people still wonder whether the autopsy remains relevant in the twenty-first century.

There are many postulated reasons for the decline in the autopsy rate (**Box 1**).

Joint Commission Eliminates Minimum Autopsy Rate

Many persons point to the 1971 decision of the Joint Commission on Accreditation of Hospitals to eliminate a minimum autopsy requirement for hospital accreditation. Although that decision may be a contributing factor, the reality is that the hospital autopsy rate was already declining prior to 1971, raising the question as to whether the Joint Commission decision was their reaction to a perceived change in the value of the autopsy within the health care community.

Clinicians' Better Diagnostic Skills

Another explanation for the decrease in the autopsy rate is greater diagnostic confidence by

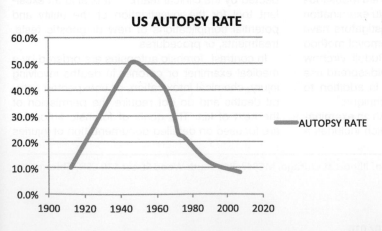

US AUTOPSY RATE

Fig. 1. Changes in the US autopsy rate: 1910–2010. (*Data from* Refs.[6–8])

Fig. 2. Percent distribution of cause of death for autopsied deaths: United States, 1972 (*A*) and 2007 (*B*). (*From* Hoyert DL. The changing profile of autopsied deaths in the United States, 1972–2007. NCHS data brief, no. 6. Hyattsville (MD): National Center for Health Statistics; 2011; with permission.)

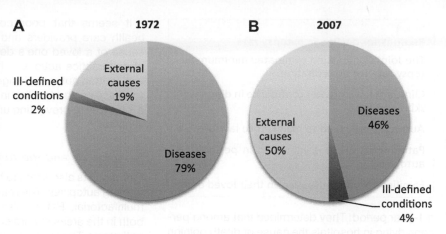

clinicians, primarily due to the increase in the quantity and quality of medical diagnostic tools. There have been many studies over the decades studying the rate at which autopsies reveal previously unknown diagnoses, which helps address the question of whether "high-tech diagnostic medicine" has actually improved diagnostic capability. The overwhelming evidence is that although there may have been some improvements, autopsies still regularly discover significant diagnoses and conditions not recognized prior to death.

A retrospective study of 100 randomly selected autopsies from 1960, 1970, and 1980 revealed 1 of 10 deaths in each of the 3 decades contained 1 or more class I major missed diagnoses, in which "detection before death would in all probability have led to a change in management that might have resulted in cure or prolonged survival" (**Fig. 4**).[3] A more extensive review and analysis of 53 autopsy series over a 40-year period looked at both major missed diagnoses (missed diagnoses involving the primary cause of death) and class

I discrepancies. They concluded that although there were statistically significant decreases in both rates from decade to decade, in 2003 a US hospital with an autopsy rate of 5% could observe a major missed diagnosis rate of 24.4% and a class I discrepancy rate of 6.7%. This represents 71,400 deaths per year, with up to half of these patients surviving to discharge had these diagnoses been known prior to death.[4] A more recent study of patients dying in an ICU of a tertiary cancer center with an autopsy rate of 13% discovered a major missed diagnosis rate of 26%, with more than half representing class I discrepancies. Opportunistic infections and cardiac complications were the most commonly missed class I discrepancies. The authors concluded, "The autopsy remains an invaluable tool for retrospective diagnostic understanding of difficult cases, medical education and quality assurance."[5]

Discrepancies between clinical diagnosis and autopsy findings are not limited to natural deaths. A study analyzed trauma-related deaths in Utah for

Fig. 3. Percent distribution of age for autopsied deaths: United States, 1972 (*A*) and 2007 (*B*). (*From* Hoyert DL. The changing profile of autopsied deaths in the United States, 1972–2007. NCHS data brief, no. 6. Hyattsville (MD): National Center for Health Statistics; 2011; with permission.)

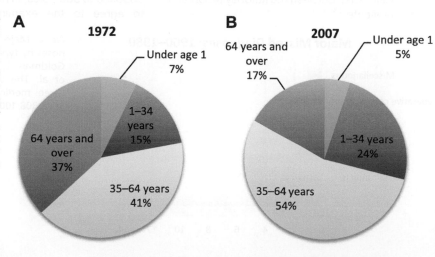

a 1-year period. They determined that among persons dying in hospitals the cause of death opinion based on clinical findings was changed after autopsy in 13% of these hospital deaths.[11] Although this study does not directly measure major or class I discrepancies, the changes in the cause of death indicate significant missing information from the clinical evaluation of these trauma victims and confirms the value of the autopsy in the forensic setting.

Autopsy Only Leads to Malpractice Lawsuits

Another misconception by clinicians is that obtaining autopsies only reveals information that can be used to initiate and support malpractice lawsuits. The College of American Pathologists studied state court records of malpractice actions over 30 years. They discovered that in 61% of cases where the autopsy favored the plaintiff (revealed major discrepancies that would have affected treatment) and 100% of cases where the autopsy favored the defendant, the defendant physicians were acquitted of malpractice.[12] The autopsy only becomes a point of contention in malpractice actions when there are issues over the quality of the autopsy, delays in generating autopsy reports, or inconsistencies between the autopsy report and death certificate.[13]

It seems that poor communication between health care providers and families regarding the cause of a loved one's death is one major driver of malpractice actions.[14] If true, then a thorough well-written autopsy designed to provide answers to clinicians and families in a timely manner will go a long way to preventing unnecessary malpractice litigation.

Pathologists and the Autopsy

Pathologists also seem to have lost interest in performing autopsies. The reasons for this change are multifactorial. Pathologists are busier than ever both in the areas of surgical pathology and clinical pathology. The lower numbers of autopsies mean that fewer pathologists have sufficient autopsy expertise to be able to perform an autopsy efficiently. Busy pathologists simply do not have sufficient time in their schedule to perform autopsies. Autopsies do not generate revenue and represent a cost center to pathology departments and hospitals.[15] There is also the perception that clinicians do not appreciate autopsies and may be antagonistic if an autopsy reveals missed diagnoses or technical errors in procedures. As a result, the few autopsies that are obtained are treated with low priority within pathology departments, contributing to a negative feedback cycle between clinicians and pathologists. This attitude is not shared by resident physicians in pathology, who believe that autopsies are important for education, answer clinical questions, have value for medical research, and are important for quality control in medicine.[16]

Family Misconceptions Regarding the Autopsy

Families, although commonly believed to be opposed to autopsies, in reality tend to be inclined to agree to the examination despite several

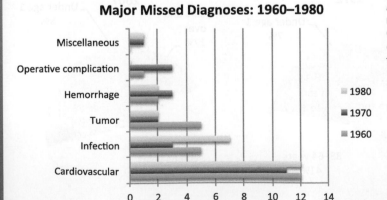

Major Missed Diagnoses: 1960–1980

Fig. 4. Major missed class I and II diagnoses by type: 1960–1980. (*Data from* Goldman L, Sayson R, Robbins S, et al. The value of the autopsy in three medical eras. N Engl J Med 1983;308:1002.)

misconceptions regarding the autopsy among the general public. These misbeliefs include that autopsies do not add anything of value, the deceased has suffered enough, the patient is too young or old for autopsy, autopsy mutilates the body and prevents open-casket viewing, and autopsy creates delays until burial or cremation.[17,18] A large part of this misunderstanding involves poor communication between health care providers and families regarding the autopsy and poor consent processes.[19]

The issue of religious objections also frequently arises as a barrier to autopsy. It is commonly believed that there are well-established broad prohibitions to autopsy in several of the major religions, notably Islam and Judaism. The reality is more complicated depending on the different subdivisions of each religion.[20] Although the religious prohibition to autopsy among Orthodox Jews is perhaps one of the more commonly known and accepted, even within this group there is disagreement as to whether the prohibition to autopsy is superseded by the greater commandment of saving of a life, when the autopsy may result in the saving of other lives.[21] In the end, it is typically the personal religious beliefs of the next of kin, rather than the specific religion to which they belong and the religion's opinions on the autopsy, that is most important.

INFORMATICS APPLICATIONS TO AUTOPSY PATHOLOGY

Therefore, the question is whether to allow the hospital autopsy to die a "natural" death despite the obvious evidence that postmortem examinations remain relevant, desirable, and valuable. The alternative to continued dwindling of the hospital autopsy is to study how to "resurrect" the autopsy, taking advantage of newer medical technologies and clinical informatics to catapult the autopsy from the nineteenth to the twenty-first century and restore its prominent place in health care and quality improvement.

VALUE OF THE AUTOPSY TO ITS CUSTOMERS

To improve the autopsy, the potential value of the autopsy from the point of view of the consumers of the autopsy must first be better understood. In cases of hospital autopsies, there are families and clinicians. In the forensic world, the criminal justice and public health systems also need to be considered. What these very different groups expect from the autopsy, what they are currently receiving, and which of their needs are currently not being met need to be asked. Once this gap is identified, which informatics techniques and tools might eliminate this gap can be examined.

Clinicians' Needs from the Autopsy

Despite evidence that clinicians still value the autopsy, their inclination to order one is at its lowest level in a century (Box 2, Table 1). A 1996 study exploring the factors that influence clinicians' decisions to request an autopsy revealed that the benefits of requesting an autopsy include confirming clinical diagnoses, increasing a clinician's medical knowledge, aiding medical research, and the autopsy's educational value, whereas the drawbacks are the request is time consuming, concern that relatives may be distressed by the request, and discomfort of the requestor.[22] A survey of internal medicine residents confirms the factors that discourage physicians from ordering autopsies, with their top 3 reasons for not obtaining autopsy consent being the family is distraught/extremely agitated, the clinician perceives that the family is unwilling, and requesting an autopsy is unpleasant.[16] These residents also agree that autopsies are important to medical education, answer clinical questions, and are valuable for medical research, quality control, and public health. They believe that having a brochure explaining autopsies that can be provided to families would be most helpful in obtaining more autopsies.[16] Better training of health personnel in requesting autopsies as well as education of the general public on the importance of autopsies is also believed to be important in increasing the autopsy rate.[23]

Looking at the attitudes of physicians to current autopsy reports gives insight into their needs. A survey of general practitioners revealed that a majority find autopsy reports useful to both themselves and families, yet only a minority plan to discuss reports with families. Overwhelming majorities agree that the clinical circumstances were clearly summarized; the reports were clearly written and interesting to them. A majority stated that an autopsy report was the first indication they received of how their patient died and more

---

Box 2
Why clinicians value the autopsy

- Confirm clinical diagnoses
- Increase own medical knowledge
- Educational value for residents and students
- Quality control/assurance in medical practice
- Important for medical research

Table 1
Influencing physician behavior

Encourage Ordering Autopsies	Discourage Ordering Autopsies
Training in requesting autopsies	Requests are time consuming
Brochure about autopsies for families	Requests are unpleasant to perform
Better communication with pathologist throughout autopsy process	Families may be distraught or angry regarding request

than 20% agreed that the cause of death was a complete surprise, representing a missed opportunity by pathologists to improve communications with clinicians.[24] Better communication between clinicians and pathologists and quicker turnaround times for autopsy reports will help increase the autopsy rate.[23]

Communications between clinicians and pathologists need to be bidirectional. Pathologists require the input of clinicians to provide the clinical history, and a conversation often reveals details and nuances that are not easily obtained from medical records. It is valuable for pathologists to know what questions a clinical team has for the pathologist to answer, and it is incumbent on pathologists to provide those answers clearly. One study looking at 125 autopsies found that specific reasons for autopsies are provided by clinicians only 55% of the time. Of the 103 clinical questions asked, only 88% of the questions were answered in the autopsy report and more than 10% of those answers were not in the final anatomic diagnosis summary, but in another part of the report, with the implication that the clinician would have to search for these answers.[25]

Families' Needs from the Autopsy

It is no surprise that families are also interested in wanting answers to questions regarding how their loved ones died. Families are interested in better understanding the cause of death of their loved ones, have a desire to learn about any infectious or inheritable conditions that could have an impact on the health of surviving family members, and are open to the concept that autopsy findings can help the health of society at large.[2,26,27] The general public has a generally positive attitude toward autopsy, and family members are likely to consent to autopsy when its value is presented to them sufficiently, their questions are answered, and their

concerns are allayed.[18,28] As with clinicians, it is apparent that an autopsy report that can be read by or discussed with families, provided in a timely manner with respect for their needs at a time of great loss, can go a long way to increasing the autopsy rate.

The Public's Needs from the Autopsy

Public health surveillance is collecting, analyzing, interpreting, and disseminating data for specific public health needs. Although the basic purposes and goals of public health surveillance have not significantly changed, they are being transformed in the twenty-first century by the evolution of electronic methods of storing health information, the rapid increase in the quantity of data to analyze, and new challenges.[29] Syndromic surveillance can have a significant impact on protection of the public health as has been documented with infectious diseases and heat-related illness/mortality.[30,31]

The National Violent Death Reporting System (NVDRS), although currently limited to 32 states, is an excellent example of how the collection of data from forensic autopsies can be successfully used for public health.[32] The National Missing and Unidentified Persons System (NamUs) is another successful application of using informatics to match unidentified bodies with missing persons.[33] Both of these systems, unfortunately, do not pull information directly from autopsy reports or medical examiner databases but require the forensic offices to enter this information directly into the respective NVDRS or NamUs databases. Creating systems surrounding autopsies, both hospital and forensic, that permit direct mining of information would greatly enhance the utility of the treasure trove of information collected through the autopsy.[34]

INFORMATICS SOLUTIONS TO ADDRESS NEEDS

Workflow Analysis

Autopsies are complex procedures with many different steps and stages, each of which represents a potential source of delay. Although most people think of the autopsy as a procedure that starts with the first incision on the body and ends when the body is sewn closed, the entire autopsy procedure includes many facets both before and after the examination of the body. Just as in other areas of pathology and laboratory medicine, there are preanalytical, analytical, and postanalytical phases.

The preanalytical phase includes confirming the autopsy permit, reviewing the medical history, discussing the case with a clinician, and identification of the body. The analytical phase, in addition to the autopsy procedure itself, includes obtaining images, tissue for histology, and specimens for other associated testing. After the examination of the body is the generation of the provisional anatomic diagnoses (PAD), preparation and review of microscopic slides, performance and review of other laboratory tests, and additional dissection of organs that have been fixed and saved, such as the brain, culminating in the completion and dissemination of the final autopsy report. In the forensic world, chain of custody also needs to be maintained.

Accreditation standards exist for the production of the PAD and final autopsy report. The College of American Pathologists accreditation standards require the PAD be submitted to the attending physician and medical record within 2 days and the final autopsy completed for all cases within 60 working days.[35] The Joint Commission standards require the PAD be recorded in the medical record within 3 days and the autopsy report included in the medical record within 60 days.[36]

In the world of forensic pathology, the requirements for autopsy report production are even less stringent. The National Association of Medical Examiners (NAME) Inspection and Accreditation Checklist from 2009 required that 90% of nonhomicide autopsy reports be produced within 60 days and 90% of homicide autopsy reports be produced in 90 days.[37] Those standards were loosened in the 2014 revision of the NAME accreditation checklist so that the 90% in 90-day requirement applies to all autopsy report and not just homicide cases.[38] The NAME Autopsy Performance Standards makes no mention of any report turnaround time.[39] The International Association of Coroners and Medical Examiners accreditation checklist has the same standard, 90% of reports completed in 90 days, as NAME.[40]

It can be easily argued that these accreditation standards in both the hospital and forensic autopsy environments are not sufficient for reporting of the results of an autopsy.

Hospital autopsy results can and should be made available to clinicians in a more timely fashion. Families likely contact clinicians looking for answers from the autopsy within a short period of time, and it is important that pathologists support their colleagues by providing them with this information quickly.[41] Timely feedback to clinicians when a case is fresh in their minds is also important in order for these cases to be used effectively for quality improvement and patient safety. Supporting clinicians' conversations with families by providing them autopsy results when they require them instead of when pathologists can get around to producing them will encourage clinicians to request more autopsies.

Forensic autopsy reports are used by law enforcement and district attorneys in making decisions regarding criminal charges as part of their investigations. These forensic reports are also increasingly important for monitoring risks to public health and safety by myriad government agencies at local, state, federal, and international levels. Families are also looking for answers and closure. Timely completion of forensic autopsy reports should also be encouraged, not discouraged. Complaints by families or government agencies regarding unacceptable delays in the production of autopsy reports can lead to negative media reports and political difficulties for forensic offices.[42–46]

The production of timely autopsy reports is not as difficult as it may seem. Lean production is a well-studied system to eliminate waste in production. Lean's basic assumption is that anything that does not add value to the customer is waste and should be eliminated from the production process. Although commonly associated with the Toyota Production System, lean is believed by many people to have had its first practical applications by Henry Ford as far back as 1927.[47,48]

The principles of lean production have been applied to the production of an autopsy report. A system that defined and evaluated 12 essential steps in the autopsy process and increased their priority reduced the autopsy completion time from a mean of 57 days to a mean of 4.8 days.[49] Another study that formally applied lean principles identified a total of 77 steps and multiple queues that introduced delays in their autopsy process. This pathology department was able to reduce the number of steps by 8% and minimize queues. The department's autopsy turnaround time was reduced from a mean of 53 days to 25 days. They increased the percentage of final reports completed within the 60-working-day CAP guideline from 71% to 100% and the percentage of PADs completed within 2 days from 26% to 87%. Most significantly, 85% of surveyed clinicians stated they were receiving reports sooner and 71% believed the autopsy service was functioning better.[50]

Autopsy Report

Autopsy reports are the main method by which autopsy and forensic pathologists communicate their work and thus their value to their clinical colleagues and the larger community. So it is not only the timeliness but also the content of the autopsy report by which pathologists are judged. The importance of reports has been long recognized in radiology, a field of medicine similar in many ways to pathology. Radiologists list the attributes of a good radiology report as the 8 Cs: clarity, correctness, confidence, concision, completeness, consistency, communication, and consultation, along with timeliness and standardization.[51]

The autopsy report has changed little over the years. In both the hospital and forensic worlds, the autopsy report is basically narrative, with some sections in outline form, notably the PAD and final anatomic diagnoses. The length of the report can vary greatly depending on the level of detail and the thoroughness of the descriptions. Features that are incorporated into other pathology and medical reports, such as coding, structured reporting, and images, have not yet been adopted into the autopsy report.

The organization of an autopsy report also varies greatly. The specific locations of different sections of the report vary from hospital to hospital or medical examiner to coroner office. For example, the clinical correlation, a major feature of hospital autopsy reports, may be placed at the beginning or end of the autopsy report. In other cases, a section contained within one institution's autopsy report, such as the microscopic description, may be a separate report in another institution. Some stillborn autopsy reports contain the description of the placenta whereas others have a separate surgical case report referenced by the autopsy report.

The Autopsy Committee of the College of American Pathologists recommended a set of consistently used headings for all autopsy reports. They opined that these headings would be useful by reducing of errors of omission, facilitating the location of information from the report by pathologist and third parties, and enhancing electronic data analysis.[52]

Structured reporting

As the era of paper medical records moves to electronic medical records, many areas of medicine are taking advantage of the opportunities inherent in digital documents. In this new era of electronic medical records, an autopsy report needs to be more than a text dump or a pdf file transferred into an electronic health record or e-mailed to a local law enforcement agency. Relevant data within autopsy reports need to be structured, which will facilitate searching, analyzing, and researching these invaluable data in numerous ways.

Radiologists have recognized the opportunities and advantages offered by structured reporting compared with the traditional free text reporting in the new era of pay for performance, evidence-based medicine and the physician quality reporting initiative. They are actively investigating structured reporting to add value to radiology reports and their profession.[53] Similarly, there are numerous articles related to synoptic or structured reporting in surgical pathology, especially with regard to cancer.[54–57]

In contrast, there are no articles identified in the summer of 2014 when searching for different combinations of the terms, *autopsy report*, *structured*, and *synoptic*. Yet there is no doubt that structuring autopsy reports would have similar benefits for autopsy and forensic pathologists that structuring surgical pathology reports have had for pathology and radiology reports for radiology.

For example, in an evaluation of suicide risk assessment, it was recognized that a structured, systematic approach toward collecting information is critical to formulating suicide risk.[58] The integration of this historical data with results of autopsy reports on persons who have successfully committed suicide (including method used, evidence of prior attempts, significant medical diagnoses, and so forth) could be invaluable in helping to identify those at highest risk and in most need of intervention and treatment.

Images

The incorporation of images is another area where the value of autopsy reports can be greatly enhanced. Digital images are being included in surgical pathology reports, especially among private pathology groups that are focused on providing services to their clinician customers. These are typically digital snapshots from a microscopic slide showing relevant diagnostic information that frequently is not adequately annotated. In these cases, the image is little more than a marketing tool and not a value-added educational tool to assist clinicians in treating patients.

Properly annotated images can add value to an autopsy report, creating an image-enhanced report (IER) that can serve as an invaluable educational tool. Clinicians who were surveyed after the institution of IER perceive the inclusion of properly annotated images as adding value to the autopsy report and assisting them in understanding the death.[59] When using digital images in medical reports, it is important to use appropriate guidelines in how these images are selected, edited, annotated, and used.[60]

Issues involving the use of images in forensic autopsy reports are complicated by the frequently sensitive nature of these images, the fact that many states consider autopsy reports public record whereas other states specifically restrict the release of digital forensic autopsy images, and the needs of public safety during the investigation of deaths. The public reaction to the publication of autopsy images showing the gunshot wounds on a person shot by law enforcement or a reaction of a family member to an image of a loved one in a state of advanced decomposition can be imagined. Yet even within forensics, the use of properly prepared and annotated images could add great value to the narrative report of a forensic pathologist in helping to explain the death (Fig. 5).

The Virtual or Minimally Invasive Autopsy

This discussion has involved how changes in the reporting of autopsy findings through the use of informatics might have a significant positive impact on the practice of autopsy pathology, help restore the value and importance of the autopsy, and lead to an increase in the autopsy rate. Attention is turned to how applying modern technology and informatics might change the autopsy procedure itself.

A

Spleen:

<u>Gross</u>: The spleen is enlarged and weighs 1720 g. The capsule is gray-blue, smooth, and glistening with 2 superficial lacerations measuring 3.0 and 2.5 cm in length, respectively. The cut surface is dark red with multiple tan to brown ill-defined patches in a geographic pattern, the largest of which measures 10 × 5 cm.

<u>Microscopic</u>: The capsule is unremarkable. There are nodular expanded foci of extramedullary hematopoiesis that contains all 3 hematopoietic cell lines. There are increased numbers of enlarged megakaryocytes with bizarre-shaped nuclei. Myeloid and erythroid lines are present but due to poor preservation the extent of maturation could not be determined. There are foci of autolysis.

B   **C**

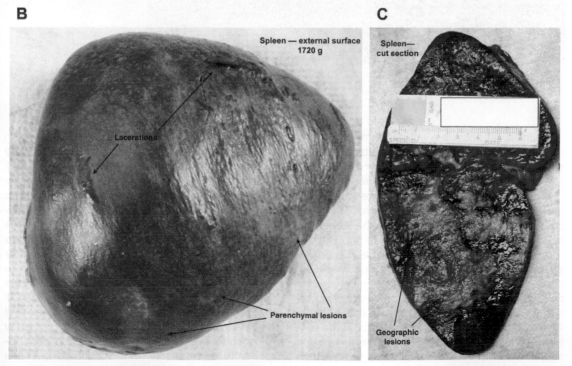

Fig. 5. (A) The gross and microscopic text description for a spleen from an autopsy. (B, C) Annotated gross images showing the surface and cut section of the spleen.

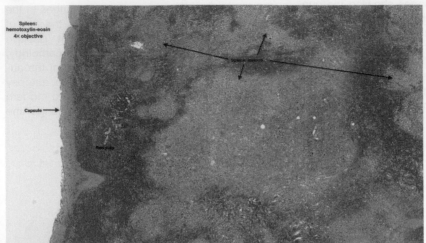

Spleen:
hemotoxylin-eosin
4× objective

Capsule →

Red pulp

Splenic trabecula

Fig. 5. (continued). (D, E)
Annotated low- and
high-power microscopic
images of the spleen.

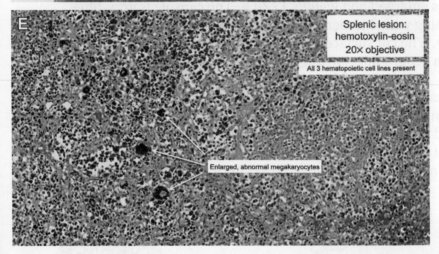

E

Splenic lesion:
hemotoxylin-eosin
20× objective

All 3 hematopoietic cell lines present

Enlarged, abnormal megakaryocytes

A virtual autopsy is a nondestructive or minimally destructive examination of the body utilizing scanning modalities, such as CT or MRI scans. The promise of a virtual autopsy is that equivalent or superior information can be gathered as a result of the examination without the destruction of the physical evidence or damage to the deceased body.

Virtual autopsies to date have been primarily involved with the practice of forensic medicine. In Europe, virtual autopsies were first used in academically situated forensic offices to study alternatives to the traditional autopsy. In the United States, the virtual autopsy got its start in the military setting with the use of these techniques to support, not replace, the traditional autopsy. There are only a few examples of virtual autopsies being studied for nonforensic hospital deaths.

Virtopsy project
The Institute of Forensic Medicine of the University of Bern, Switzerland, has been one of the early leaders of the study of virtual autopsy in Europe. It is this group that created and trademarked the term, *Virtopsy*. The group started their revolutionary work in the 1990s with a study of 3-D photogrammetry-based optical scanning of the external surfaces of the body as a way to better document external injuries and compare them to alleged weapons or mechanisms of injury. Within a few years they began using both multislice CT (MSCT) and MRI scans of deceased bodies and compared them with conventional autopsy. They discovered that MSCT is equivalent and even superior to conventional forensic autopsies in the evaluation of skeletal injuries, the detection of pneumothorax or gas emboli, and the location

and recovery of foreign bodies. MRI is well suited for the evaluation of soft tissue injuries but is not nearly as effective for documenting the common causes of sudden natural death, especially cardiac.[61]

Postmortem angiography has been performed for many years, primarily by infusing the coronary arteries after removal of the heart at autopsy; however, the ability to properly perfuse a deceased body using methods similar to living patients has been technically difficult.[62] The Institute of Forensic Medicine investigated different methods to perfuse the vascular system with contrast, finally discovering an adequate method through the use of a modified heart-lung machine. They demonstrated that this method was able to detect not only significant coronary artery disease with the same accuracy as conventional autopsy but also other vascular diseases, such as aortic dissection, pulmonary emboli, and aneurysms of the major vasculature (**Fig. 6**).[63]

The Institute of Forensic Medicine also studied the use of image-guided biopsy to obtain specimens to document disease histologically. In the same study in which they studied CT angiography in sudden deaths due to chest pain, they also obtained biopsies of the heart, lungs, and blood clots from the pulmonary arteries under CT guidance. In 2 of 3 cases, the myocardial biopsy was concordant with the histologic sections obtained from conventional autopsy. Sampling error was responsible for instances where the biopsy did not reveal the histopathology. This method was also adequate in distinguishing a pulmonary embolus from postmortem clot in the pulmonary artery and a pulmonary neoplasm.[63]

Studies have also demonstrated that postmortem CT scans are comparable to autopsy in the evaluation of free blood in the abdomen,[64] pericardial effusion, and hemopericardium[65] and in organ volume measurements for most internal organs in infants dying of sudden unexpected death (**Figs. 7 and 8**).[66]

The Institute of Forensic Medicine has combined this technology into a virtual autopsy system, called the *Virtobot*. This system can perform automated 3-D surface documentation of injuries and image-guided robotic needle biopsies. Surface scanning has recently been reduced from 30 minutes to 10 minutes per side of the body, although the complete documentation takes between 2 and 3 hours. They have used this system to surface scan a variety of blunt, sharp, and gunshot injuries. Needle biopsy accuracy currently averages 1.4 mm from the target.[67]

Armed Forces Medical Examiner virtual autopsy

In the United States, the Office of the Armed Forces Medical Examiner (OAFME), responsible for the postmortem examination of all active duty military personnel, began to use multidetector CT

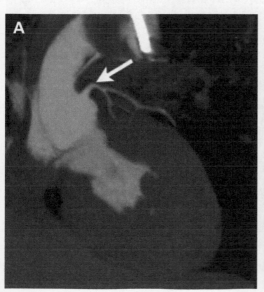
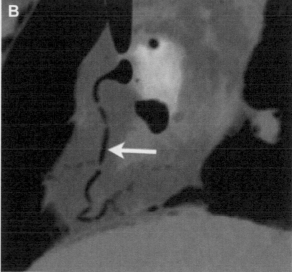

Fig. 6. Postmortem CT angiography showing a normal left coronary artery (*arrow*) opacified by contrast (*A*) and right coronary artery (*arrow*) filled with air (*B*). (*From* Saunders SL, Morgan B, Raj V, Rutty GN. Post-mortem computerized tomography angiography: past, present and future. Forensic Sci Med Pathol 2011;7:276; with permission.)

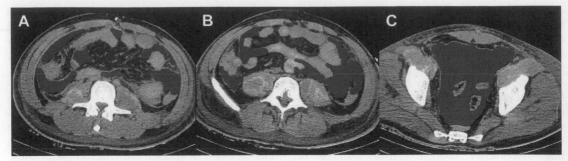

Fig. 7. Axial CT images of the abdomen at 3 distinct levels (*A–C*). The free abdominal blood is manually marked during segmentation (*red colored areas*). (*From* Ampanozi G, Hatch GM, Ruder TD, et al. Post-mortem virtual estimation of free abdominal blood volume. Eur J Radiol 2011;81:2134; with permission.)

(MDCT) scanning to detect unexploded ordinance in military personnel prior to autopsy. They quickly realized that CT scans combined with autopsy have the potential to provide better evaluation of the nature of wounds sustained by military personnel in combat. They were able to better define wound tracks and locate metallic fragments from high-velocity gunshot wounds.[68]

Once combat wounds were better characterized, it became easier to retrospectively evaluate these injuries for potential survivability, separating these injuries into not survivable (NS) and potentially survivable (PS). Understanding the nature of these injuries will allow the military to not only

identify injuries that are PS so they can quickly receive life-saving medical treatment but also develop techniques and equipment to minimize exposure to wounds that are NS.[69,70]

The OAFME has also studied the implications of using postmortem MDCT for nonmilitary situations. During the response to January 2010 Haiti earthquake, the OAFME had the responsibility to examine and repatriate US citizens who were victims of that mass fatality disaster. They discovered that using MDCT in combination with digital radiographs and external examination allowed them to triage cases for virtual or conventional autopsy.[71] This has the potential to greatly improve the

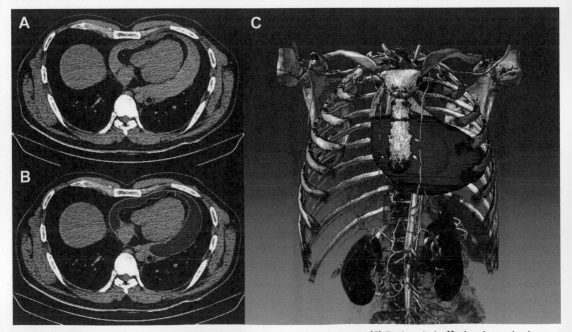

Fig. 8. (*A*) Volume measurement by segmentation using axial CT images. (*B*) Pericardial effusion is marked manually for each slice or resampled slices. (*C*) 3-D reconstruction of segmented pericardial effusion. (*From* Ebert LC, Ampanozi G, Ruder TD, et al. CT based volume measurement and estimation in cases of pericardial effusion. J Forensic Legal Med 2012;19:127; with permission.)

efficiency of the response of medical examiners to mass fatality incidents, directing appropriate levels of scarce resources to where it is most needed.

Virtual autopsies in the hospital setting

Virtual autopsies have been studied in the hospital setting. Similar to the studies in forensic practice, the use of a single modality (CT or MRI) revealed significant deficiencies in the accuracy of virtual autopsy compared with conventional autopsy.

When compared with the gold standard of the traditional autopsy, major discrepancy rates of 32% for CT alone, 43% for MRI alone, and 30% for combined CT-MRI have been reported, with the most common missed diagnoses ischemic heart disease, pulmonary emboli, and pneumonia. Radiologists in this study identified cases in which they thought traditional autopsy would not be necessary, and in those cases the major discrepancy rate fell to 16% for CT, 21% for MRI, and 16% for CT-MRI imaging.[72] The approximately one-third major discrepancy rate for postmortem CT was confirmed in another study, which determined the positive predictive value for cause of death by postmortem CT at 75%. Demonstrating the potential value of using postmortem CT as an adjunct to autopsy instead of a replacement, the same study reported a combined diagnostic yield of 133% compared with autopsy alone.[73]

The ability of ultrasound-guided needle biopsy to increase the accuracy of virtual autopsy in hospital autopsies yielded a sensitivity of 94% and specificity of 99% compared with conventional autopsy, with agreement on the cause of death in 77% of cases. The major area of deficiency in this study was related to cardiac deaths.[74]

These studies show some promise for the use of CT and/or MRI to either increase the value of the autopsy or replace it in selected cases. One potential advantage of a virtual autopsy is the increased likelihood that families will consent to a non- or minimally invasive procedure, especially in cases of religious objections.[75] Adapting some of the techniques pioneered in the forensic Virtopsy project, especially the use of postmortem angiography and image-guided needle biopsies, has the potential to raise the accuracy of the virtual procedure to near that of the conventional autopsy. Intelligent triaging of cases through the use of scanning to determine which deaths require a conventional autopsy can also help to increase efficiency in ever busier pathology departments.

The potential downside of adoption of virtual autopsy involves the logistics and expense of providing this service. Given that there are currently no government or private insurer reimbursements for conventional autopsies, it is unlikely that there will be reimbursements for virtual autopsy. The costs for CT and MRI scanners are significant. They require specially shielded rooms as well as properly trained technicians to operate them. In contrast, the cost of autopsy space, equipment, and personnel is considerably less. Either radiologists will provide the interpretations or pathologists will have to be trained to interpret them.

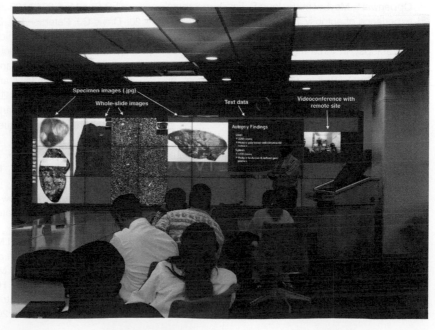

Fig. 9. An autopsy case presentation on a pathology department's multitiled high-resolution display running the scalable adaptive graphics environment (SAGE). Autopsy data, gross images, and whole-slide images can be viewed simultaneously and discussed with participants both in the space and through videoconferencing.

SUMMARY

The hospital autopsy, despite the decline in autopsy rates over the past 3 decades, still has a significant role to play in patient care. Even in the twenty-first century world of high-tech medicine, the autopsy discovers unexpected findings on a regular basis. As an era of personalized medicine and accountable care is entered, the autopsy is well positioned to provide insight and evidence to support new therapies and enhance patient safety.

The autopsy cannot remain unchanged from how it has been practiced for more than a century. It needs to adapt to the changing demands of medicine by adopting informatics and new technology to keep pace with the rest of clinical care and pathology. For example, at the University of Illinois at Chicago, the Department of Pathology and the Electronic Visualization Laboratory (EVL) in the Department of Computer Science developed an application to display whole-slide images within EVL's collaborative SAGE, expanding SAGE's existing capacity to simultaneously display and share a variety of high-resolution images, video, and data (**Fig. 9**).

Pathologists need to take leadership of the evolution of the autopsy, document the value of the autopsy to patient care, and advocate for appropriate financial reimbursement for this medical procedure.

REFERENCES

1. McPhee SJ, Bottles K. Autopsy: moribund art or vital science. Am J Med 1985;78:107–13.
2. Oppenwal F, Meyboom-de Jong B. Family members' experience of autopsy. Fam Pract 2001;18:304–8.
3. Goldman L, Sayson R, Robbins S, et al. The value of the autopsy in three medical eras. N Engl J Med 1983;308:1000–5.
4. Shojania KG, Burton EC, McDonald KM, et al. Changes in rates of autopsy-detected diagnostic errors over time: a systematic review. JAMA 2003;289:2849–56.
5. Pastores SM, Dulu A, Voigt L, et al. Premortem clinical diagnoses and postmortem autopsy findings: discrepancies in critically ill cancer patients. Crit Care 2007;11:R48.
6. Roberts WC. The autopsy: its decline and a suggestion for its revival. N Engl J Med 1978;299:332–8.
7. Landefeld CS, Chren MM, Myers A, et al. Diagnostic yield of the autopsy in a university hospital and a community hospital. N Engl J Med 1988;318:1249–54.
8. Hasson J, Schneidermann H. Autopsy training programs. To right a wrong. Arch Pathol Lab Med 1995;119:289–91.
9. Hoyert DL. The changing profile of autopsied deaths in the United States, 1972-2007. NCHS data brief, no. 6. Hyattsville (MD): National Center for Health Statistics; 2011.
10. Lundberg GD. Low-tech autopsies in the era of high-tech medicine: continued value for quality assurance and patient safety. JAMA 1998;280:1273–4.
11. Esposito TJ, Sanddal T, Sanddal N, et al. Dead men tell no tales: analysis and use of autopsy reports in trauma system performance improvement activities. J Trauma Acute Care Surg 2012;73:587–90.
12. Bove KE, Iery C, Autopsy Committee of CAP. The role of the autopsy in medical malpractice cases, I. Arch Pathol Lab Med 2002;126:1021–31.
13. Bove KE, Iery C, Autopsy Committee of CAP. The role of the autopsy in medical malpractice cases, II. Arch Pathol Lab Med 2002;126:1032–5.
14. Fielding SL. When patients feel ignored: study findings about medical liability. Acad Med 1997;72:6–7.
15. Sinard JH, Autopsy Committee of CAP. Accounting for the professional work of pathologists performing autopsies. Arch Pathol Lab Med 2013;137:228–32.
16. Hull MJ, Nazarian RM, Wheeler AE, et al. Resident physicians opinions on autopsy importance and procurement. Hum Pathol 2007;38:342–50.
17. Brown HG. Perceptions of the autopsy: views from the lay public and program proposals. Hum Pathol 1990;21:154–8.
18. Oluwasola OA, Fawole OI, Otegbayo AJ, et al. The autopsy: knowledge, attitude and perceptions of doctors and relatives of the deceased. Arch Pathol Lab Med 2009;133:78–82.
19. Henry J, Nicholas N. Dead in the water-are we killing the hospital autopsy with poor consent practices? J R Soc Med 2012;105:288–95.
20. Davis GJ, Peterson BR. Dilemmas and solutions for the pathology and clinician encountering religious views of the autopsy. South Med J 1996;89:1041–4.
21. Goodman NR, Goodman JL, Hoffman WI. Autopsy: traditional Jewish laws and customs "Halacha". Am J Forensic Med Pathol 2011;32:300–3.
22. Birdi KS, Bunce DJ, Start RD, et al. Clinician beliefs underlying autopsy requests. Postgrad Med J 1996;72:224–8.
23. Hagestuen PO, Aase S. The organization and value of autopsies. Tidsskr Nor Legeforen 2012;132:152–4.
24. Karunaratne S, Benbow EW. A survey of general practitioners' views on autopsy reports. J Clin Pathol 1997;50:548–52.
25. Bayer-Garner IB, Fink LM, Lamps LW. Pathologists in a teaching institution assess the value of the autopsy. Arch Pathol Lab Med 2002;126:442–7.
26. Alabran JL, Hooper JE, Hill M, et al. Overcoming autopsy barriers in pediatric cancer research. Pediatr Blood Cancer 2013;60:204–9.

27. Heazell AE, McLaughlin MJ, Schmidt EB, et al. A difficult conversation? The views and experiences of parents and professionals on the consent process for perinatal postmortem after stillbirth. BJOG 2012; 119:987–97.

28. Tsitsikas DA, Brothwell M, Aleong JC, et al. The attitudes of relatives to autopsy: a misconception. J Clin Pathol 2011;64:412–4.

29. Smith PF, Hadler JL, Stanbury M, et al, CSTE Surveillance Strategy Group. "Blueprint version 2.0": updating public health surveillance for the 21st century. J Public Health Manag Pract 2013;19(3):231–9.

30. Paterson BJ, Durrheim DN. The remarkable adaptability of syndromic surveillance to meet public health needs. J Epidemiol Glob Health 2013;3:41–7.

31. Kovats RS, Ebi KL. Heatwaves and public health in Europe. Eur J Public Health 2006;16(6):592–9.

32. Campbell R, Weis MA, Millet L, et al. From surveillance to action: early gains from the National Violent Death Reporting System. Inj Prev 2006;12(Suppl II):ii6–9.

33. Ritter N. Missing persons and unidentified remains: the nation's silent mass disaster. NIJ J 2007;256. Available at: http://www.nij.gov/journals/256/pages/missing-persons.aspx. Accessed August 15, 2014.

34. Savel TG, Foldy S. The Role of Public Health Informatics in enhancing public health surveillance. MMWR 2012;61(Suppl):20–4.

35. College of American Pathologists. Commission on Laboratory Accreditation Anatomic Pathology Checklist. Available at: http://www.cap.org. Accessed July 30, 2014.

36. Joint Commission on Accreditation of Healthcare Organizations (JCAHO). Accreditation manual for Hospitals. Oakbrook Terrace (IL): Joint Commission on Accreditation of Healthcare Organizations; 2001.

37. National Association of Medical Examiners. NAME Inspection and Accreditation Checklist Second Revision Adopted September 2009. Available at: https://netforum.avectra.com/temp/ClientImages/NAME/069196e4-6f95-437c-a2be-47649a70685e.pdf. Accessed July 30, 2014.

38. National Association of Medical Examiners. NAME Inspection and Accreditation Checklist Second Revision Adopted February 2014. Available at: https://netforum.avectra.com/temp/ClientImages/NAME/de7871b6-1a1f-403c-9c23-d6d623e7a4a8.pdf. Accessed July 30, 2014.

39. The National Association of Medical Examiners Inspection and Accreditation Committee. Forensic Autopsy Performance Standards. Available at: https://netforum.avectra.com/temp/ClientImages/NAME/eed6c85d-5871-4da1-aef3-abfc9bb80b92.pdf. Accessed July 30, 2014.

40. International Association of Coronrs & Medical Examiners Accreditation Checklist. Available at: http://iacme.orainc.com/help/checklist. Accessed July 30, 2014.

41. Hutchins GM, Berman JJ, Moore GW, et al. Autopsy Committee of the College of American Pathologists. Practice Guidelines for autopsy pathology: autopsy reporting. Arch Pathol Lab Med 1995;119:123–30.

42. Shenoy R. Report: Varied reasons for delays in state Medical Examiner's Office. The Sun Chronicle. June 8, 2014. Available at: http://www.thesunchronicle.com/devices/news/local_news/report-varied-reasons-for-delays-in-state-medical-examiner-s/article_c868ed3a-eedc-11e3-aefb-0019bb2963f4.html. Accessed August 25, 2014.

43. Gutman D. Lack of pathologists backlogs W. Va. Medical Examiner's Office. Sunday Gazette-Mail. 2014. Available at: http://www.wvgazette.com/article/20140713/GZ01/140719793. Accessed August 25, 2014.

44. Editorial Board. Family of football player who died last year still seeking answers on cause. Fayette Observer. August 17, 2014. Available at: http://www.fayobserver.com/opinion/editorials/our-view-office-of-chief-medical-examiner-must-answer-for/article_f42d9ad2-f50e-5f00-a575-6991d435629c.html. Accessed August 25, 2014.

45. Monahan B. Medical examiner delays lead to court delays, frustrations. WGGB. March 3, 2014. Available at: http://www.wggb.com/2014/03/03/medical-examiner-delays-lead-to-court-delays-frustations/. Accessed August 25, 2014.

46. Huet E. S.F. medical examiner lags in rulings on deaths. SF Gate. November 23, 2013. Available at: http://www.sfgate.com/bayarea/article/S-F-medical-examiner-lags-in-ruling-on-deaths-5006771.php. Accessed August 25, 2014.

47. Shah R, Ward PT. Defining and developing measures of lean production. J Operations Management 2007;25:785–805.

48. Holweg M. The genealogy of lean production. J Operations Management 2007;25:420–37.

49. Adickes ED, Sims KL. Enhancing autopsy performance and reporting. A system for a 5-day completion time. Arch Pathol Lab Med 1996; 120(3):249–53.

50. Siebert JR. Increasing the efficiency of autopsy reporting. Arch Pathol Lab Med 2009;133:1932–7.

51. Reiner BI, Knight N, Siegel EL. Radiology reporting, past, present and future: the radiologist's perspective. J Am Coll Radiol 2007;4(5):313–9.

52. Hanzlick RL, Autopsy Committee College of American Pathologists. The autopsy lexicon: suggested headings for the autopsy report. Arch Pathol Lab Med 2000;124:594–603.

53. Reiner BI. The challenges, opportunities and imperative of structured reporting in medical imaging. J Digit Imaging 2009;22(6):562–8.

54. Larn E, Vy N, Bajdik C, et al. Synoptic reporting for thyroid cancer: a review and institutional experience. Expert Rev Anticancer Ther 2013;13(9): 1073–9.

55. Becher MW. Practical neuropathology synoptic reporting for central nervous system tumors. Arch Pathol Lab Med 2011;135(6):789–92.

56. Epstein JI, Srigley J, Grignon D, et al. Recommendations for the reporting of prostate carcinoma. Hum Pathol 2007;38(9):1035–9.

57. Ibarra JA. The pathologist in breast cancer: contemporary issues in the interdisciplinary approach. Surg Oncol Clin N Am 2000;9(2):295–317.

58. Menon V. Suicide risk assessment and formulation: an update. As J Psych 2013;6:430–5.

59. Pritt B, Gibson P, Cooper K, et al. What is a picture worth? Digital imaging applications in autopsy reports. Arch Pathol Lab Med 2004;128:1247–50.

60. Pritt BS, Gibson PC, Cooper K. Digital imaging guidelines for pathology: a proposal for general and academic use. Adv Anat Pathol 2003;10(2): 96–100.

61. Bolliger SA, Thali MJ, Ross S, et al. Virtual autopsy using imaging: bridging radiologic and forensic sciences. A review of the Virtopsy and similar projects. Eur Radiol 2008;18:273–82.

62. Saunders SL, Morgan B, Raj V, et al. Post-mortem computerized tomography angiography: past, present and future. Forensic Sci Med Pathol 2011;7: 271–7.

63. Ross SG, Thali MJ, Bolliger S, et al. Sudden death after chest pain: feasibility of virtual autopsy with postmortem CT angiography and biopsy. Radiology 2012;264:250–9.

64. Ampanozi G, Hatch GM, Ruder TD, et al. Post-mortem virtual estimation of free abdominal blood volume. Eur J Radiol 2011;81:2133–6.

65. Ebert LC, Ampanozi G, Ruder TD, et al. CT based volume measurement and estimation in cases of pericardial effusion. J Forensic Leg Med 2012;19: 126–31.

66. Prodhomme O, Seguret F, Martrille L, et al. Organ volume measurements: comparison between MRI and autopsy findings in infants following sudden unexpected death. Arch Dis Child Fetal Neonatal Ed 2012;97:F434–8.

67. Ebert LC, Ptacek W, Breitbeck R, et al. Virtobot 2.0: the future of automated surface documentation and CT-guided needle placement in forensic medicine. Forensic Sci Med Pathol 2014;10:179–86.

68. Levy AD, Abbott RM, Mallak CT, et al. Virtual autopsy: preliminary experience in high-velocity gunshot wound victims. Radiology 2006;240(2):522–8.

69. Eastridge BJ, Mardin M, Cantrell J, et al. Died of wounds on the battlefield: causation and implications for improving combat casualty care. J Trauma 2011;71:S4–8.

70. Eastridge BJ, Mabry RL, Seguin P, et al. Death on the battlefield (2001-2011): implications for the future of combat casualty care. J Trauma Acute Care Surg 2012;73:S431–7.

71. Berran PJ, Mazuchowski EL, Marzouk A, et al. Observational case series: an algorithm incorporating multidetector computerized tomography in the medicolegal investigation of human remains after a natural disaster. J Forensic Sci 2014;59(4): 1121–5.

72. Roberts IS, Benamore RE, Benbow EW, et al. Post-mortem imaging as an alternative to autopsy in the diagnosis of adult deaths: a validation study. Lancet 2012;379:136–42.

73. Westphal SE, Apitzsch J, Penzkofer T, et al. Virtual CT autopsy in clinical pathology: feasibility in clinical autopsies. Virchows Arch 2012;461:211–9.

74. Weustink AC, Hunink MG, van Dijke CF, et al. Minimally invasive autopsy: an alternative to Conventional autopsy? Radiology 2009;250:897–904.

75. Cannie M, Votina C, Moerman PH, et al. Acceptance, reliability and confidence of diagnosis of fetal and neonatal virtoupsy compared with conventional autopsy: a prospective study. Ultrasound Obstet Gynecol 2012;39:659–65.

Laboratory Automation and Middleware

Michael Riben, MD

KEYWORDS

- Laboratory automation • Middleware • Anatomic pathology • Workflow optimization
- Histology automation

ABSTRACT

The practice of surgical pathology is under constant pressure to deliver the highest quality of service, reduce errors, increase throughput, and decrease turnaround time while at the same time dealing with an aging workforce, increasing financial constraints, and economic uncertainty. Although not able to implement total laboratory automation, great progress continues to be made in workstation automation in all areas of the pathology laboratory. This report highlights the benefits and challenges of pathology automation, reviews middleware and its use to facilitate automation, and reviews the progress so far in the anatomic pathology laboratory.

OVERVIEW

First coined in the mid-1940s by an engineer who worked for Ford Motor Company, the term automation is often used to describe the substitution of human/manual effort and intelligence with mechanical, electrical, or computerized processes.[1] Laboratory testing, which began as an entirely manual "hands-on" complex workflow process that demanded highly skilled personnel, represented an ideal candidate for the application of automation given the meticulous and repetitive nature of the work. The first demonstration of an automated testing instrument occurred in New York City at the first international congress of clinical chemistry in 1956: a small sample of blood was loaded into a blood analyzer, manufactured by Technicon and invented by pathologists at Western Reserve University School of Medicine, and 2.5 minutes later, it produced results for levels of sugar, calcium, and urea.[2] The first commercial automated clinical laboratory instrument, the Autoanalyzer I, in 1957, used continuous-flow analysis, which dramatically increased instrument throughput capacity compared with manual processes available at the time. Since its introduction, pathologists have been striving to apply the tools of automation throughout the entire clinical laboratory.[3] Although this transition initially began with the development of instruments in the chemistry and hematology laboratory, all areas of the clinical laboratory have been impacted by automation technology. The focus of this article is limited to a review of laboratory automation and middleware as it applies to the practice of surgical pathology.

LABORATORY TEST CYCLE

The laboratory test cycle is a common framework for understanding the different aspects of the laboratory testing process (**Fig. 1**). Unlike the clinical pathology laboratory, where this framework is easily applicable, the steps of the surgical pathology workflow have much more overlap between the phases, depending on established local laboratory workflows. For easy comprehension, we have developed a simplified workflow and categorized them according to test cycle phase (**Table 1**). In addition, for the preanalytic, analytical, and postanalytic phases of the surgical pathology testing workflow, a few examples of automation tools that have been applied to these workflow steps are noted.

STRATEGIC ADVANTAGES AND CHALLENGES FOR AUTOMATION FOR SURGICAL PATHOLOGY

For surgical pathology, laboratory automation has been applied to processes and information related

Department of Pathology, University of Texas M.D. Anderson Cancer Center, 1515 Holcombe Blvd, Houston, TX 77030, USA

E-mail address: mriben@mdanderson.org

Surgical Pathology 8 (2015) 175–186

http://dx.doi.org/10.1016/j.path.2015.02.012

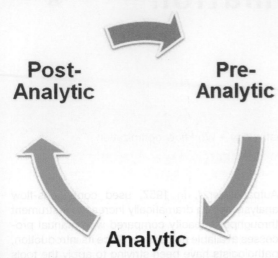

Fig. 1. The laboratory test cycle.

to all aspects of the laboratory testing cycle. The catalyst for applying automation tools for surgical pathology is multifactorial. Over the years, and continuing today, these factors have included demands for increased volume throughput, demands for faster turnaround times, economic billing and reimbursement factors that mandate cost savings with a "do more with less" mantra, demands for higher quality, demands for safer work environments, and patient safety initiatives to prevent laboratory errors that directly affect patient care. More recently, the aging pathology laboratory workforce along with increasing requirements for secondary uses of the assets acquired and produced in the laboratory are driving innovation.

Automation offers significant strategic benefits over manual processes (**Table 2**). Specifically, automation addresses tasks that directly impact

---

Table 1
Workflow steps in surgical pathology and associated automation tools

Test Cycle Phase	Workflow Steps	Automation Tools
Preanalytic	Electronic order in the AP-LIS	
	Specimen acquisition	
	Specimen label and identification	Barcode and RFID tracking
	Specimen transport and delivery	Real-time location systems
	Specimen receipt and verification	
	Specimen accessioning	Preaccessioning middleware
Analytical	Tissue examination and grossing	
	Prosection dictation and transcription	Voice recognition and synoptic
	Gross image capture and annotation	Automated wireless photo capture
	Tissue block processing	Automated and microwave processors
	Tissue block embedding	Automated tissue embedders
	Block sectioning and slide creation	Automated microtomes, robotic slide instruments
	Slide hematoxylin and eosin staining	Automated hematoxylin and eosin stainers
	Slide coverslipping	Automated slide coverslippers
	Histochemistry slide-based testing	Automated special stain stainers
	Immunohistochemistry slide-based testing	Automated immunocytochemistry stainers
	In situ hybridization slide-based testing	Automated in situ hybridization
	Tissue Homogenate Molecular testing	Automated laser capture
	Diagnostic evaluation and workup	Synoptic reporting, voice recognition
	Diagnostic transcription	Voice recognition
	Slide scanning	High-throughput whole-slide scanners
Postanalytic	Report verification and release	
	Report delivery	Automated faxing, interfaces
	Archival and storage of block and slides	
	Image management for postanalytical processes	PACS for pathology
	Block and slide retrieval	Barcode and RFID tracking

Abbreviations: PACS, Picture Archiving and Communications System; RFID, Radio Frequency Identification.

Table 2
Automation benefits and challenges

Benefits	Challenges
Decreases turnaround time	Lack of standards
Decreases pathology errors	Space
Increases system throughput	Middleware functional gaps
Replacement for aging workforce	Shifts technical skill sets required
Decreases exposure to hazardous chemicals	Change management
Reduces repetitive stress injuries	Costs
Decreases risk for injuries (hands)	Dealing with downtime issues
Increases employee satisfaction	Inability to automate every task
Supports economic growth	

quality and errors, sometimes referred to as "3-D tasks" or "dull, dirty, and dangerous."[4] By reducing the potential for injuries, such as repetitive stress or cuts from knife blades, and by reducing direct exposure to hazardous chemicals, there is a positive impact on employee satisfaction. In the hospital environment, employee satisfaction is an important contributing factor to the quality of patient care.[5] Most importantly, automation, along with workflow optimization, offers benefits for decreasing total testing turnaround time and increasing system throughput capacity, resulting in economic growth for the laboratory. Lastly, automation offers a solution for the aging histology laboratory workforce, of which almost half are predicted to reach retirement age by this year.[6]

There are, however, numerous challenges to overcome (see **Table 2**). These include physical space constraints for sophisticated devices, financial costs that must be overcome to get started, changes in the technical skills required for employees, downtime planning and training issues that might be radically different from traditional processes, and change management issues related to paradigm shifts in workflow and process. Because not all tasks can be automated, there is a significant challenge to integrating automation workcells due to functional gaps in the software solutions currently available in the laboratory. A significant challenge to total laboratory automation in the anatomic pathology laboratory is an absence of standards essential to allowing disparate devices and software systems to interconnect. With the proliferation of automation systems in the clinical pathology laboratory, pathologist and industry leaders recognized the requirement for standards to allow for interoperability of different instruments, devices, and software from different vendors, resulting in what today are the AUTO standards by the Clinical Laboratory Standards Institute (formerly National

Accrediting Agency for Clinical Laboratory Sciences).[7] Their initial efforts included standards for specimen containers, bar codes for specimen containers, communication between instruments, devices, automation software and the laboratory information system (LIS), electromechanical interfaces, and operational requirements, characteristics, and information elements.[8] Since their initial release, additional standards addressing managing and validating LISs, Internet access to diagnostic devices, Autoverification, IT security of diagnostic instruments and software, and label standard addressing content, location, font, and orientation have also been developed.[9] Unfortunately, consideration for anatomic pathology was not included. Successful total laboratory automation will be dependent on industry and pathology leaders coming together to either modify the current standards and apply them to anatomic pathology, or create anatomic pathology–specific standards that could be used by device manufacturers and software developers. Fortunately, there are recent efforts to build the standards needed to support information system integration, championed by the Integrating the Healthcare Enterprise international initiative. Leveraging current Health Level Seven (HL7) and Digital Imaging and Communication in Medicine industry standards, this group has been defining standard-based informatics transactions to support basic diagnostic workflow and a technical framework to manage semantically rich reports, whole-slide image management, and integration with research systems, such as biobanking systems.[10,11] As an example of what is still required, a standard for barcode label format and content, would facilitate different devices using the same barcode for different functions, which might allow the immunohistochemistry device to initiate the proper program, while simultaneously allowing the whole-slide imaging device to initiate scanning and provide annotation of the whole-slide image representation, without relabeling in-between. To overcome these challenges, a focus on middleware solutions is required.

MIDDLEWARE

In the broadest sense of the term, middleware is an automation tool consisting of software that connects 2 otherwise separate "applications."[12] A simple way to think of it is that it allows software to interact.[13] In reality, there are very specific definitions for, and types of, middleware constructs, depending on different computing use-cases. The overall goal of middleware is to provide interoperability, adaptiveness, and re-configurability.[14] Colloquially, middleware is sometimes referred to as "plumbing" because it is often unseen by the end-user, but works to connect different applications/hardware devices that need to interact with each other (Fig. 2). In the clinical laboratory, Roche Diagnostics originated the term "middleware solution," referring to software that acted between instruments (analyzers) and the LIS. However, as laboratories and testing underwent radical changes at a pace that the LIS s were unable to

keep up with, laboratory middleware now refers to all kinds of software solutions that facilitate expanded and advanced functionality, not typically offered by the LIS (Table 3). Today, typical functional capabilities of laboratory middleware include autoverification, reflex test ordering based on results, automatic dilutions, rule-based decision support, real-time interactive quality control, real-time monitoring of moving averages, quality assurance system integration, multi-instrument/workcell integration, and sample storage and retrieval management.[15] Whereas these software solutions are standards of practice for most clinical pathology laboratories, the approach and penetrance of middleware for anatomic pathology lags significantly behind, but is starting to catch up.

The modern histology laboratory possesses numerous stand-alone systems and technologies, provided by a variety of vendors, most of which work in isolation of all other devices and systems. Only rarely do these devices connect to the anatomic LIS directly to automate processes or integrate tracking of assets along the production of materials. In most cases, these workstations are isolated, with no software or hardware tools

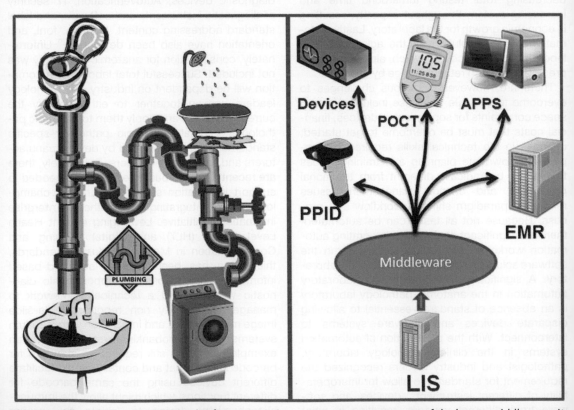

Fig. 2. Middleware: just as plumbing is often unseen, but connects numerous areas of the house, middleware sits between devices and applications to facilitate interaction with the LIS. APPS, Applications; EMR, Electronic Medical Records; POCT, Point of Care Testing; PPID, Positive Patient Identification System.

Table 3
Laboratory middleware

Category	Function	Examples
Instrument middleware	Sits between laboratory devices and LIS	Remisol Advance (Beckman Coulter), Instrument Manager (Data Innovations) TD Harmony (Technidata), WAM (Sysmex)
Laboratory-link software	Provides access for remote order entry and results review	Labworks (Atlas Medical), Copia (Orchard Software), ITF Portal (Halfpenny Technologies)
EMR laboratory-link software	Connects LISs to electronic medical records	iON (Atlas Medical), Copia (Orchard Software)
Positive-patient ID software	Patient ID confirmation and workflow management	Bridge (Cerner), SoftID (Soft), Mobilab (Iatric)
POCT-link software	Connects point-of-care devices to the LIS or EMR	QML (Telcor), RALS (Alere Informatics)
Application integration system	Integrates the LIS with enterprise applications	PathStation (M.D. Anderson)
Specimen-tracking software	Provides real-time asset tracking of specimens from the patient to the laboratory and within the laboratory	GPS for the Lab (Tagent), ColdTrack (Biotillion) Easyspecimen (ODIN)
Pathology asset tracking	Track histology blocks and slides in the laboratory	Vantage (Roche), Cerebro (Leica), HTS (General-Data)
Image management	Manages whole-slide images between the LIS and PACS	DP3 (Corista), PathXL Clinical (PathXL) VisualShare (VisualShare) PathPACS (Apollo)
Business analytics	Aggregate views of laboratory data	Viewics

Abbreviations: EMR, electronic medical record; LIS, laboratory information system; POCT, Point of Care Testing.
Beckman Coulter - Indianapolis, IN; Data Innovations - South Burlington, VT; Technidata - America Software LLC, Tucson, AZ; Sysmex - Kobe, Japan; Atlas Medical - Calabasas, CA; Orchard Software - Camel, IN; Halfpenny Technologies - Blue Bell, PA; Cerner - North Kansas City, MO; Soft - Clearwater, FL; Iatric - Boxford, MA; Telcor - Lincoln, NE; Alere Informatics - Charlottesville VA; Tagent - Mountain View, CA; Biotillian - LLC, Slillman, NJ; ODIN - San Diego, CA; Roche - Tuscon, AR; Leica - Buffalo Grove, IL; General-Data - Cincinnati, OH; Corista - Concord, MA; PathXL - Belfast, Ireland; VisualShare - Salt Lake City, UT; Apollo - Falls Church, VA; Viewics - Sunnyvale, CA.

to orchestrate and command control of movement between these different workstations, resulting in manual intervention and traditional "sneaker-net" (physically carrying assets and information from one device to another).[16] In recent years, this has led to the development of both commercial and "home-grown" middleware software solutions to fill the gaps in functionality. These systems are designed to sit between the LIS and either the laboratory devices and its software applications, or enterprise software systems for which the laboratory needs to communicate information. Examples of these supplemental laboratory application modules, or SLAMS (coined by Dr Bruce Friedman) include the following: (1) Specimen-tracking, location, storage, retrieval, and discard systems to manage the specimen from the moment it is acquired in the clinical setting, arrives in the laboratory, and eventually gets discarded. The use of barcodes and radiofrequency ID tags along with real-time location systems makes this possible. (2) In-laboratory asset (eg, slides, trays, blocks, containers) comprehensive tracking and management systems also rely on the same technologies, in conjunction with quality manufacturing programs, such as LEAN and Six Sigma. (3) Image management and annotation systems using technologies such as machine vision and picture archiving and communication software. (4) Positive-patient/asset ID systems that leverage barcode-driven checking and confirmation for ensuring the right tissue, from the right patient, is being placed in the correctly labeled cassettes, from which the correct slides are manufactured. (5) Immunohistochemistry/specialized testing management and integration software to control the ordering of studies on different devices, particularly in multidevice environments. (6) Synoptic reporting for cancer protocol data collection. (7) Business analytics and data mining systems that use standard database technologies, natural language parsing for textual data, and rules engines for sophisticated decision support. (8) Billing system decision support to better detect duplicate billing, uncorrelated or undocumented ancillary procedures billing, automatic procedural diagnostic and procedural coding, and fee schedule errors. Other functional gaps that have yet to be developed include reliable and complete anatomic specimen remote electronic ordering with automatic specimen accessioning, rare-event error detection systems for both the manufacturing of assets and diagnostic workflows, real-time decision support systems for diagnosis, such as content-based image retrieval, and clinical/research biobanking workflow integration software. These are just a few examples, and the functional gaps are expected to increase with the advent of molecular testing of tissue specimens.

ANATOMIC PATHOLOGY AUTOMATION

Until recently, the anatomic pathology laboratory consisted of workstations where work processes relied on batch workflow, controlled by paper/clerical-based processes, which are inherently error-prone. The recent development of a framework for classifying errors in anatomic pathology has helped raise awareness of the types of errors that can exist in pathology, and is an essential step in developing error-reduction solutions, as well as representing excellent targets for automation solutions.[17] Whereas in the clinical pathology laboratory, the middleware, robotics, communication standards, and LIS s have coalesced to allow for what is commonly referred to as total laboratory automation, the anatomic pathology laboratory is still primarily focused on workstation or workcell automation. Only rare laboratories have attempted any kind of robotic specimen handling or distribution automation for specimens, tissue blocks, or glass slides. Although the anatomic laboratory still lacks interoperability standards for barcoding, labeling, or data formatting, significant automation has occurred throughout all phases of the testing cycle.

PREANALYTIC PHASE

Several aspects of the preanalytic phase of the testing cycle are amenable to automation. Specimen collection has been traditionally the purview of the clinician, although somewhat assisted by the laboratory by specifying handling, packaging, and data requirements. This was followed by in-

laboratory accessioning and order entry in the LISs. However, misidentification of specimens continues to plague this practice, which has prompted efforts to push remote order entry/clinician order entry with either automated or preaccessioning so that specimens arrive to the laboratory with an identification number that the LIS recognizes and/or generated. This eliminates transcription errors downstream from the patient into the laboratory systems. Along with positive-patient identification checking, and specimen real-time location systems that use barcode or radio frequency identification tags, this facilitates the intake of material to the anatomic laboratory. One challenge that limits total laboratory automation in the preanalytic phase is the need to manually confirm the actual tissue acquired and received is equivalent to the data that exist in the LIS. Future systems using machine vision and image analysis could possibly assist with this functional gap.

ANALYTICAL PHASE

Each of the different work centers in the anatomic pathology (histology) laboratory has been amendable to some automation. (**Table 4**) We briefly review each area of the laboratory.

GROSSING AUTOMATION

The act of grossing remains a laborious and meticulous process that is key to rendering accurate and complete diagnostic evaluations. Initial automation applications have included voice recognition and report production systems, positive specimen/cassette verification software to ensure the right tissue is placed in the right cassette, barcode-driven just-in-time block printing, and automated gross image capture. However, unlike the clinical laboratory, there is a lack of standardized specimens that arrive into the grossing laboratory.[18] One exception to this is the biopsy specimen, which usually consists of a single piece or multiple small portions of tissue, of somewhat characteristic form, such as a cylindrical core, punch, or wedge portion of tissue. As such, there is great potential for automating both the steps of grossing and cassette submission using robotics, machine vision applications, and image analysis. One proposed system would use specimen containers typically used for blood collections, hardware (track system, robotics) typically used in the clinical laboratory, "specimen tubes" with the same form factor as blood collection tubes, and tissue bags used for biopsy specimens: clinicians would place the acquired biopsy into a tissue bag, and then place

Table 4
Histology laboratory automation: workstations and examples

Work Center	Technology	Examples
Grossing	Grossing tools, sectionable cassettes	Accu-Edge Grossing Fork (Sakura), ProCut, CutMAte (Milestone), Tissue-Tek Paraform (Sakura)
Processing	Automatic processors	Peloris II (Leica), VIP6 (Sakura)
Processing	Microwave processors	LOGOS (Milestone), Tissue-Tek Express 120
Embedding	Automatic embedders	Synergy (Milestone), Tissue-Tek AutoTEC (Sakura)
Microtomy	Automatic microtomes	RM2265 (Leica), Tissue-Tek AutoSection (Sakura)
Mounting	Automatic slide mounter	PaceSetter (Aquaro Biosystem)
Microtomy and mounting	Robotic microtomy/slide mounting	AS-400 (Kurabo)
Staining	Automatic hematoxylin and eosin stainers	ST5010 (Leica) CoverStainer (Dako)
Coverslipping	Automatic coverslippers	Coverslipper (Dako) CV5030 (Leica)
Staining/ coverslipping	Robotic combined staining and coverslipping	Symphony (Roche), Tissue-Tek Prisma/Film (Sakura)
Histochemistry	Automatic histochemistry	ST5020 (Leica), Benchmark SpecialStain (Ventana/Roche)
Immunohistochemistry	Automatic immunohistochemistry devices	BOND-III (Leica), ULTRA (Ventana/Roche)
In situ hybridization	Automatic in situ hybridization	BOND-III (Leica), ULTRA (Ventana/Roche)
Scanning	High-throughput, high-speed whole-slide scanning	UFS (Philips), AT2 (Leica) NanoZoomer 2 (Hamamatsu)

Vendors: Sakura Finetek USA Inc, Torrance, CA; Leica Biosystems, Buffalo Grove, IL Milestone Inc, Shelton, CT; Aquaro Biosystems, Ann Arbor, MI; Kurabo, Osaka, Japan; Dako North America Inc, Carpinteria, CA; Philips Healthcare, Andover, MA; Hamamatsu, Shizuoka Pref, Japan; Roche Ventana, Tuscon, AR.

this into the "specimen" tube with formalin.[19] On arrival, these tubes could be placed on a track system for distribution to the grossing station where a barcode-driven workflow could initiate cassette printing, a robot would transfer the bag from the tube to the cassette, followed by cassette closure, cassette stacking, and loading into a basket for processing.[19] A second proposal hopes to automate the grossing of biopsies by using machine vision and image analysis: the specimen is inserted into the device, and an image is captured to facilitate specimen quantification, dimension detection, size measurement, color detection, and reporting of anomalous colors, resulting in a complete gross description. (Lyman Garniss, personal communication, August 2014).

SPECIMEN PROCESSING

Specimen processing involves the dehydration and clearing with infiltration of paraffin for sectioning. The process includes the use of hazardous chemicals and solutions. Over time, the process has gone from a laborious and time-consuming process, which took up to 28 hours and comprised almost 80% of the histology work time, to a fully automated process that averages 4 to 11 hours, depending on the tissue.[20] Since the introduction of the first automatic tissue processor, the Autotechnicon, in the 1940s, the devices have not only transformed processing by yielding reliable consistency and improved time reduction, improvements have focused primarily on infiltration and further time reductions.[20] More recently, the introduction of microwave-assisted tissue processing has further reduced this processing time to 1 to 2 hours, resulting in the ability for the first time to do same-day diagnosis, while producing slides with comparable histology, and histochemical and immunohistochemical properties to traditional methods.[21–24] This newer technology has the added benefit of eliminating traditional exposure to the hazardous chemicals associated with traditional processing.[25] Note, it is important to realize that the device itself must be coupled with workflow optimization, typically in small continuous batches of tissue cassettes, as tissue processing accounts for only a percentage of the total work process.[20,26,27]

TISSUE-EMBEDDING AUTOMATION

Tissue embedding has always been seen as the most critical step in ensuring proper orientation for sectioning of the tissue for examination. As such, it relies on information gathered during the grossing process and communicated based on how the specimen was sectioned, via markings on the cassette, inking of the specimen, grossing log notes, or slips of paper in the cassette. To automate embedding, a paradigm shift was required: block creation without any manual embedding at all.[28] The first commercial device to do this is the Sakura AutoTEC (Sakura Finetek USA, Inc. Torrance CA), which uses the Tissue-Tek Paraform sectionable cassette inserts with accompanying cassette frames. These flouropolymer sectionable cassette inserts survive tissue processing to be cut on the microtome. There are 6 varieties of inserts to accommodate a variety of tissues types and sizes.[29] The AutoTEC device is used to infiltrate the tissue with paraffin and prepare the tissue block for sectioning. Initial studies have shown that there may be slight increases in time required for grossing specimens and preparing the cassettes, and additional time required at microtomy for sectioning, but no overall increase in the number of blocks required to be submitted.[30]

MICROTOMY AUTOMATION

The rotary microtome is the universal histology laboratory device responsible for cutting the sections that get placed onto slides. If you exclude tissue processing, microtomy tasks, including trimming, sectioning, and mounting of slides on to slides, exhausts the preponderance of histotech time.[31,32] Although automated microtomes have existed for some time, they have been underused because experienced histotechnologists can operate the manual rotary microtomes with the same speed. In the past, block depth trimming and block alignment still required manual intervention. New devices, however, are now able to trim the block to the appropriate depth and precisely orient the block.

In reality, the advantages of microtomy automation can be realized only in combination with the mounting of the sections to the slides. A new device, the PaceSetter from Aquaro biosystems (Ann Arbor, MI, USA), automates the section mounting onto slides by using a hands-free process consisting of a gentle flowing fluid-filled track to catch the section, move the section onto a glass slide, and complete mounting of it on the slide.[33] This device can be connected essentially to any microtome, which allows for a low barrier to implementation. The most complete automation system for tissue block sectioning and slide mounting is the Kurabo AS-200s (Kurabo Industries LTD, Osaka, Japan), a robotic device that combines all of the steps and requires no manual intervention after blocks have been loaded into the device. A recent evaluation showed that the slide sections were comparable with manual or semi-automated sectioning, including difficult tissues like bone, and it shines in situations where multiple sections of the same block are required.[34] However, there were increases in cost related to embedding temperature, and a doubling of required time needed to section an equivalent number of blocks as humans, which makes implementation in the laboratory in its current configuration unlikely.[34]

STAINING AND COVERSLIPPING AUTOMATION

There are enumerable automated staining devices available that can be programmed to perform desired hematoxylin and eosin stains. Once stained, these slides can be transferred to automated coverslippers that apply either a glass or film coverslip. This automation paradigm so greatly facilitates these processes that it is almost impossible to justify doing these steps manually, with the exception of frozen sections in which there is increased urgency to interpret the sections, and there is increased difficulty to prevent sections from "slipping" off the glass during staining.[35] More recently, devices have been introduced that combine the 2 steps, allowing for input of unstained slides and an output of a stained and coverslip slide ready for review. These continuous-flow high-throughput devices allow for more effective workflow management and load balancing, enabling efficient scaling of output without increasing staffing while decreasing variability and errors.[14]

HISTOCHEMISTRY, IMMUNOHISTOCHEMISTRY, AND IN SITU HYBRIDIZATION AUTOMATION

Slide-based testing typically involves testing for specific proteins, although new technologies are allowing for DNA-based and RNA-based tests. Because histochemistry, immunohistochemistry, and in situ hybridization all localize tissue molecules at the microscopic level and comprise well-defined sequential steps at specific temperatures and time intervals, they are amenable to complete automation.[35] Ideally, integration with the LIS so as to automate order exchange and data exchange and eliminate relabeling events, enhances their impact on patient safety initiatives in the laboratory and yields greater efficiency.

SURGICAL PATHOLOGY SAMPLE PREPARATION AUTOMATION FOR MOLECULAR TESTING

Molecular testing typically requires tissue homogenates derived from surgical pathology material and assets. However, pathology specimens and tumors are complex mixtures of both normal and abnormal cell types, as well as supportive cells such as blood vessels, interstitial tissues, and inflammatory cells. To derive pure cell populations from tissue, newer automated platforms for microdissection have been introduced.

DIAGNOSTIC AUTOMATION AND DIGITAL PATHOLOGY

The case examination, workup, and diagnostic decision process has traditionally relied on nonautomated clerical methods, even though the workflow steps tend to be a data-intensive process, often requiring information from the medical record, radiology, and the clinical laboratory, as well the current pathology information. Movement of case worksheets, coordination of slides and slide folders, as well as transfers of this material have been manually performed and tracked in the past. Examples of diagnostic automation include in-laboratory physician order entry, voice recognition for automated report generation, synoptic reporting and data entry templates for discrete data capture and data reuse, and microscopic image capture for pathology report construction. At M.D. Anderson, a workflow integration engine called PathStation (developed by Department of Pathology, Section of Pathology Informatics) (**Fig. 3**) automates disparate information system access (ie, the medical record, the clinical LIS , the dictation system, and the image management application) and sets patient context in all of them to facilitate data aggregation and allow for barcode-driven workflow efficiencies, at the time of case evaluation. The rise of digital pathology is now enabling additional automation around image analysis and stain scoring, and mitoses counting for precise quantitation of markers and morphologic features. Digital pathology also can automate

difficult case expert consultation requests, real-time frozen section consultations, and distribution of case materials over geographically large areas.[36]

POSTANALYTICAL PHASE

The LIS traditionally has facilitated automated delivery of reports. The days of actually printing a report and mailing it to a clinician have evolved to automatic faxing of reports to clinicians, direct exchange of either feature-poor, text-based electronic reports or formatted feature-rich portable document formatted reports that limit data reuse, with their electronic medical records (EMRs) using HL7 interfaces, or laboratory-link software portals to distribute reports via the Web on an on-demand basis. The national initiatives (Office of the National Coordinator for Health Information Technology's meaningful use initiative) to incentivize adoption of EMRs by all clinicians will mandate automation of electronic transfer for most pathology reports in the near future. Our challenge is to address the functional gaps that currently exist that limit the ability of the pathology report to add value to the EMR. Examples include, but are not limited to, rules engine–based surgical pathology report analysis of report completeness and coding compliance, automated distribution of information and feature-rich formatted reports that still facilitate data reuse by our clinician customers, automated and robotic asset (block and slide) archival storage and retrieval management in the file room, and automation of pathology critical results notification with closed loop communications with the responsible clinicians in a manner similar to what currently exists for the clinical pathology laboratory.

TOTAL LABORATORY AUTOMATION AND SURGICAL PATHOLOGY

A definition of what could be considered total laboratory automation for anatomic pathology is yet to be clearly defined. Perhaps the minimum criteria might include an integrated workflow solution and tracking system that connects and communicates with workstation devices that exist across aspects of the preanalytic, analytical, and postanalytic phases of the surgical pathology workflow.[18] The core laboratory at BML Laboratories in Tokyo, Japan, represents the most comprehensive implementation of laboratory automation for surgical pathology, having automated nearly the complete workflow, including tissue acquisition, sample processing, and slide

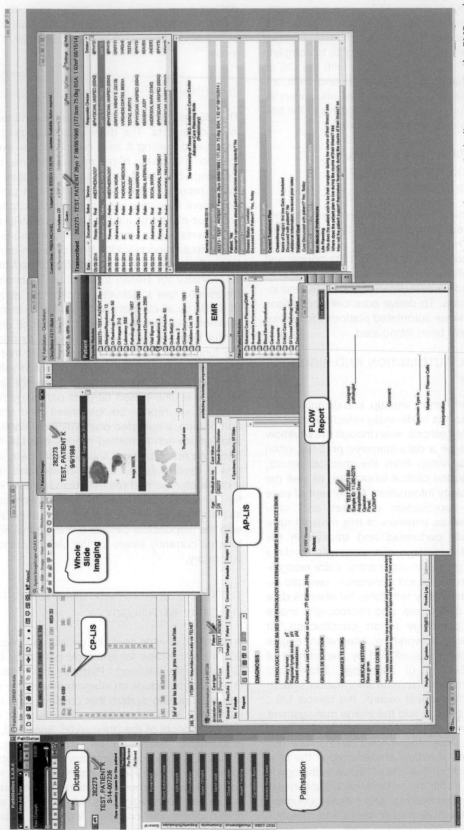

Fig. 3. Diagnostic sign-out automation. The PathStation integrates all of the key applications needed to evaluate and dictate the case, including access to the EMR and the image management application. AP-LIS, Anatomic Pathology Laboratory Information System; CP-LIS, Clinical Pathology Information System; EMR, Electronic Medical Record.

generation by using an integrated tracking system with advanced robotics.[14]

SUMMARY

Great strides have been made in automating the practice of surgical pathology. The drivers for these changes show no signs of decreasing, particularly in the unsettled economic environment affecting practices with health care reform and the accountable care act. Meeting that challenge involves developing innovative solutions for integrating existing and new workcell automation devices, creating middleware that targets functional gaps, applying tracking and robotics for material processing workflows, and creating usable standards that industry and pathologists can implement. Digital pathology, analytical diagnostic tools, data integration, decision support, and predictive analytics will greatly automate diagnostic evaluations and enhance reporting to the EMR, creating exponential value for patient care.

REFERENCES

1. Merriam-Webster Dictionary. Available at: http://www. merriam-webster.com/dictionary/automation. Accessed August 9, 2014.
2. Olsen K. The first 110 years of laboratory automation: technologies, applications, and the creative scientist. J Lab Autom 2012;17(6):469–80.
3. Nolen JD. The power of laboratory automation. MLO Med Lab Obs 2014;46(1):12–3. Available at: http://www.ncbi.nlm.nih.gov/pubmed/24527521.
4. Hoffmann GE. Concepts for the third generation of laboratory systems. Clin Chim Acta 1998;278(2):203–16. Available at: http://www.ncbi.nlm.nih.gov/pubmed/10023828.
5. The Relationship Between Employee Satisfaction and Hospital Patient Experiences. Cust News 2012. Available at: http://customercarenews.com/the-relationship-between-employee-satisfaction-and-hospital-patient-experiences/. Accessed June 9, 2014.
6. Buesa RJ. Histology aging workforce and what to do about it. Ann Diagn Pathol 2009;13(3):176–84.
7. Hawker CD, Schlank MR. Development of standards for laboratory automation. Clin Chem 2000;750:746–50.
8. Hawker C. Standards in lab automation:enabling plug and play. Adv Adm Lab 2006;15(9):20.
9. Clinical and Laboratory Standards Institute. Automation and informatics standards. CLSI Cat 2014. Available at: http://shop.clsi.org/automation-documents/. Accessed April 2, 2015.
10. Daniel C, García Rojo M, Bourquard K, et al. Standards to support information systems integration in anatomic pathology. Arch Pathol Lab Med 2009;133(11):1841–9.
11. Daniel C, Rojo MG, Klossa J, et al. Standardizing the use of whole slide images in digital pathology. Comput Med Imaging Graph 2011;35(7–8):496–505.
12. Middleware. Webopedia. Available at: http://www.webopedia.com/TERM/M/middleware.html. Accessed June 9, 2014.
13. What is Middleware. Middlew Resour Cent. Available at: http://web.archive.org/web/20120629211518/http://www.middleware.org/whatis.html. Accessed June 9, 2014.
14. Pantanowitz L, Balis U. Laboratory auatomation. In: Pantanowitz L, Tuthill JM, Balis UG, editors. Pathology informatics: theory and practice. 1st edition. Chicago: ASCP Press; 2012. p. 147–56.
15. Bagwell H. Redefining middleware: maximize your investment and increase quality. Med Lab Obs 2011;43(12):18–20.
16. Harten B. The middleware revolution: bridging automation gaps in laboratory processes. MLO Med Lab Obs 2012;44(2):35. Available at: http://search.ebscohost.com/login.aspx?direct=true&db=rzh&AN=2011459634&site=ehost-live.
17. Sirota RL. A framework for error in anatomic pathology. Pathol Case Rev 2009;14(2):53–6.
18. Paxton A. Seamless automation within in reach for AP? CAP Today 2014;1:44–50 59.
19. Sharma SG, Singh M. Automating grossing in anatomic pathology in pathology informatics 2012 abstracts. J Pathol Inform 2013;4:S46.
20. Buesa RJ. Microwave-assisted tissue processing: real impact on the histology workflow. Ann Diagn Pathol 2007;11(3):206–11.
21. Evaluation F, Pegolo E, Pandolfi M, et al. Implementation of a microwave-assisted tissue-processing system and an automated embedding system for breast needle core biopsy samples: morphology, immunohistochemistry, and FISH evaluation. Appl Immunohistochem Mol Morphol 2013;21(4):362–70.
22. Morales AR, Nadji M, Livingstone AS. Rapid-response, molecular-friendly surgical pathology: a radical departure from the century-old routine practice. J Am Coll Surg 2008;207(3):320–5.
23. Leong AS, Price D. Incorporation of microwave tissue processing into a routine pathology laboratory: impact on turnaround times and laboratory work patterns. Pathology 2004;36(4):321–4.
24. Morales AR, Nassiri M, Kanhoush R, et al. Experience with automated microwave-assisted rapid tissue processing: method validation of histologic quality and impact on the timeliness of diagnostic surgical pathology. Am J Clin Pathol 2004;121(4):528–36.
25. Smith T. Automating the art of histology. Adv Adm Lab 2006;15(9):34.

26. DeSalvo W. The pathology/histology automation must continue to further innovation. Adv Adm Lab 2010;19(12):8.

27. Felder RA. Automation meets anatomic pathology. Adv Adm Lab 2005;14(8):28.

28. Dimenstein I. From manual to automatic embedding in surgical pathology. Grossing Technol Surg Pathol. Available at: http://grossing-technology.com/newsite/home/perspectives-in-grossing-technology/from-manual-to-automatic-embedding-in-surgical-pathology/. Accessed June 9, 2014.

29. Dimenstein IB. Sectionable cassette for embedding automation in surgical pathology. Ann Diagn Pathol 2010;14(2):100–6.

30. Phelan SM. Impact of the introduction of a novel automated embedding system on quality in a university hospital histopathology department. J Histol Histopathol 2014;1(1):3.

31. Cuddihy MJ, Garrity AG. Automation in the histology lab. 2014. Available at: http://aquarobio.com/white-papers/.

32. Buesa RJ. Productivity standards for histology laboratories. Ann Diagn Pathol 2010;14(2):107–24.

33. What is the PaceSetter. Available at: http://aquarobio.com/pacesetter/. Accessed September 9, 2014.

34. Onozato ML, Hammond S, Merren M, et al. Evaluation of a completely automated tissue-sectioning machine for paraffin blocks. J Clin Pathol 2013;66(2):151–4. Available at: http://ovidsp.ovid.com/ovidweb.cgi?T=JS&PAGE=reference&D=medl&NEWS=N&AN=21900334.

35. Morales A, Nassiri M. Automation of the histology laboratory. Lab Med 2007;38(7):405–10.

36. Lynn K. Digital pathology and imaging: past, present and future. Med Lab Obs 2011;43(3):40–1.

Molecular Pathology Informatics

Somak Roy, MD

KEYWORDS

- Molecular informatics • Next-generation sequencing • Clinical informatics • Bioinformatics

ABSTRACT

Molecular informatics (MI) is an evolving discipline that will support the dynamic landscape of molecular pathology and personalized medicine. MI provides a fertile ground for development of clinical solutions to bridge the gap between clinical informatics and bioinformatics. Rapid adoption of next generation sequencing (NGS) in the clinical arena has triggered major endeavors in MI that are expected to bring a paradigm shift in the practice of pathology. This brief review presents a broad overview of various aspects of MI, particularly in the context of NGS based testing.

OVERVIEW

Molecular pathology has emerged as a major arsenal for promoting and sustaining personalized health care in modern medicine. In contrast to other ancillary diagnostic tools, molecular pathology delivers a wide spectrum of theranostic information starting from as little as a minute fragment of tissue or a simple blood draw. The results of molecular testing are significantly more complex than a simple numerical value or a binary outcome (yes/no). The post–Human Genome Project era has witnessed the most significant developments in genomics that has impacted the way clinical medicine is practiced today. Personalized medicine, which enables patient-specific therapeutic and disease management protocols, is being increasingly boosted and supported by the results of molecular testing performed on tissue biopsies and resections. In addition, it also serves as a valuable diagnostic tool in morphologically challenging cases. Genomic profiling of certain cancers, such as lung, colon, and melanoma, are now considered to be the standard of care for guiding appropriate treatment protocols. Very recently, a global molecular testing guideline was published for molecular testing of lung cancers by the collaborative efforts of College of American Pathologists, International Association for the Study of Lung Cancer, and Association for Molecular Pathology.[1] The Cancer Genome Atlas project (http://cancergenome.nih.gov/) over the past few years has released a wealth of genomic profiling information about major tumor types that had significantly fueled the discovery of potential actionable biomarkers for routine clinical use.[2–8]

A wide array of assay methodologies and platforms are used in laboratories for performing molecular testing, such as Sanger sequencing, real-time polymerase chain reaction (PCR), allele-specific PCR, DNA and RNA in situ hybridization (ISH), multiplex ligation-dependent probe amplification, microarray technology, and, more recently, next-generation sequencing (NGS) technology. The choice of platform depends on the question(s) answered by the clinical test and its appropriate applicability to patient care.

MOLECULAR INFORMATICS

Given the increasing popularity and relevance of high-complexity molecular testing in surgical pathology, where does informatics fit into the equation? To answer this question, it is important to understand the major operational domains of informatics, namely bioinformatics (BI) and clinical informatics (CI). Bioinformatics is a dynamic and rapidly evolving multidisciplinary field of informatics that has emerged out of the application of computational, mathematical, and statistical methods to investigate biological phenomena. BI dates back to as early as the 1960s, when fundamental

Department of Pathology, Molecular and Genomic Pathology, University of Pittsburgh Medical Center, 3477 Euler way, Pittsburgh, PA 15213, USA
E-mail address: roys@upmc.edu

Surgical Pathology 8 (2015) 187–194
http://dx.doi.org/10.1016/j.path.2015.02.013
1875-9181/15/$ – see front matter © 2015 Elsevier Inc. All rights reserved.

discoveries in molecular biology were made. With more recent data deluge and development of massive repositories of biological and genomic data, the symbiotic relationship between molecular biology and BI has fueled mutual exponential growth.[9–11] Large and complex data (so-called big data), data-driven analytics, statistical modeling, development of new algorithms, and discovering meaningful and relevant information from raw biological data is inherent to BI.[10] In contrast, CI is a more established discipline that has developed and matured over a longer period of time with rigorous testing and validation in a clinical environment. CI implementations in health care systems are typically on an enterprise scale, using industry standard software and hardware with principal focus on secure and reliable data transmission, storage, retrieval, and interoperability between information systems and wide variety of medical devices rather than data-driven analytics and discovery. One of the key differences between BI and CI is application development environment and life cycle, which gives rise to several other differences between the two disciplines. Application development in BI is centered on a fundamental genomic or biological phenomenon that is under investigation in a given research project. The pace of design, testing, implementation, and troubleshooting (software patches) is typically coupled with the progress of the research project. If a BI application is successful and is usable across a wider user community, further improvement and maintenance is supported by open-source software development. The overall life cycle is fast paced but with variable support, documentation, and version control. CI applications (such as electronic medical record [EMR], laboratory information system [LIS]), in contrast, have a much tighter and longer development and implementation life cycle. Vendors usually provide formal application support, tight version control, and extensive documentation. Updates for feature enhancements and patches for troubleshooting are relatively infrequent and often expensive.

This conceptual distinction has existed for several years in clinical laboratories with minimal interactions between the two disciplines. With conventional molecular testing instrumentation, vendors were able to mask the complexity of underlying BI with a point-and-click user interface. However, with the speedy introduction of NGS testing in clinical laboratories, molecular pathology has finally broken this barrier, forming a unique collaborative environment for development of informatics solutions that bridge the gap between BI and CI. The term molecular informatics (MI) is often loosely used to refer to various informatics principles and operations in a molecular laboratory. The rapid advance in this domain during a short period of time has manifested its presence in the practice of molecular pathology.

Conceptually, MI forms the core conduit for generating, processing, porting, and management of the molecular data points from each step of every assay performed in the molecular laboratory. With increasing sophistication of the assay platform and workflow elements, the magnitude and complexity of the generated information increases exponentially. Surprisingly, MI has largely been an unrealized and neglected part of laboratory workflow, until the introduction of NGS technology in clinical laboratories.

Even a basic quantitative PCR instrument performs significant computation for generating and displaying results that the user is typically unaware of. The practice of conventional molecular laboratories has been centered on paper-based manual data management for targeted analysis and low complexity testing for several years. However, the colossal data surge as a result of NGS based testing breaks the capacity of this conventional system. As a consequence, the critical role of MI has been realized on a global scale, initiating several large-scale efforts across different organizations to develop principles and guidelines for developing information systems that can appropriately manage, present, and share molecular data.[12–15] Although MI encompasses a wide range of functions across the entire workflow for different testing platforms in the molecular laboratory, because of the limited scope of this article, only a broad overview of the different aspects of MI that pertains mostly to NGS testing is presented to the readers, given its significant impact and clinical relevance.

NEXT-GENERATION SEQUENCING

After the invention of Sanger sequencing in 1977[16] and PCR in 1985,[17] several important technological developments were witnessed that improved the practice of molecular pathology significantly. However, NGS has been a revolutionary change that has not only transformed the concepts and practice of molecular pathology testing but also affected the paradigm of disease management in clinical medicine and oncology. NGS enables very large-scale measurements of the genome, yielding an unprecedented amount of potentially valuable information.[18] This is unlike any other conventional molecular testing technology that has been in existence. For example, to perform a complete molecular profiling of a lung adenocarcinoma using conventional methods, DNA sequence variations (mutations) are detected using Sanger sequencing, real-time PCR, and other modalities. Gene fusions and copy number changes are detected using ISH technologies. Gene expression, if indicated, is typically detected using reverse-transcriptase PCR coupled with quantitative real-time PCR. Information on gene methylation, such as *MGMT* and *MLH1*, is obtained by methylation-specific PCR. In contrast, all of this testing can be performed using NGS on a single platform.

NGS testing can not only to detect sequence variations, but also gene fusions, copy number changes, gene expression, methylation profile, and large structural alterations from a single run on a single platform, making it a very efficient technology in clinical medicine. The high capacity of NGS sequencers allows multiplexing of several patient samples on a single run in a cost-effective way using DNA barcodes.[13,19] The underlying massively parallel sequencing of millions to billions of DNA fragments and subsequent preservation of information on every individual sequencing reads leverages extracting such a wide repertoire of genomic information.[18] The sequence reads can be manipulated and measured using diverse algorithms to derive the appropriate information.

Not surprisingly therefore, the scope for clinical application of NGS testing is expansive to include pharmacogenomics, somatic tumor profiling, minimal residual disease monitoring, and inherited diseases testing. Clinical NGS testing has been most applicable (and somewhat economically viable) to somatic profiling of solid and hematologic tumors using targeted resequencing of regions or genes of interest.[20–23] NGS-based molecular testing in surgical pathology has unraveled the next level of diagnostic and therapeutic stratification that is highly relevant for targeted therapy, subsequent management, and follow-up of patients. Cytology and tissue biopsies are a critical triage point for rendering an immediate diagnosis and subsequent submission of appropriate tissue for molecular testing.

NEXT-GENERATION SEQUENCING INFORMATICS

As mentioned briefly in the preceding section, discrete preservation of sequencing reads is a critical aspect of NGS technology that leverages a wealth of information about the interrogated genome. NGS data processing involves several sequential steps that are performed by different software applications in tandem, which is commonly referred to as a "pipeline." **Fig. 1** illustrates a simplified version of an NGS pipeline.

Depending on the NGS platform used, the raw sequencing data are represented as a high-definition image file or as electrical signal trace with embedded features.[18] This information is unusable for detecting abnormalities in the genome as is, and therefore requires further processing to generate sequence information in a more appropriate format for consumption by downstream processes. This is also referred to as primary data processing and involves signal processing to generate raw sequence reads and subsequent alignment to the reference genome. An important feature to note is the magnitude and complexity of the data generated by a typical NGS instrument. The size of an individual sequencing file is roughly proportional to the number of sequencing reads contained in them and range in size from approximately 0.2 GB to 200 GB, depending on the scope of genomic measurements performed. During a pipeline execution, several intermediate files of significant magnitude also are generated that contribute to the total bulk of NGS data. The standard processes in an analytical pipeline, such as sequence alignment and variant detection on aligned sequence reads, are resource hungry. Multiple CPU cores and large amounts of Random Access Memory in a high-performance desktop workstation or a compute cluster environment are prerequisites. In terms of software, most of these analytical pipelines are optimized to run on a Unix or Linux operating system (OS).[24]

Subsequent to the primary data analysis of NGS data, secondary and tertiary downstream analyses are essential components of the global analytical pipeline in a clinical laboratory environment. The secondary analysis involves detection of variants (genomic alterations) using different algorithms (see **Fig. 1**). Tertiary analyses involve variant annotation, filtering, prioritization, variant and other public database lookups, data visualization tools, literature review, and knowledge-based management. These analytical steps can be performed by a combination of a wide variety of software, many of which are in active development and require constant support and improvement by the developer.[24] From a laboratory management standpoint, it is critical to understand the need for validating software pipelines in general to ensure highly accurate and reliable molecular test results due to their significant impact on therapeutic management.[12]

BIG DATA AND CLOUD COMPUTING

With increasing use of NGS and constant improvement in software algorithms, data processing and generation is voluminous but faster

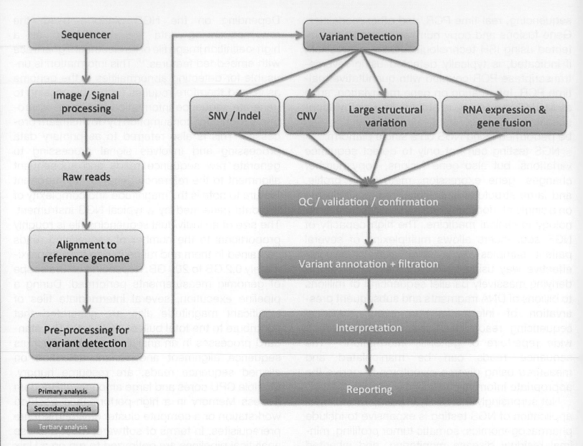

Fig. 1. A simplified workflow for NGS data analysis, regardless of the type of sequencing technology used. The workflow is broadly categorized into primary (*orange*), secondary (*purple*), and tertiary (*blue*) analysis steps. A wide repertoire of software applications can perform the individual steps in the workflow. It is important to note that for accuracy of clinical test results, each of the components of the analytical pipeline should be appropriately optimized and validated. CNV, copy number variation; QC, quality control; SNV, single nucleotide variant.

and more productive. This has led to rapid accumulation of datasets that are of astronomical scale (typically several terabytes to petabytes) that defy the conventional computational capacity for processing and storage. Data with this property is commonly referred to as big data. The concept of big data is relatively recent and there exists no widely accepted threshold or definition, as "big" is quite relative. The National Institute of Standards and Technology and other major enterprises, such as Google, Oracle, and Microsoft, have proposed their own definitions of big data.[25] Terabytes of data may not be "big" for an organization with access to enterprise data centers or a cloud computing environment, but may be "big" for organizations with a small to medium-scale information technology (IT) infrastructure. Big data existed in health care systems even before its true realization in the post-genome era. Rapid introduction of NGS testing has led to confrontation with many challenges in

implementation, but in parallel has also initiated innovation on a global scale to improve health care IT infrastructure to support genomics-driven personalized health care.[26,27] The 4 V's that define the elements of big data from a digital marketing perspective are velocity, volume, variety, and veracity.[28] NGS testing generates large amounts of data in a short period of time that contains a wide variety of information, which is often unpredictable at the initiation of testing and therefore confirms to the 4 elements of big data. Handling "big" genomic data and integrating with clinical data points in LISs and EMRs is an enormous task that will require significant collaboration among various stakeholders in health care.[26,28] The benefit of big data analytics is the power to predict clinical outcomes based on insight into archived clinical data in LISs and EMRs.[26] As NGS testing continues in health care, archived data will be enriched with genomic information, which when subjected to big data analytics will reveal potentially highly relevant information for cost-effective clinical decision-making. Such data-driven clinical decision support systems are under active research and development.

Intertwined with big data analytics is the concept of cloud computing. Cloud computing hosts a wide variety of functions, which are rendered as services to consumers for storing and processing data. Because hardware and software infrastructure is instantly scalable (up or down) based on the needs of the end user, it is a valuable and cost-effective resource for storing large data sets and performing complex data analysis. Cloud computing provides an ideal environment for data analytical requirements for NGS testing.[29–31] Laboratories do not require large capital investment on setting up and maintaining hardware and software infrastructure and still reap the benefits at a relatively low cost. Maintenance functions, such as data backup, redundancy generation, data security, and troubleshooting without downtime, are typically inclusive in the subscription fee.[31]

INFORMATICS CHALLENGES FOR NEXT-GENERATION SEQUENCING–BASED CLINICAL TESTING

Despite the various advantages of NGS testing, big data and cloud computing in molecular pathology, the real-world implementation of NGS poses several informatics challenges and concerns. The principal bottlenecks are centered on genomic data management, data security, and systems interoperability. There may be additional informatics challenges that are specific to an organization's local circumstances and therefore not included in this discussion.

DATA STORAGE

NGS instruments generate a tremendous volume of data per sample per run. The magnitude scales are proportional to the scope of genomic measurements (targeted sequencing, whole exome, whole genome).[18] Data storage in external hard disk drives is not practical or reliable. It is recommended that clinical genomic data be backed up automatically into a secure off-site storage facility (such a disaster recovery center) with enough redundancy to allow minimum downtime for data recovery after a catastrophic event. Data storage should also allow use of alternate analytical pipelines on the archived data for validation and development. Thankfully, the cost per MB of data has dramatically decreased to sustain increasing storage requirements.[31] However, the initial capital investment to

set up or use large-scale data backup facilities may be prohibitive depending on the institution's existing IT infrastructure. Given the increasing adaptation of high-throughput sequencing platforms in clinical laboratories, appropriate forecasting and budgeting of computing resource requirements is critical to avoid unexpected downtime in clinical testing. Unplanned data management also may increase the cost of storage (eg, storing raw sequencing data indefinitely). It is therefore important for molecular laboratories to set up reasonable retention policies for high-volume data. Unfortunately, there are no recommendations or guidelines available as of date that can be used by clinical laboratories, which adds to the complexity for forecasting resources.

NETWORKING INFRASTRUCTURE

One of the critical elements of handling NGS data, that is often overlooked until confronted with, is appropriate network connectivity for moving NGS datasets. It is an integral component of data archiving, data sharing across multiple users, and reusing the primary data for alternative analysis. A typical 10/100 Mbps local area network infrastructure that exists by default in most institutions cannot support the movement of massive NGS datasets and often affects other critical network-dependent hospital operations, such as EMR and LIS transactions. It is therefore imperative to include appropriate network requirements as part of the discussion with the IT team when implementing NGS in clinical laboratories.

COMPUTING INFRASTRUCTURE

As described previously, NGS data processing is resource intensive. That being said, the actual requirements are highly variable depending on the sequencing platform used and the scope of measurements desired. Constant improvements in algorithms for NGS data processing have allowed optimized use of memory and CPU cores allowing high-throughput analysis on desktop workstations. Although such a setup is not ideal in a production (clinical) environment for several reasons, including limited room for scaling up, it is often the most immediately practical and affordable solution. More appropriate and long-term solutions require setting up high-performance compute cluster or distributed compute grid with the flexibility of scaling up or down based on the laboratory's requirement.[28,31] This however requires technical expertise, involvement of the institution's IT group, and significant capital investment. The final decision for a given institution requires striking a balance and involvement of a multidisciplinary team of molecular pathologists, pathology informatics, bioinformaticians, and clinical IT personnel.

DATA SECURITY

Cloud computing provides the "next-generation" environment for cost-effective data analytics and management. Cloud computing environments are broadly classified into private (institutional), public, and hybrid depending on the access profile and relationship to an institution's firewall.[28,32] Public clouds are maintained by large commercial companies, which offer a wide variety of computing services without significant upfront capital investment. However, the principal concern in use of public clouds for health care data is data privacy and compliance with appropriate federal and institutional regulation.[32] Breach of hospital-managed clinical data is detrimental to its clients (patients), as well as the reputation of the institution itself. The clinical laboratory community with the current state of cloud computing is hesitant to use such services, despite all the technical and economic advantages. This is a domain of active development and there is drive toward appropriate auditing of public cloud services to ensure compliance with health care data privacy laws, albeit with the possibility of increase in associated cost of such services.[32]

Institutional cloud (private) setup is more attractive from a clinical laboratory perspective because it provides all the advantages of cloud computing but in a highly secure environment where the clinical data stays behind the firewall. The major limitation in implementing a private cloud is the significant capital, manpower, and infrastructure investment that may not be practical for many if not all organizations.

Privacy concerns surrounding genomic data in health care have been a matter of active discussion and fueled more recently by clinical NGS testing. The Health Insurance Portability and Accountability Act (HIPAA), enacted in 1996, enforces the adoption of privacy protection modalities by the federal government across all entities that hold protected health information (PHI).[33] There has been subsequent modification to HIPAA and enactment of additional laws (HITECH, 2009) and the Patient Protection and Affordable Care Act (ACA, 2010) to strengthen PHI security. With the adoption of new rules for privacy, security, and breach notification, in the final "HIPAA Omnibus Rule" (2013), genomic information has been designated as PHI.[34] This significantly impacts the storage and management of large-scale genomic information in clinical laboratories, including options for using cloud-based services.

INTEROPERABILITY

A typical molecular pathology laboratory houses different analytical instruments that generate data and require some form of integration with existing informatics resource pool within the laboratory (custom database, Excel spreadsheets, LIS, shared pool for data storage). Unlike conventional molecular analytical instruments, NGS instruments allow network connectivity for bidirectional data transfer and sequence data archiving. However, NGS instruments by default do not support messaging protocols to interoperate between other CI systems or software. Additionally, significant technical challenges arise when interoperating NGS instruments that run on a UNIX-based OS with a hospital informatics infrastructure that typically runs on a Windows-based OS. IT support for a UNIX-based system may often be a significant bottleneck in deploying and maintaining NGS instruments. This necessitates development of middleware solutions to optimize NGS operations. Due to the substantial learning curve associated with establishing common grounds with the 2 disciplines, it is critical for molecular laboratories to involve bioinformaticians in active clinical NGS operations to foster collaborative development with CI.

Downstream (tertiary) NGS data analytics pose additional interoperability challenges. There are several applications (freeware, proprietary and custom developed) that are available or are in constant development to facilitate downstream data analysis, including interoperability with existing clinical systems using standard messaging protocols.

FUTURE PERSPECTIVE

Massively parallel sequencing technology has significantly impacted the traditional practice of clinical medicine and has led to a paradigm change in diagnostic and therapeutic principles of various diseases. Despite the promising outcomes of using NGS-based clinical testing, some of the critical bottlenecks (described previously), as well as the general constraining economic and regulatory environment, threatens full-scale implementation in clinical laboratories. Implementing NGS assays not only requires capital investment for purchase of appropriate hardware and reagents but also demands significant investment in acquiring skilled technical personnel, bioinformaticians, full-time employees for managing billing and customer service relationships, and a strong informatics infrastructure that is flexible enough to scale on demand and bridge the gap between BI and CI and support laboratory operations. Interestingly enough, despite these perplexing challenges, there is an increasing trend in adopting NGS testing across clinical laboratories. As NGS technology is maturing in the clinical domain, MI is going to play a key role in setting a stable ground.

REFERENCES

1. Lindeman NI, Cagle PT, Beasley MB, et al. Molecular testing guideline for selection of lung cancer patients for EGFR and ALK tyrosine kinase inhibitors: guideline from the College of American Pathologists, International Association for the Study of Lung Cancer, and Association for Molecular Pathology. J Mol Diagn 2013;15:415–53.
2. Cancer Genome Atlas Research Network. Comprehensive molecular profiling of lung adenocarcinoma. Nature 2014;511:543–50.
3. Cancer Genome Atlas Research Network. Comprehensive molecular characterization of gastric adenocarcinoma. Nature 2014;513:202–9.
4. Cancer Genome Atlas Research Network. Comprehensive molecular characterization of urothelial bladder carcinoma. Nature 2014;507:315–22.
5. Cancer Genome Atlas Research Network, Kandoth C, Schultz N, et al. Integrated genomic characterization of endometrial carcinoma. Nature 2013;497:67–73.
6. Cancer Genome Atlas Research Network, Weinstein JN, Collisson EA, et al. The Cancer Genome Atlas Pan-Cancer analysis project. Nat Genet 2013;45:1113–20.
7. Davis CF, Ricketts CJ, Wang M, et al. The somatic genomic landscape of chromophobe renal cell carcinoma. Cancer Cell 2014;26:319–30.
8. Hoadley KA, Yau C, Wolf DM, et al. Multiplatform analysis of 12 cancer types reveals molecular classification within and across tissues of origin. Cell 2014; 158:929–44.
9. Pantanowitz L, Tuthill JM, Balis UGJ. Pathology Informatics: Theory and Practice. Canada: ASCP Press; 2012.
10. Hogeweg P. The roots of bioinformatics in theoretical biology. PLoS Comput Biol 2011;7:e1002021.
11. Yu U, Lee SH, Kim YJ, et al. Bioinformatics in the postgenome era. J Biochem Mol Biol 2004;37:75–82.
12. Gargis AS, Kalman L, Berry MW, et al. Assuring the quality of next-generation sequencing in clinical laboratory practice. Nat Biotechnol 2012;30:1033–6.
13. Rehm HL, Bale SJ, Bayrak-Toydemir P, et al. ACMG clinical laboratory standards for next-generation sequencing. Genet Med 2013;15:733–47.
14. Mattocks CJ, Morris MA, Matthijs G, et al. A standardized framework for the validation and verification of clinical molecular genetic tests. Eur J Hum Genet 2010;18:1276–88.
15. Praxton A. CAP leads way with next-gen checklist. CAP Today 2012.
16. Sanger F, Nicklen S, Coulson AR. DNA sequencing with chain-terminating inhibitors. Proc Natl Acad Sci U S A 1977;74:5463–7.
17. Mullis KB, Faloona FA. Specific synthesis of DNA in vitro via a polymerase-catalyzed chain reaction. Methods Enzymol 1987;155:335–50.
18. Mardis ER. Next-generation sequencing platforms. Annu Rev Anal Chem (Palo Alto Calif) 2013;6:287–303.
19. Xuan J, Yu Y, Qing T, et al. Next-generation sequencing in the clinic: promises and challenges. Cancer Lett 2013;340:284–95.
20. Cottrell CE, Al-Kateb H, Bredemeyer AJ, et al. Validation of a next-generation sequencing assay for clinical molecular oncology. J Mol Diagn 2014;16:89–105.
21. Nikiforov YE, Carty SE, Chiosea SI, et al. Highly accurate diagnosis of cancer in thyroid nodules with follicular neoplasm/suspicious for a follicular neoplasm cytology by ThyroSeq v2 next-generation sequencing assay. Cancer 2014;120(23):3627–34.
22. Pritchard CC, Salipante SJ, Koehler K, et al. Validation and implementation of targeted capture and sequencing for the detection of actionable mutation, copy number variation, and gene rearrangement in clinical cancer specimens. J Mol Diagn 2014;16:56–67.
23. Singh RR, Patel KP, Routbort MJ, et al. Clinical validation of a next-generation sequencing screen for mutational hotspots in 46 cancer-related genes. J Mol Diagn 2013;15:607–22.
24. Pabinger S, Dander A, Fischer M, et al. A survey of tools for variant analysis of next-generation genome sequencing data. Brief Bioinform 2014;15:256–78.
25. Ward JS, Barker A. Undefined by data: a survey of big data definitions. ArXiv e-prints; 2013. Available at: http://arxiv.org/abs/1309.5821. Accessed October 9, 2014.
26. Schneeweiss S. Learning from big health care data. N Engl J Med 2014;370:2161–3.
27. Miriovsky BJ, Shulman LN, Abernethy AP. Importance of health information technology, electronic health records, and continuously aggregating data to comparative effectiveness research and learning health care. J Clin Oncol 2012;30:4243–8.
28. Merelli I, Perez-Sanchez H, Gesing S, et al. Managing, analysing, and integrating big data in medical bioinformatics: open problems and future perspectives. Biomed Res Int 2014;2014:134023.
29. Grossman RL, White KP. A vision for a biomedical cloud. J Intern Med 2012;271:122–30.
30. Heath AP, Greenway M, Powell R, et al. Bionimbus: a cloud for managing, analyzing and sharing large genomics datasets. J Am Med Inform Assoc 2014; 21(6):969–75.
31. Stein LD. The case for cloud computing in genome informatics. Genome Biol 2010;11:207.

32. Dove ES, Joly Y, Tasse AM, et al. Genomic cloud computing: legal and ethical points to consider. Eur J Hum Genet 2014. [Epub ahead of print].

33. U.S. Department of Health and Human Services: Health Information Privacy Rule. Available at: http://www.hhs.gov/ocr/privacy/hipaa/administrative/privacyrule/. Accessed October 9, 2014.

34. Modifications to the HIPAA Privacy, Security, Enforcement, and Breach Notification rules under the Health Information Technology for Economic and Clinical Health Act and the Genetic Information Nondiscrimination Act; other modifications to the HIPAA rules. Fed Regist 2013; 78:5565–702.

Pathology Gross Photography
The Beginning of Digital Pathology

B. Alan Rampy, DO, PhD[a], Eric F. Glassy, MD[b],*

KEYWORDS

- Gross photography • Digital pathology • Electronic medical record • Diagnostic report
- Anatomic pathology

ABSTRACT

The underutilized practice of photographing anatomic pathology specimens from surgical pathology and autopsies is an invaluable benefit to patients, clinicians, pathologists, and students. Photographic documentation of clinical specimens is essential for the effective practice of pathology. When considering what specimens to photograph, all grossly evident pathology, absent yet expected pathologic features, and gross-only specimens should be thoroughly documented. Specimen preparation prior to photography includes proper lighting and background, wiping surfaces of blood, removing material such as tubes or bandages, orienting the specimen in a logical fashion, framing the specimen to fill the screen, positioning of probes, and using the right-sized scale.

OVERVIEW: SETTING THE STAGE

Today, digital pathology equates to whole-slide imaging (WSI). But before high-priced scanners and computer-assisted diagnoses, there were static images of microscopic slides and gross surgical pathology specimens. This is where digital pathology started. Photomicrography has given way to WSI but capturing and documenting gross surgical pathology specimens is just as important and, the authors argue, a key component of the pathology report and the electronic medical record.

AP is a visual discipline and photographic documentation of clinical specimens is an essential element of the effective practice of pathology. Because photography is not a fundamental subject of medical training, pathology residents most often have little experience with photography as it applies to the AP setting. Moreover, whereas there seems to be broad consensus that basic digital gross pathology competency should be considered a requisite component of pathology education[1] and is accordingly included in the list of training objectives and residency handbooks of most major residency programs, available learning resources are scant. Of the publications with regard to gross pathology photography, most address the logistics of image acquisition, transfer, and storage or the relative benefits of select hardware/software advances.[2–6] As such, only a few articles serve as essential guides to understanding the importance of hands-on strategies and techniques for quality gross photography.[7–10] The aim of this article is to describe informally, through a variety of examples, many of the important concepts that underlie quality gross pathology photography.

GROSS PHOTOS IN PRACTICE

Quality gross specimen photographs are a fundamental element of AP practice. Such images not only are part of patient medical records but also are often reviewed at conferences, used as educational material, and integrated into professional publications. The value of thoughtful, complete, and first-rate image support cannot be overstated. Photos obtained by a prosector assigned to a

Disclosures: Dr B.A. Rampy: Medical Advisory Board: Xifin, Inc; Dr E.F. Glassy: Consultant: Leica Biosystems, PersonalizeDx; Advisory Board: Definiens; and Minority cOwnership: Pathology, Inc (reference laboratory).
a Department of Pathology, University of Texas Medical Branch, 301 University Boulevard, Mail Route 0747, Galveston, TX 77555-0747, USA; b Affiliated Pathologists Medical Group, 19951 Mariner Avenue #155, Torrance, CA 90503, USA
* Corresponding author.
E-mail address: efglassymd@affiliatedpath.com

Surgical Pathology 8 (2015) 195–211
http://dx.doi.org/10.1016/j.path.2015.02.005

surgpath.theclinics.com

particular case are often the only permanent record of specimen features and associated anatomic landmarks, prior to histopathologic sampling. As pathology practices merge and cases are handed off to others at sign-out, the need for visual documentation of complicated surgical specimens becomes even more critical. A related benefit of gross photography may be realized at microscopic examination, whereupon photographic review may be used to map sites of histologic sections. In addition to multidisciplinary review of digital pathology WSI at tumor board conferences in select institutions, it is expected that relevant gross pathology photographs will be available for assessment as well. Pathology practice is also part of the broad realm of patient-centered care, health information sharing, and electronic medical records, and, with ever increasing frequency, pathology gross photography is considered for integration into AP laboratory information systems, electronic medical records, and pathology diagnostic reports.[11] This guide for gross pathology imaging would not be complete without mention of the critical importance of associated specimen/patient information. Just as many experienced pathologists have desk drawers full of 35-mm photographic slides identified only by a specimen accession number, quality digital gross images are only of value if they are stored and archived along with appropriate metadata. Given these considerations, along with thoughtful attention to optimized patient care, clinical concerns, and associated educational opportunities, any pathology laboratory may establish a standard of excellence for gross specimen photography.

THE DECISION TO SHOOT

Not every gross specimen needs to be photographed. A good guideline to determine whether a specimen should be photographed is simple—all grossly evident pathology should be documented. Following this basic rule, if and when a clinical request for gross presentation of a particular specimen is received, the relevant pathology images may be reliably and readily provided. But that is not quite all. The photos should be taken to best show any and all associated disease processes, and the photos should be aimed to address all relevant clinical questions and concerns. Additionally, all grossly absent yet expected pathologic features should be documented in the photo records. Moreover, when the issue may be of particular clinical importance, photos should document the appearance of the specimen as it was received in pathology, before any further

manipulations have taken place. For clarity, it is generally a good idea to orient a series of photographs of the same specimen in the same way. Consider photographing specimens that have sutures or other surgical markings in a manner that corresponds to the description, such as "short suture superior" at the top of the photo. Each set of images should tell a story, so that the final composite leads to a conclusion.

Because gross-only specimens, by definition, have no tissue submitted for histology, and hence no associated histologic diagnosis, complete quality photo documentation is imperative. This means that gross-only specimens should be photographed from all perspectives and all clinically relevant details should be included. Explanted medical devices, such as breast implants, intrauterine devices, and catheters, are a special subset of gross-only specimens and should be treated as such. These devices should be examined thoroughly and additional photos should document all identifying features like brand name and serial number as well as any probable sites of defect. As with medical devices, any specimens that, based on clinical history, likely will have medicolegal action should be documented thoroughly. They should be photographed from all perspectives, with attention to any clinically relevant details. If the specimen is patient derived and associated with trauma, thoroughly document associated pathologic changes, which may include such features as hemorrhage, lacerations, and so forth as well as any foreign material present (bullets, grass, gravel, and the like). Last but certainly not least, thoroughly document all unusual or rare specimens with photos from all perspectives, and be certain to include characteristic features of the pathology involved, because these shots may serve as valuable material for students, pathologists in training, and clinicians.

Although a vermiform appendix is most often considered a simple and routine surgical specimen, photos should document the associated grossly evident pathology. As shown in **Fig. 1**, with markedly congested vessels along the serosa and a tan to olive-green suppurative exudate, this gross image readily supports the diagnosis of acute gangrenous appendicitis and periappendicitis. **Fig. 2** is a gross image of another vermiform appendix submitted to surgical pathology with the clinical diagnosis of acute appendicitis. This specimen should likewise be well documented with photographs. There is no evident pathology present. Yet, because the appendix was submitted with clinical diagnosis of acute appendicitis, this discrepancy must be clearly demonstrated in the associated gross photos. A segment of rib

Fig. 1. Appendix: acute gangrenous appendicitis and periappendicitis.

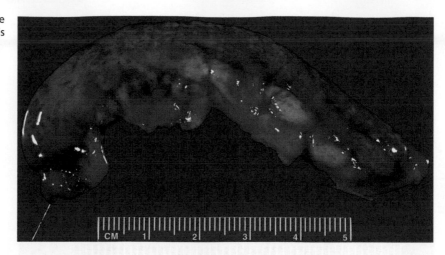

submitted as a gross-only specimen is presented in **Fig. 3**. This segment of rib was received in surgical pathology as a routine, incidental element of a radical nephrectomy. As such, the rib is considered a gross-only specimen. Whereas there is no grossly evident pathology, other than that associated with the surgical manipulation, it should be photographed from both anterior and posterior perspectives to document the essentially normal appearance. An explanted breast implant specimen is a special type of gross-only specimen, because it is considered a medical device (**Fig. 4**). Hence, it should be handled with the routine protocol for such items—photographed from all perspectives to fully document the appearance of the device and with additional images to record any identifiers, such as the "225" text seen on one aspect. The pathology evident in the specimen of **Fig. 5** is exclusively that associated with trauma and should be thoroughly documented, because such images support the

clinical history of traumatic amputation—a history that potentially raises the probability of subsequent medicolegal concerns. The specimen presented in **Fig. 6** is a remarkable example of a solitary fibrous tumor, as seen in a transverse section of lung. Appearance during gross handling may suggest that a specimen warrants particularly comprehensive gross photography. This most often occurs when a specimen appears, through gross examination, to be unusual or rare or, in contrast, is a classic example of a common pathologic finding.

THE SETUP

If at all possible, a small room should be dedicated to the gross pathology photography setup. Specific photographic equipment, accessories, and configuration will no doubt be driven by space and budgetary constraints, but a few guidelines are suggested. Almost without exception, the

Fig. 2. Appendix: no pathologic change.

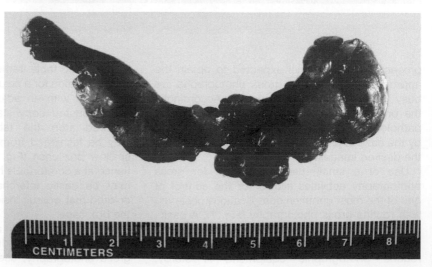

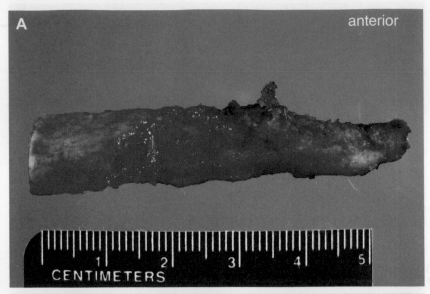

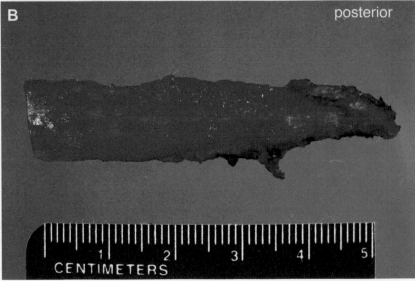

Fig. 3. (*A*) Anterior and (*B*) posterior aspects of gross-only rib specimen.

prosectors or personnel expected to obtain the appropriate, high-quality gross photographs are busy with other clinical demands. Accordingly, the probability of long-term excellence in gross pathology photography is most strongly predicted by the ease of use and time required for obtaining the desired images.

Use of a small, dedicated room for gross photography activities allows for the control of one of the most common complications observed with routine gross photography (**Fig. 7**). A basic, user-friendly gross pathology photography stand may be configured with only a few pieces of routine photographic equipment. A sturdy,

broad-based table frame may serve as an excellent foundation for a column copy stand of at least 40 inches with an adjustable camera arm and table-mounted copy stand lights with diffusion. Secured atop the table, a specimen stage may be fashioned from a strong, glass-topped, shallow box case (**Fig. 8**). With this case positioned at a comfortable height, background colors may be easily interchanged by placement of colored mat boards inside the open front face of the box case.

To minimize vibration and image blur, as well as to minimize direct handling of the camera during gross photography, use a shutter release cable

Fig. 4. Breast implant gross-only medical device.

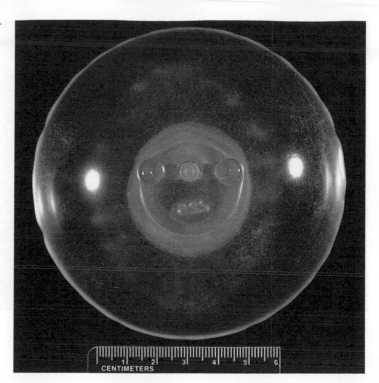

or a wireless remote shutter control. Moreover, as a means of real time quality control, always review the just-captured images of gross specimens, so that if necessary, adjustments may be made and new photos obtained while the material is readily available. To achieve this end, a remote monitor for the camera greatly simplifies the tasks of image review for framing, focus, and exposure compared with appraisal using the small camera screen.

In the setting of AP photography, it is imperative to regularly clean the camera lens with lens cleaning solution and a cleaning cloth. This section through a pneumonectomy specimen (**Fig. 9**) documents a good example of squamous cell carcinoma, except that the area just left of center is visually soft and somewhat blurred due to a smudge on the camera lens. Likewise, prepare any specimen to be photographed. Surfaces should be wiped clean of blood, and other material, such as tubes or bandages, should be removed. In **Fig. 10**, the photo stand glass, often called the specimen stage, is smeared such that it distracts from this photo of a lumpectomy

Fig. 5. Finger status post traumatic amputation.

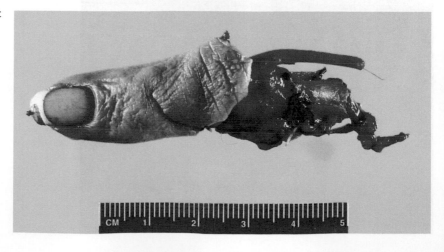

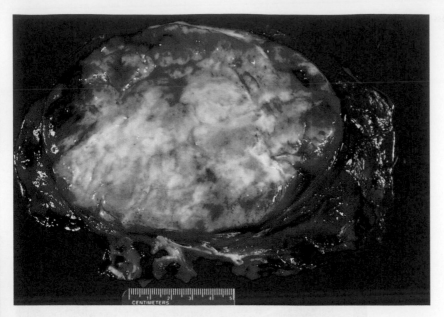

Fig. 6. Left lung: solitary fibrous tumor (transverse section).

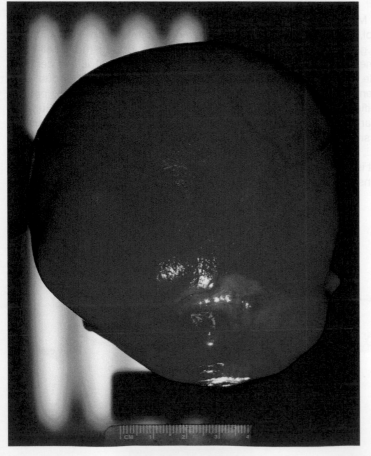

Fig. 7. Reflection of overhead fluorescent lights is a distraction in this external image of a markedly enlarged ovary.

Fig. 8. Glassed-topped box with open front slot for easy placement of background mat boards.

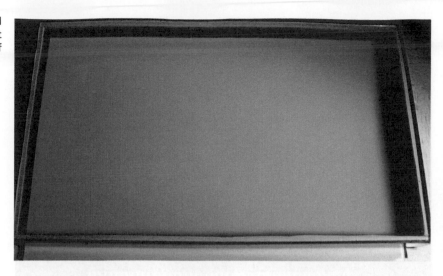

specimen, which exhibits a tan irregular mass subsequently diagnosed as ductal carcinoma in situ. Similarly, the quality presentation of this example of a cross-section through a neurofibroma (**Fig. 11**) is greatly diminished by the presence of a surgical suture draped across the cut surface. Whereas routine specimen preparation is an essential step for general photo quality, if clinically relevant, additional photo documentation may be essential to record the state of a specimen as it was received in pathology. This photo of a segment of umbilical cord with a true knot (**Fig. 12**) demonstrates the state of the specimen "as is" or as it was received in pathology and illustrates a clinically relevant feature. Regardless of specimen type, clinical concerns, or questions, always aim to capture as much detail as possible,

and, accordingly, take the time and effort to position a specimen and the camera such that the entire specimen (or particular regions of interest) fills most of the available frame. Failure to attend to this exceedingly important facet of photographic documentation often results in images of little or no value to patients or any of the associated stakeholders (**Fig. 13**). A collection of poor photo techniques is shown in **Fig. 14**.

THE TOOLS

Choose an appropriate background to highlight specimen details. Black is a reasonable choice for many specimens (**Fig. 15**) and moreover may mask small smudges or drops of fluid on the specimen stage. Black, however, is typically a poor

Fig. 9. A smudge on the camera lens results in image blur (left of center) for this cross-section of pneumonectomy specimen.

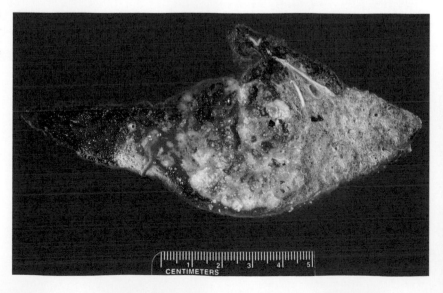

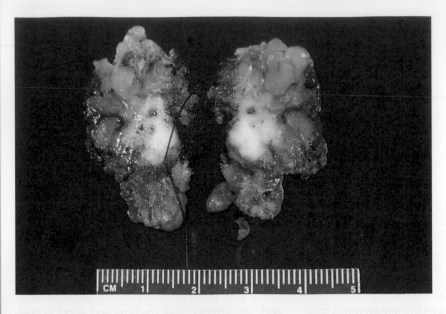

Fig. 10. The specimen stage is smeared in this image of a lumpectomy specimen.

choice for dark brown or dark red specimens, like liver and spleen or any specimens that exhibit blood covered surfaces. In general, red, yellow, and brown are most often poor background selections for routine specimens, whereas, in contrast, light blue (**Fig. 16**) and light green (**Fig. 17**) are colors that enhance overall image presentations. But red may be a good choice for slices of fixed brain sections (see **Fig. 18**). If using just a cloth background, consider wetting the cloth first to enhance the contrast and reduce the texture of the cloth. Given these recommendations, in pathology practice, background selections are often driven by personal preference, resources, or particular camera characteristics.

It is generally accepted that most pathology gross photos should include a scale and label, identified with the specimen accession number. In the frame of the image, the scale should be placed inferior to yet near the specimen. Not only does such placement contribute to an ease of interpretation for specimen gross morphology but also this arrangement simplifies the task of photo editing (removing accession number or other identifiers), if the image is to be shared in presentation or publication. The scale should not be placed on the specimen or obstruct the view of any part of the specimen (**Fig. 18**). To further assist the viewer of gross pathology photos, employ the following sensible

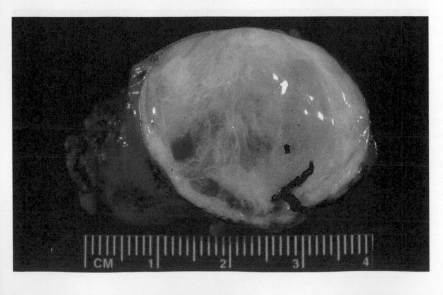

Fig. 11. Lack of specimen preparation results with a surgical suture across the surface of this cross-section of a neurofibroma.

Fig. 12. A segment of umbilical cord is photographed as is.

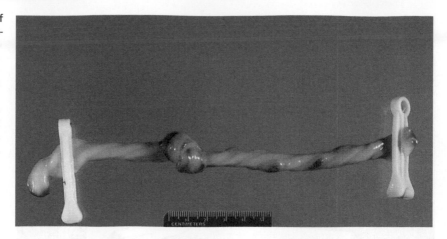

guidelines. If a specimen is large, use an entire standard 15-cm scale for reference (**Fig. 19**). Whereas, if a specimen is small, just a few centimeters or less, cut the scale to a length slightly longer than the specimen (**Fig. 20**). This greatly aids with visually approximating specimen-related dimensions. And, as another service to the viewer, be sure to include the zero point and the unit of measure designation, usually centimeters, in the segments of the scale cut to size. As nearly as can be approximated, place the scale with the associated label in the plane of focus for the specimen. This may be readily accomplished with the use of a "third hand" (**Fig. 21**) to hold the scale with label at the appropriate plane of focus while remaining out of the image frame. A plastic pointer or metal probe may also be attached to indicate a particular area of interest (discussed later). Such a device was used during the capture of many of the images for this article. Another option is to use a wooden holder, made from a slide box, that allows the height of a ruler and label attached to a glass slide to be readily adjusted (**Fig. 22**). Once a gross photo appropriately identifies a specimen with a scale and label, any additional close-up photos or macrophotos of a portion of the same field of view need not be accompanied by the label and scale. As for rulers, it is important not to include any logos or marketing text that distract from the effective presentation of the specimen. Rolls of disposable rulers that may be attached to a glass slide are also available.

The number and wide variety of digital cameras available for gross imaging are remarkably

Fig. 13. A poorly framed image of a mildly enlarged ovary results from the camera at too great distance from the specimen and lacks morphologic detail.

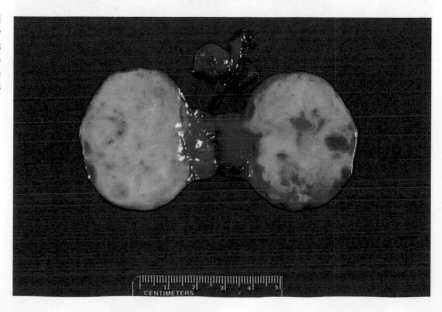

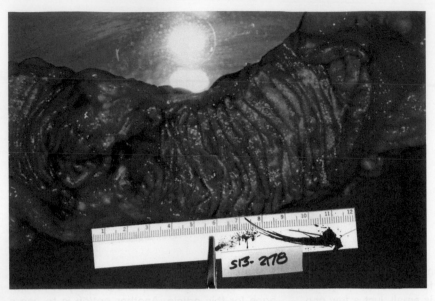

Fig. 14. This gross photo suffers from multiple composition errors. The background is marred by reflected lighting, the label and ruler are askew, the ruler has a prominent logo and is smeared with blood, and the alligator clip from the third hand (see **Fig. 20**) is also visible, the scale overlies and obscures part of the specimen. The specimen label is handwritten and legible, but a printed label is preferable.

extensive and a detailed discussion is not possible in this article. Some of these cameras capture images that may be readily and directly imported into an AP laboratory information system, whereas others require wireless or manual transfer from a memory card. An LED lighting system often yields superior images compared with flash photography. Even without a dedicated photo setup, the best camera is the one with ready access, which often may be a mobile smartphone. These multiuse devices often have the capacity to capture excellent macroimages, usually without a

flash, derived through use of the built-in camera or by attaching high-quality lenses, such as the Olloclip, to smartphones. Waterproof cases are also available for many cameras and smartphones, which may offer the benefit of keeping the phone clean.

THE CLUES

As specimens are handled and processed, attention must be directed to the associated clinical concerns and questions, such that important

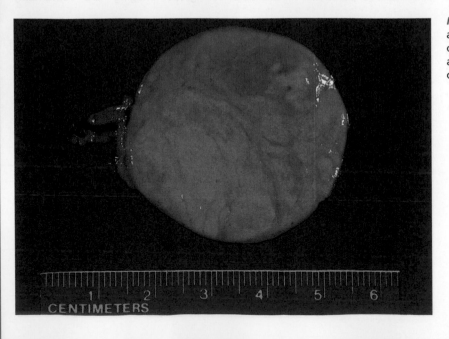

Fig. 15. Black serves as an excellent background of this section of an amber/orange adrenal cortical adenoma.

Fig. 16. Light blue serves as an excellent background for most specimen types and colors and provides a nice contrast to the dark red tissue of this section of kidney with a small tan/pink angiomyolipoma positioned near the upper left.

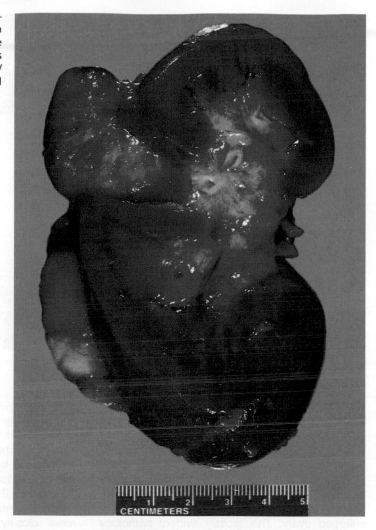

Fig. 17. Light green is a suitable background for the variety of colors seen in this section of a dermatofibrosarcoma protuberans, which exhibits a darkly pigmented skin surface, a light tan neoplasm, yellow adipose tissue, and specimen margin inks, including black along the deep margin and orange to the right.

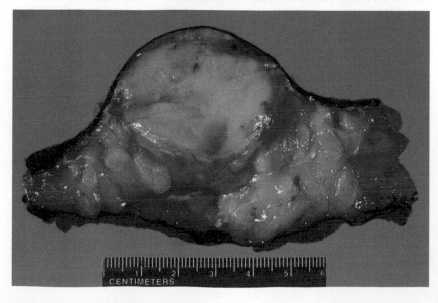

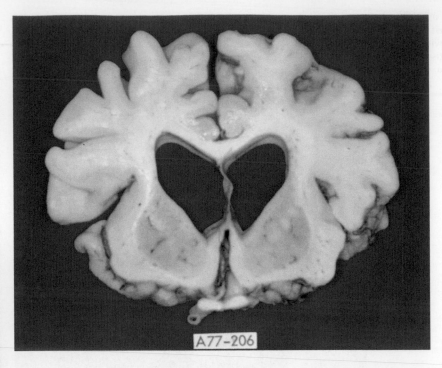

A77-206

Fig. 18. Brain section showing hydrocephalus. Normally red is a poor background for gross surgical pathology specimens, but for brain slices, the red cloth background creates a pleasing contrast to the pale neural tissue. The cloth was first wetted down and smoothed out before laying the brain section on top.

photos are obtained at various stages of sectioning. Often, intact organs reveal little of the pathologic changes that lie deep within the specimen. Always remember to photograph the appropriate cut surfaces, which reveal specimen structural architecture, and associated relations to any evident pathologic features. Fig. 23A reflects a perfectly adequate image of a markedly enlarged ovary. This grossly evident pathology should be photographed, yet little detail with regard to the associated specific pathologic process may be determined from this superficial

photograph. A cross-section of the ovary (see Fig. 23B) does much to reveal diagnostic features of this neoplasm. The solid, yellow-tan whorled cut surface is characteristic of a fibrothecoma and thus should be included in the photographic history for this specimen. When shooting a sectioned specimen, if 2 or more slices exhibit essentially the same features, photograph 1 individually, so as to more closely frame the specimen and best demonstrate the gross pathology. Note again, in Fig. 23B, this lesion is homogeneous throughout; hence, photographing this one-half of the

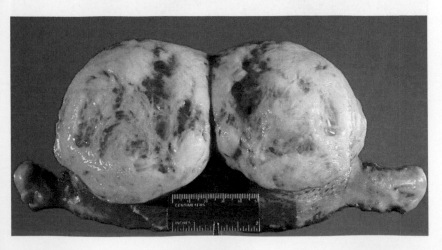

Fig. 19. A scale obscures the view of a portion of the uterine wall in this bivalved hysterectomy specimen with a large leiomyoma.

Fig. 20. For this longitudinal cross-section of a deeply invasive adenocarcinoma of the distal esophagus, the segment of scale is not even as long as the lesion of interest and certainly too short to readily estimate overall gross dimensions.

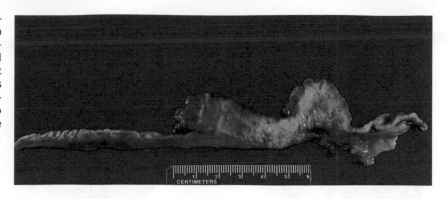

specimen is, in this instance, more effective than presenting both (essentially identical) cut surfaces side by side.

To draw attention to a focal region of interest, an appropriately positioned probe may be used to highlight the significant area while minimally obstructing the view of the overall specimen. Such an approach is used to great effect in **Fig. 24**, wherein a localization needle, submitted with a breast lumpectomy specimen, serves to direct attention to a small focus of ductal carcinoma in situ. Moreover, such an approach is particularly useful for demonstrating narrow channels through specimens, such as sinus tracts, perforations, and so forth (**Fig. 25**). Another method to best emphasize the gross architecture of delicate specimens is to photograph them floating in saline. The liquid helps support delicate tissue architecture, as is often present with small papillary and cystic structures. With this approach, the best images are obtained with the specimen transilluminated from below or from the sides (**Fig. 26**). In certain circumstances the best gross photo may not be derived from a customary camera mounted on a photo stand. A seldom-used yet often effective alternative technique for gross photography is derived through the use of a digital flatbed scanner. With limited specimen preparation and scanner configuration to optimize lighting and background,[12,13] specimens with intricate 3-D structure and depth (field of view) of up to a 0.5 cm or more may yield high-quality detailed images (**Fig. 27**). A final strategy is sometimes useful in the unfortunate incidence that an important photograph of a specimen was not obtained in the fresh state. To somewhat restore or refresh the original colors of a specimen that has been formalin fixed, place it from 1 to a few hours in 100% ethanol. Results vary greatly depending on the tissue type and the duration of

Fig. 21. This well-framed and well-demonstrated section of breast fibroadenoma is accompanied by a scale segment that affords easy translation to the overall specimen and internal elements.

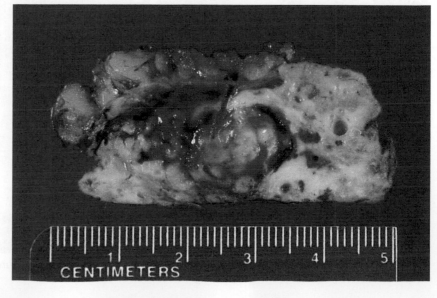

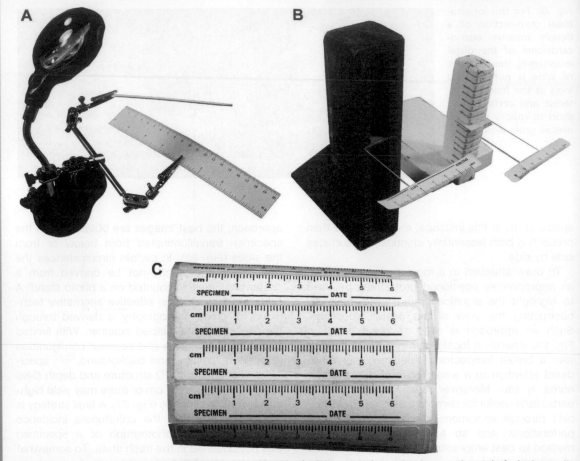

Fig. 22. The image on the top left (*A*) shows a third hand, which consists of movable arms at the end of which are alligator clips. The clips can hold a scale, a probe, or other item at an appropriate position. At the top right (*B*) are 2 wooden slide holders. The glass slide can be positioned within the grooves to put the ruler and label at the correct focal point. Also, the glass slide is not visible if it is in the frame of the photograph. On the bottom (*C*) is a roll of paper rulers.

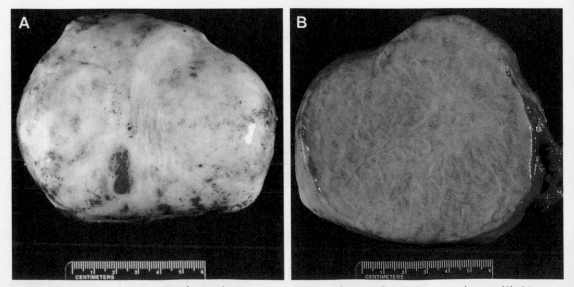

Fig. 23. (*A*) External photograph of an enlarged ovary reveals only superficial features, whereas (*B*) this cross-section of the ovary reveals the characteristic gross features of a fibrothecoma.

Fig. 24. A localization needle submitted with this lumpectomy is included to direct attention to a small focus of ductal carcinoma in situ.

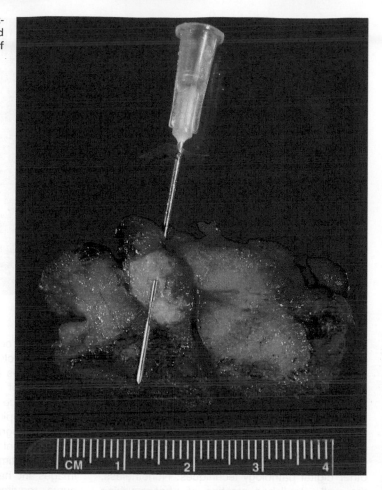

Fig. 25. A fundamental element of this photo of a vermiform appendix with gangrenous appendicitis is the placement of a probe that localizes an associated site of perforation.

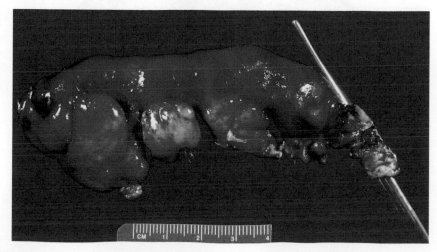

Fig. 26. The specimen for this striking photo is a complete hydatidaform mole, which is floated in saline to better demonstrate the innumerable, delicate, cystic grapelike villi, which are a characteristic feature.

prior fixation, but for obtaining a gross image for special circumstances, the protocol is usually worth a try (**Fig. 28**).

THE POINT

Contemporary AP practice is abuzz with the many exciting new opportunities associated with WSI, quantitative image analysis, telepathology, and other digital pathology techniques. Nonetheless, the well-established practice of photographing AP specimens, whether from surgical pathology or autopsy, continues to be of invaluable benefit to patients, clinicians, pathologists, and students. As such, this time-honored convention—the true beginning of digital pathology—will continue to afford unique advantages alongside the newer and developing imaging solutions. The widespread integration of digital photography into routine pathology workflow has almost eliminated turnaround time for availability of gross pathology images and has also greatly flattened the learning curve required for users to obtain excellent photos. With a limited set of hardware resources

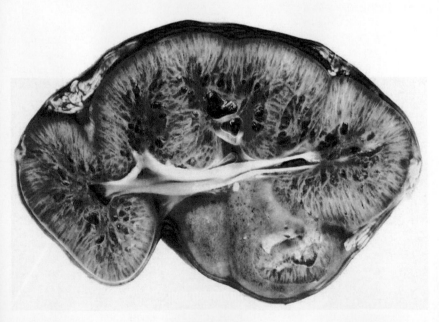

Fig. 27. Remarkable morphologic detail is exhibited in this image acquired with a commercial flatbed scanner of a longitudinal hemisection of formalin-fixed kidney with infantile polycystic kidney disease.

Fig. 28. This photo illustrates the result of an attempt to simulate the fresh appearance of this slice from a previously formalin-fixed ovarian mass, a Sertoli-Leydig cell tumor. After several hours in 100% ethanol, the tan-brown fixed section refreshed with a more tan-pink to red appearance, somewhat similar to the original fresh appearance. Because this was a previously sectioned specimen, note the territory of absent tissue in the upper right.

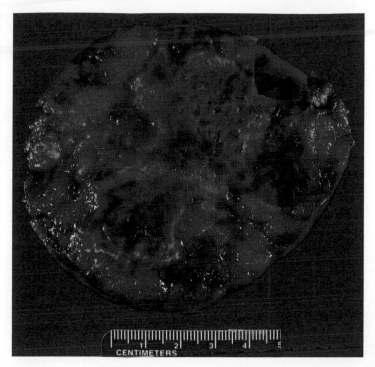

and effort, and following a few basic guidelines as set forth in this article, any AP practice may expect a standard of excellence in gross pathology photography.

REFERENCES

1. Wright JR, Spitalnik SL. Digital Pathology Workshop Proceedings from the Association of Pathology Chairs 2002 Annual Meeting. Available at: http://www.apcprods.org/Meetings/2002/index.cfm. Accessed March 5, 2015.
2. Campbell GA. Imaging, image analysis and computer-assisted quantitation: applications for electronic imaging in pathology. In: Cowen D, editor. Informatics for the clinical laboratory: a practical guide for the pathologist. New York: Springer; 2002. p. 251–67.
3. Hamza SH, Reddy VV. Digital image acquisition using a consumer-type digital camera in the anatomic pathology setting. Adv Anat Pathol 2004;11(2): 94–100.
4. Park RW, Eom JH, Byun HY, et al. Automation of gross photography using a remote-controlled digital camera system. Arch Pathol Lab Med 2003;127: 726–31.
5. Leong FJ, Leong AS. Digital photography in anatomic pathology. J Postgrad Med 2004;50(1): 62–9.
6. Riley RS, Ben-Ezra JM, Massy E, et al. Digital photography: a primer for pathologists. J Clin Lab Anal 2004;18:91–128.
7. Finkbeiner WE, Ursell PC, Davis RL. Autopsy photography and radiology. In: Finkbeiner WE, Ursell PC, Davis RL, editors. Autopsy pathology: a manual and atlas. 2nd edition. Philadelphia: Saunders Elsevier; 2009. p. 81–6.
8. Lester SC. Microscopy and photography. In: Lester SC, editor. Manual of surgical pathology. 3rd edition. Philadelphia: Saunders Elsevier; 2010. p. 215–6.
9. Rosai J. Gross techniques in surgical pathology. In: Rosai J, Ackerman L, editors. Rosai and Ackerman's surgical pathology. 10th edition. Edinburgh (United Kingdom): Mosby Elseveir; 2011. p. 31.
10. Barker N. Photography. In: Westra WH, Hruban RH, Phelps TH, et al, editors. Surgical pathology dissection: an illustrated guide. 2nd edition. New York: Springer; 2003. p. 26–32.
11. Amin M, Sharma G, Parwani AV, et al. Integration of digital gross pathology images for enterprise-side access. J Pathol Inform 2012;3:10.
12. Mai KT, Stinson WA, Burns BF, et al. Creating Digital Images of Pathology Specimens by using a Flatbed scanner. Histopathology 2001;39:323–5.
13. Matthews TJ, Denney PA. Digital imaging of surgical specimens using a wet scanning technique. J Clin Pathol 2001;54:326–7.

and effort, and following a few basic guidelines as set forth in this article, any AP practice may expect a standard of excellence in gross pathology photography.

REFERENCES

Advanced Imaging Techniques for the Pathologist

Jeffrey L. Fine, MD

KEYWORDS

- Advanced imaging • Digital pathology • Optical coherence tomography • OCT • Digital pathology
- In vivo microscopy • Ex vivo microscopy

ABSTRACT

Advanced imaging refers to direct microscopic imaging of tissue, without the need for traditional hematoxylin-eosin (H&E) microscopy, including microscope slides or whole-slide images. A detailed example is presented of optical coherence tomography (OCT), an imaging technique based on reflected light. Experience and example images are discussed in the larger context of the evolving relationship of surgical pathology to clinical patient care providers. Although these techniques are diagnostically promising, it is unlikely that they will directly supplant H&E histopathology. It is likely that OCT and related technologies will provide narrow, targeted diagnosis in a variety of in vivo (patient) and ex vivo (specimen) applications.

OVERVIEW

This article discusses a group of novel imaging techniques that are exciting because they may disrupt traditional pathology diagnosis. Such technologies permit direct tissue imaging without delays for histology preparation or for slide scanning, which may mean that turnaround time for pathology diagnosis could radically diminish even if a pathologist is off-site. In vivo imaging is also a possibility, which might blur or diminish traditional boundaries between pathology and other medical specialties. Finally, this might represent a fabulous opportunity to fundamentally re-evaluate current surgical pathology practice, with more emphasis placed on creating clinically valuable tests versus traditional all-inclusive histopathology examination. There are unprecedented pressures related to simultaneously increasing clinical expectations and decreasing access to resources. It is the author's opinion that traditional pathology diagnosis may not continue to be feasible for all applications; brightfield microscopy may not be rapid enough or inexpensive enough despite its current status as gold standard for most histopathology diagnosis. Furthermore, nonpathology specialties are vigorously developing new clinical applications based on advanced imaging; if pathologists wish to be involved in such diagnostic efforts then proactive involvement is essential. Rather than present an exhaustive list of the various advanced imaging modalities,[1] an in-depth presentation of OCT is chosen. The aim is to present a pathologist-friendly introduction, so that interested pathologists will be better able to participate in these advanced imaging efforts.

OPTICAL COHERENCE TOMOGRAPHY

OCT was originally developed more than 20 years ago and found its first application in ophthalmology,[2] with additional early work with blood vessel and gastrointestinal imaging.[3,4] There are many variants of OCT but it is generally understand that these mean differences in speed, resolution, tissue depth, and image orientation. Specifics are less important than understanding the general idea of what OCT is and how it could be used in a particular situation. Briefly, a specimen is illuminated and the reflected light is used to create a 2-D image or a stack of 2-D images that are virtual slices of the tissue (**Fig. 1**). An

Disclosure: No conflicts of interest to report.
Subdivision of Advanced Imaging and Image Analysis (Pathology Informatics) Department of Pathology, University of Pittsburgh School of Medicine, 200 Lothrop Street, Pittsburgh, PA 15213, USA
E-mail address: finejl@upmc.edu

Surgical Pathology 8 (2015) 213–221
http://dx.doi.org/10.1016/j.path.2015.02.004

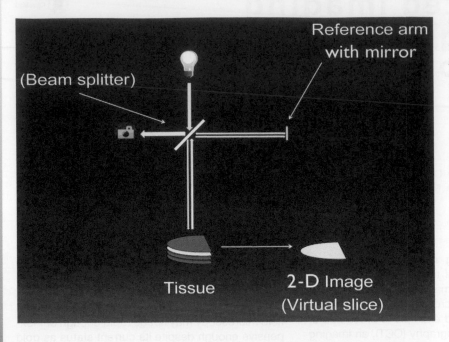

Fig. 1. OCT explained. Light is emitted from a source (*light bulb* and *yellow arrows*) and passes through a beam splitter. Some light travels along a reference arm and is reflected from a mirror back into the beam splitter (*more yellow arrows*). Some light travels into the tissue (*yellow arrow*), interacts with the tissue, and is then reflected back into the beam splitter (*white arrow*). Reflected light, both from reference arm and from tissue, combines in the beam splitter and undergoes interference. This interference pattern is imaged (*blue camera icon*) and is a 2-D image of the tissue due to the interaction of light with tissue. By varying the length of the reference arm, the imaged depth into the tissue can be varied. Depth is limited by the amount of reflected light; infrared light permits deeper imaging but offers less resolution than broad-spectrum visible light.

OCT image shows differences in reflectivity; nearly transparent tissues (eg, fat) reflect little light and are contrasted with other shinier tissues (**Fig. 2**). OCT can be simplistically explained by comparison with 3 other imaging techniques that may be more familiar: ultrasound, phase-contrast microscopy, and CT. The ultrasound similarity is easily understood, and that is reflection;

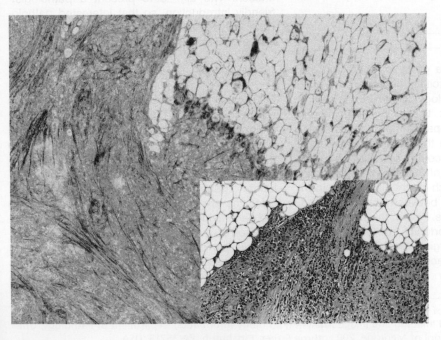

Fig. 2. Example OCT image (invasive lobular carcinoma of breast). The larger image is an OCT image of invasive lobular breast carcinoma with infiltration into fat. Fat is perhaps the most easily identified tissue due to the difference in reflectivity between cell membranes and cytoplasm of individual fat cells. The sharpness of the cell membranes visually conveys the high resolution of the image (approximately 1 μm per pixel in the original image). The inset H&E photomicrograph is derived from a WSI of the same tissue (approximately 0.5 μm per pixel, ×20 objective magnification). In the OCT image, individual tumor cell nuclei are visible as white spots in the gray background.

ultrasound derives images from reflected sound, whereas OCT is based on light (Table 1). Unlike sound, light travels too quickly for direct time-based imaging so OCT images use interferometry, which is also used in phase-contrast microscopy. Although phase contrast is different from reflectivity, the overall configuration of an imager or microscope with a reference light path and interference-based imaging is similar.[5] OCT also features a variable-length reference path for light, which means that variable tissue depths can be imaged into a tissue's surface. Imaging a series of images at different depths results in a stack of 2-D images, which can be viewed in sequence or can be reconstructed into a 3-D data set. This is like CT imaging, in that CT produces a stack of virtual slice radiographs that can be viewed in 2-D in multiple orientations or that can be used to create 3-D images (Fig. 3). OCT is also like CT in that it represents a data set that is too large to be viewed directly; viewable images represent subsets of the data. CT image viewers display portions of the data, using selective viewing recipes called windows (ie, bone window, soft tissue window, sinus window, brain window, and so forth). OCT images do not yet have such windows established but only because the images are so new to pathologists.

OCT image data sets can be large, although not as large as whole-slide images (WSIs). A single 2-D OCT slice of a frozen section block–sized piece of tissue, at 1-μm resolution, can be 20,000 by 10,000 pixels in size (more than 300 megabytes of raw data per slice). Such an image can be acquired in approximately 20 minutes with a current-generation OCT system without undue difficulty, but acquiring a stack of 150 to 200 such images would be infeasible due to time and computing constraints. A compromise is a series of few (eg, 3–5) levels, much like what is done with histopathology slides. Finally, manual review of such large image sets should optimally be augmented with software that helps detect clinically important areas, such as pathologists' computer-assisted diagnosis. One investigator team uses an OCT system to image large portions

of the esophagus.[6] Such an image set is akin to totally submitting a specimen for H&E histology and then cutting many levels into each block—it would represent an enormous amount of image review if attempted manually. Therefore, the review should be targeted and augmented by computer assistance.

EXPERIENCE WITH OPTICAL COHERENCE TOMOGRAPHY

The author's earliest experience with OCT was the result of a collaboration with ophthalmologists.[7] Although this system only featured 20-μm resolution, it did not require contact with the specimen and, therefore, theoretically could be mounted vertically in a specimen grossing type of application, just as a conventional camera is deployed. Although not as good as a histology section, such OCT resolution permits seeing lesions, such as ductal carcinoma in situ (DCIS) in breast tissue, and may, therefore, be suitable for intraoperative margins assessment (Fig. 4). Furthermore, such an image does not require a cryostat, microscope, or the skill needed to obtain good frozen section histology on breast tissue. Finally, miniaturization of this type of device could eventually permit in vivo imaging from within an operating room; this should be of interest to surgeons because many procedures are now performed in outpatient surgical centers that do not have intraoperative support by pathologists, either on-site or remotely.

Another type of OCT imaging worth discussing in more detail, due to its high tissue resolution, is full-field OCT.[8] This imaging system is unique in that it is a pathology system that produces 2-D images at a 1-μm resolution, using oil-immersion microscopy on a tissue-block sized tissue piece inside a specimen holder (Fig. 5). This resolution is theoretically adequate for much diagnostic work and these images can often closely resemble medium-magnification H&E images, especially in tissues that contain cysts or lumens (Fig. 6). Such close correlation between OCT and H&E,

Table 1
Comparison of optical coherence tomography with other imaging modalities

OCT	Similarity	Difference
Ultrasound	Reflection	OCT uses light, not sound
Phase-contrast microscopy	Interferometry	OCT shows reflectivity
CT	Virtual slices and 3-D data; images a subset of data	OCT has limited penetration into tissue depth

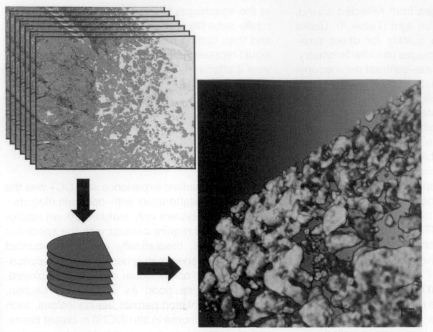

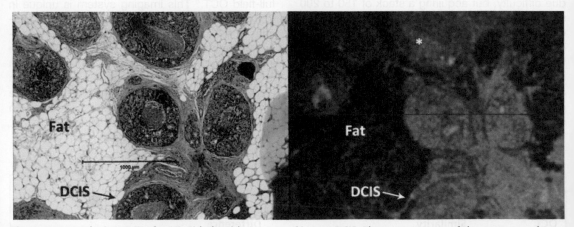

Fig. 3. 3-D OCT view of uterine papillary serous carcinoma. A series of OCT images were acquired from a hysterectomy specimen, from 1 field of view and at multiple tissue depths (*upper left corner*). These are stylistically shown as a stack of flat shapes (*lower left corner*). Using radiology (CT) software, a 3-D reconstruction view is created (*yellow/orange image to right*). Despite not being optimized for a pathology image, this clearly demonstrates the papillary architecture of the tumor.

however, represent a potential pitfall, because some lesions likely are difficult to see reliably without training and without targeted computer assistance (eg, image analysis and radiology-like windows). One good example is an image of vulvar Paget disease; if looked for, then squamous nuclei and Paget nests can easily be seen in the OCT image (**Fig. 7**). If there is not yet a diagnosis, then it is

not clear that a pathologist could confidently make the diagnosis from OCT alone. The Paget lesion is visible, however, which means there is a diagnostic pattern in the OCT image data; in the author's opinion, this means that the OCT image can be diagnostic, but it will require more work to make this a reliable process. Breast tissue is another area that has been challenging due to

Fig. 4. Low-resolution OCT of DCIS. Side-by-side images of breast DCIS. These are images of the same area from a breast specimen: (*left*) H&E and (*right*) spectral domain OCT. The H&E image is from a WSI scanned at 0.5 μm per pixel (×20 objective magnification). The OCT image was acquired at approximately 20 μm per pixel using an ophthalmology device. Although higher-resolution OCT is possible, this device could be used to image breast tissue from a benchtop vantage point without special sample preparation (ie, just as with an conventional digital camera). Fat, DCIS and necrosis (*asterisk*) can clearly be identified in the OCT image; although perhaps not adequate for initial diagnosis, such an image might be useful for intraoperative assessment of margins.

Fig. 5. Full-field OCT device. The main image is a photograph of a full-field OCT imaging system (Light-CT, LLTech, Paris, France). It use oil immersion microscopy with a ×10 objective and can image at 1 μm resolution in X, Y, and Z axes. It accommodates tissue block–sized tissue in a specimen holder (*inset, lower right corner*). Prior to OCT acquisition, a gross specimen scout image is also acquired (*inset, upper right corner*). This scout image permits driving about tissue in live mode prior to initiating a higher-quality permanent scan of the tissue.

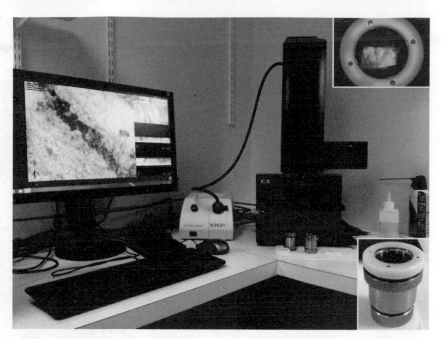

inadequate contrast out of the box and despite good tissue resolution. Even subtle tumor infiltrates can retrospectively be seen but more work is needed to make this a more reliable procedure

for detection or identification of breast tumor cell infiltrates (**Fig. 8**).

Therefore, OCT images are not likely to be a direct replacement for traditional H&E

Fig. 6. OCT example (mucinous cystic ovary). This is an example of the high image quality that can be obtained with some specimens, such as this mucinous cystadenoma in an ovary (H&E image overlaid on top of OCT image). Glands versus stroma are easily discerned, and even the glandular cells' mucinous morphology is visible. Although H&E is more detailed, that image took much more time to create due to permanent section histology and WSI time requirements. The OCT image is a portion of a larger image that typically requires 10 to 20 minutes of acquisition time in this particular system (Light-CT, LLTech, Paris, France) (H&E image scanned at 0.5 μm objective resolution).

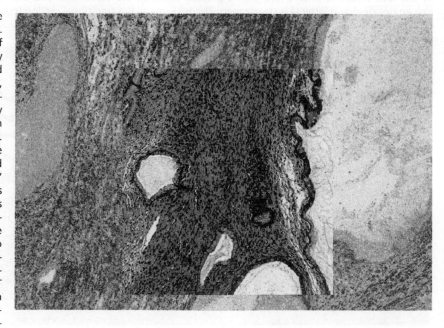

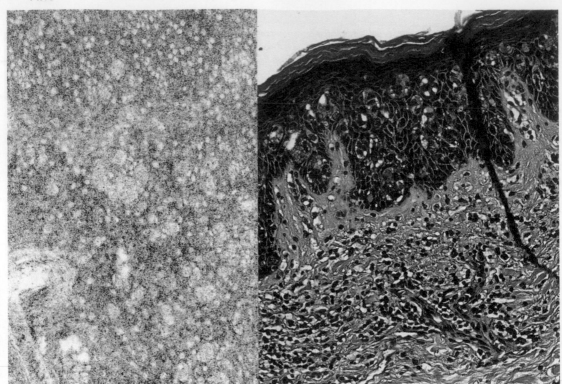

Fig. 7. Vulvar Paget disease. This is a side-by-side view of vulvar skin containing Paget disease: (*left*) OCT and (*right*) H&E. The OCT image was acquired en face from the skin surface, simulating a possible in vivo application. A population of smaller white round spots is clearly seen; these correlate with benign squamous cells. Larger irregular white blobs represent epidermal tumor nests of Paget cells. Although not well seen, in the lower left of the OCT image, a surface hair that is pressed between the vulvar skin and the imaging coverslip (shaped like an upside-down letter L) is clearly seen. The H&E image is a traditional section (eg, perpendicular to the surface) and shows the epidermis with small nests of Paget cells (H&E image scanned at 0.5 μm objective resolution).

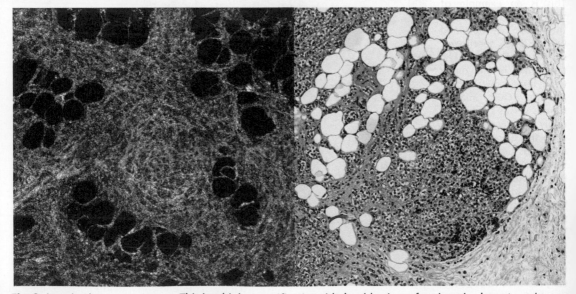

Fig. 8. Invasive breast carcinoma. This is a high-magnification side-by-side view of an invasive breast carcinoma: (*left*) OCT and (*right*) H&E. Tumor nuclei are clearly seen as small round dark shadows in the OCT image, and these correlate with the tumor nuclei in the H&E image. These are easily recognizable retrospectively, which means that pathologists and image analysis can be trained to find tumor in OCT images. This is an example of an OCT image, however, that is not ready-made for pathology diagnosis based on its superficial resemblance to the H&E image (H&E image scanned at 0.5 μm objective resolution).

histopathology for all tissues and for all clinical situations. In contrast to breast tissue, endometrium is extremely amenable to OCT imaging because there is already good contrast between glands, stroma, and myometrium without further image optimization. Although there will be a learning curve for interpretation of endometrial OCT images, it is already clear that pathologists can recognize structures just from their resemblance to known histopathology entities.[9] For example, in the author's own study, 3 pathologist subjects were able to distinguish benign versus malignant endometrium with a 10.44% discordance rate, despite having only 5 to 10 minutes of experience with an endometrial OCT image training set (Figs. 9 and 10).[10]

DISCUSSION

OCT is a powerful new imaging modality for pathologists. Although much early work took place in other medical specialties, OCT is microscopy and it produces images that are much more detailed than those typically interpreted by physicians in other specialties, such as radiology or gastroenterology. Pathologists are a natural choice for interpreting these images due to existing expertise not only with microscopy but also with test design and implementation. Although OCT images are unlikely to replace H&E histopathology, they are well suited to targeted clinical applications even with current-generation image quality (eg, intraoperative endometrial assessment). Therefore, development of advanced imaging applications may require a shift away from all-inclusive H&E diagnosis to narrower tests that address specific clinical questions. This is not without precedent; frozen section is a test that can quickly address clinical need without the

expectation of definitive diagnosis (usually). Frozen section testing is generally bundled with a traditional H&E diagnosis, just as an OCT-based depth-of-invasion assessment in endometrial cancer is tied to subsequent histopathology review of the specimen. The real practice disruption likely will be from advanced imaging tests that are not bundled with a histology review. If pathologists wish to be involved in such testing, they should be actively engaged with clinical colleagues to identify unmet needs and other opportunities for rapid imaging diagnosis.

To this end, pathologist investigators need to work on building bridges between existing H&E histopathology and these new imaging techniques. Not only will such work permit new ex vivo applications but also it should also facilitate in vivo assessment. The previous example of vulvar OCT is a good example; the ability to make diagnoses in en face vulvar images could well translate into diagnosis on in vivo images from a gynecology office setting without a need for biopsy. Biopsy seems like a trivial procedure, but it does matter to patients. In vivo breast margin assessment is another good example and one that is being driven by breast surgeons.[11] Pathologists can be valued partners in these efforts, but it requires a proactive approach.

Although current full-field OCT images may require 10 to 20 minutes of acquisition time, it is likely that refinements will lead to shorter imaging times just as has occurred with WSIs.[12] Therefore, timewise, OCT already compares favorably with frozen section, is much faster than routine histology, and does not require a separate slide-scanning step. OCT images may not require as much laboratory infrastructure to produce and could become an inexpensive method to project pathology expertise away from centralized laboratories.

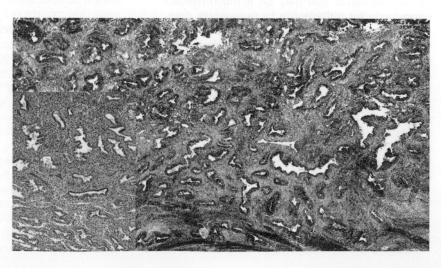

Fig. 9. Benign endometrium. This is a full-field OCT image of benign endometrial tissue (inset is an H&E image of the same tissue). The OCT and H&E images strongly resemble one another. Glands are readily seen because they contain lumens, but the glandular epithelium is also readily distinguished from endometrial stroma (H&E image scanned at 0.5 μm objective resolution).

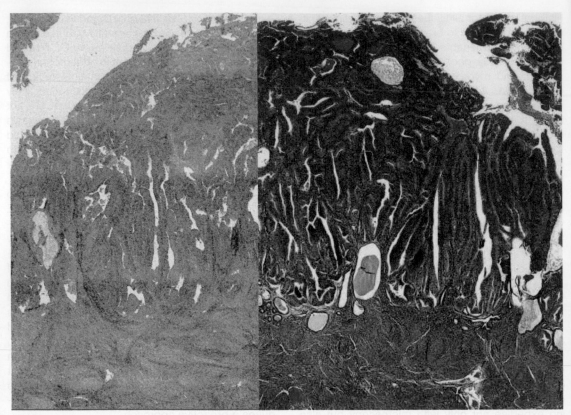

Fig. 10. Endometrial carcinoma. Low-magnification OCT (*left*) and H&E (*right*) images of the same endometrial tumor. The architecture of the glands is evident on OCT, as is the interface between endometrium and myometrium. Such images could be used for intraoperative assessment of endometrial tumor depth-of-invasion assessment and for confirmation of histology (H&E image scanned at 0.5 μm objective resolution).

Unfortunately, this short discussion cannot do justice to the ramifications of OCT and related direct tissue microscopy technologies, but these may be disruptive to the pathology status quo. In particular, in vivo diagnosis crosses into territory traditionally off-limits to laboratories. Such upending of the status quo may be a much-needed opportunity for pathologists to re-evaluate diagnostic practice fundamentally and even what it means to be a pathologist. This may already be happening as WSIs develop into clinical practice and as pathology groups seek to cope with an uncertain future.[13–15] Although H&E-based histopathology may remain a gold standard, it is possible that it will become too slow or too expensive in specific clinical situations. OCT and other advanced imaging may represent a way forward that permits responsive, excellent patient care despite decreased availability of resources.

REFERENCES

1. Chen Y, Liang CP, Liu Y, et al. Review of advanced imaging techniques. J Pathol Inform 2012;3:22.

2. Gabriele ML, Wollstein G, Ishikawa H, et al. Optical coherence tomography: history, current status, and laboratory work. Invest Ophthalmol Vis Sci 2011; 52(5):2425–36.

3. Brezinski ME, Tearney GJ, Bouma BE, et al. Optical coherence tomography for optical biopsy: properties and demonstration of vascular pathology. Circulation 1996;93(6):1206–13.

4. Tearney GJ, Brezinski ME, Bouma BE, et al. In vivo endoscopic optical biopsy with optical coherence tomography. Science 1997;276(5321):2037–9.

5. Murphy DB, Oldfield R, Schwartz S, et al. Introduction to phase contrast microscopy. Nikon microscopy U (The source for microscopy education). Available at: http://www.microscopyu.com/articles/phasecontrast/phasemicroscopy.html. Accessed September 01, 2014.

6. Suter MJ, Vakoc BJ, Yachimski PS, et al. Comprehensive microscopy of the esophagus in human patients with optical frequency domain imaging. Gastrointest Endosc 2008;68(4):745–53.

7. Fine JL, Kagemann L, Wollstein G, et al. Direct scanning of pathology specimens using spectral domain optical coherence tomography: a pilot study.

Ophthalmic Surg lasers Imaging 2010;41(Suppl): S58–64.

8. Jain M, Shukla N, Manzoor M, et al. Modified full-field optical coherence tomography: a novel tool for rapid histology of tissues. J Pathol Inform 2011; 2:28.

9. Jain M, Narula N, Salamoon B, et al. Full-field optical coherence tomography for the analysis of fresh unstained human lobectomy specimens. J Pathol Inform 2013;4:26.

10. Cucoranu IC, Fine JL. Optical Coherence Tomography (OCT) for Intra-Operative Style Interpretation of Endometrium (USCAP Abstract, Informatics). Mod Pathol 2013;26:375–83.

11. Bydlon TM, Barry WT, Kennedy SA, et al. Advancing optical imaging for breast margin assessment: an analysis of excisional time, cautery, and patent blue dye on underlying sources of contrast. PLos One 2012;7(12):e51418.

12. Pantanowitz L, Valenstein PN, Evans AJ, et al. Review of the current state of whole slide imaging in pathology. J Pathol Inform 2011;2:36.

13. Cornish TC, Swapp RE, Kaplan KJ. Whole-slide imaging: routine pathologic diagnosis. Adv Anat Pathol 2012;19(3):152–9.

14. Kothari S, Phan JH, Stokes TH, et al. Pathology imaging informatics for quantitative analysis of whole-slide images. J Am Med Inform Assoc 2013;20(6): 1099–108.

15. Robboy SJ, Weintraub S, Horvath AE, et al. Pathologist workforce in the United States: I. Development of a predictive model to examine factors influencing supply. Arch Pathol Lab Med 2013;137(12): 1723–32.

Overview of Telepathology

Navid Farahani, MD[a],*, Liron Pantanowitz, MD[b]

KEYWORDS

- Telepathology • Digital imaging • Robotic • Static • Teleconsultation • Telemicroscopy
- Virtual microscopy • Whole-slide imaging

ABSTRACT

Telepathology is the practice of remote pathology using telecommunication links to enable the electronic transmission of digital pathology images. Telepathology can be used for remotely rendering primary diagnoses, second opinion consultations, quality assurance, education, and research purposes. The use of telepathology for clinical patient care has been limited mostly to large academic institutions. Barriers that have limited its widespread use include prohibitive costs, legal and regulatory issues, technologic drawbacks, resistance from pathologists, and above all a lack of universal standards. This article provides an overview of telepathology technology and applications.

OVERVIEW

Telepathology is the practice of pathology at a distance, transmitting macroscopic and/or microscopic images using telecommunication links for remote interpretations (telediagnosis), second opinions or consultations (teleconsultation), and/or for educational purposes.[1–4] The original material (eg, glass slide) is spatially separated from the remote consultant (telepathologist) who will interpret a representative image of the material. The digital or analog image is remotely viewed on a computer monitor or cell phone screen. Ubiquitous access to the Internet, or to other broadband telecommunications linkages, facilitates nearly global image sharing. As a result, telepathology has been used to aid a growing number of laboratories around the world to deliver pathology services by allowing them to easily connect with

experts. Telepathology has even been used to enhance the efficiency of pathology services between hospitals less than a mile apart.[5,6] With increasing subspecialization in pathology, the use of telepathology to access subspecialists (eg, neuropathologists) has been extremely beneficial.[7–12] The practice of telepathology, however, is not only limited to diagnostic work but can be used in quality assurance (eg, rereview of cases), education, and research.[9,11]

The first recorded instance of "telepathology" occurred in the late 1960s, when a real-time "television microscopy" service was established between Massachusetts General Hospital (MGH) and Logan Airport Medical Station in Boston, Massachusetts.[13] Since then, there has been a proliferation of telepathology technology and services worldwide.[14,15] The number of "telepathology" citations indexed in MEDLINE has grown from the first citation listed in 1986 to 900 citations in 2015. The variety of telepathology systems developed and applications deployed continues to grow. To date, 12 distinct classes of telepathology systems have been described in the literature. These are listed in the Weinstein Telepathology System Classification, the primary modes of which are static imaging, dynamic imaging, and virtual slide telepathology.[9] Despite the low equipment start-up costs, static image telepathology was slowly replaced by dynamic methods in an attempt to improve diagnostic accuracy.[16,17] With dynamic telepathology, the telepathologist is more actively involved in glass slide field selection, typically by using robotic, remote-controlled microscopy.[18–20] Virtual slide telepathology is the most recently developed mode of telepathology. This technology is also referred to as whole-slide

[a] Department of Pathology and Laboratory Medicine, Cedars-Sinai Medical Center, Los Angeles, CA, USA;
[b] Department of Pathology, University of Pittsburgh School of Medicine, Pittsburgh, PA, USA
* Corresponding author.
E-mail address: nfarahan@gmail.com

Surgical Pathology 8 (2015) 223–231
http://dx.doi.org/10.1016/j.path.2015.02.018

imaging (WSI) telepathology. WSI systems produce giant, high-resolution, digital images of entire glass slides (ie, digital slides).[21] With disruptive WSI technology, innovative telepathology services have emerged.[12]

There are many potential uses of telepathology. Telepathology has been applied in anatomic pathology (eg, remote frozen section diagnosis, telecytology) and clinical pathology (eg, telehematology, telemicrobiology). Drawbacks to the widespread use of telepathology include cost, technology restrictions (eg, limited resolution, large image files), resistance from pathologists (eg, reluctance, skepticism, technophobia), lack of standards, and the potential threat of competition for pathology services. The development of standards for digital radiology imaging was critical to the success of teleradiology, and the same is likely to be true for telepathology. Standards for telepathology have begun to be developed, such as the recent guidelines set forth by the American Telemedicine Association.[22] The Canadian Association of Pathologists and Royal College of Pathologists also have published guidelines for telepathology.[23,24] Emerging legal and regulatory issues in telepathology also are being addressed, which will hopefully catalyze the practice of telepathology.[25]

TELEHEALTH

Telepathology falls under the broader category of telehealth. According to the Office for the Advancement of Telehealth, telehealth is defined as the use of electronic information and telecommunications technologies to support "long-distance" clinical health care, patient and professional health-related education, public health, and health administration. Telemedicine, another branch of telehealth, describes the remote transfer of clinical information via electronic communications.[3,26] Technologies used in telemedicine include the Internet, videoconferencing, store-and-forward imaging, streaming media, and wireless communications. Telemedicine can be further subdivided by specialty (eg, telepathology, teleradiology, teledermatology, telesurgery, telepsychiatry). The field of telemedicine is broad, because it also includes telerounding (eg, e-ICU "rounding"), telemonitoring (eg, home arrhythmia monitoring), televisits, tele-home care, and telemanagement of patients.[27] Currently, most telemedicine programs consist of a central medical hub with several rural spokes, so as to improve access to services in underserved areas. Telehealth initiatives are growing due to lower costs of technology, federal funds supporting such programs, and advancements in technology.[28] Although the various branches of telehealth

present unique opportunities for both patients and clinicians, they also possess distinct operational, ethical, and legal issues.[29] As the field grows, more standards and telepractice guidelines will be needed.[30]

HISTORICAL OVERVIEW

The history of telepathology has been long and eventful.[15,16,31] A list of several major milestones are provided in **Table 1**. The first telepathology

Table 1 Historical telepathology milestones	
Date	**Historical Milestones**
1968	Black-and-white photos of blood smears were sent via video from Logan Airport to the Massachusetts General Hospital in Boston
1980	Remote telepathology broadcasting demonstration on a commercial scale
1986	First video robotic telepathology system using satellite; introduction of the term "telepathology" into the English language; first telepathology patent application prepared for submission to the US Patent and Trademark Office with the patent granted in 1993
1989	Norway nationwide telepathology program established for frozen section services
1990	Published telepathology experience with more than 2200 VA hospital cases
1994	Hardware for a complete telepathology system becomes available
1995	AFIP static image consult service started
2000	WSI comes to market
2001	Dynamic telepathology used in the US Army Telemedicine Program
2005	US Army converts to WSI platform
2009	FDA panel meeting addresses the use of digital pathology for primary diagnosis
2011	Introduction of WSI dynamic-robotic/static imaging systems
2013	Telepathology guidelines developed by the Royal College of Pathologists
2014	Updated clinical guidelines for telepathology from ATA; published Canadian Association of Pathologists guidelines for establishing a telepathology service for anatomic pathology using WSI

Abbreviations: AFIP, Armed Forces Institute of Pathology; ATA, American Telepathology Association; FDA, Food and Drug Administration; VA, Department of Veterans Affairs; WSI, whole-slide imaging.

event occurred in 1968, when black-and-white real-time television images of blood smears and urine specimens were sent from Logan Airport in Boston to the MGH for interpretation. In the 1990s, the value of telepathology for diagnosis was showcased by a landmark paper involving thousands of cases remotely interpreted at the Department of Veterans Affairs (VA) hospital in the United States.[17,32] Telepathology was used by VA hospitals for both anatomic pathology (eg, frozen sections) and clinical pathology services, without having a pathologist on-site at remote locations. The VA group involved in this study used an Apollo dynamic telepathology system, based on Weinstein and colleagues' robotic telepathology patents.[17,32] Their published data showed a high diagnostic concordance of robotic telepathology with light microscopy, and decreased turnaround time for surgical pathology cases at the remote site. By 2009, Dunn's group[17,32] had reported on their experience with over 11,000 telepathology cases. Pathologist-specific discordance rates using dynamic/robotic telepathology (0.12%–0.77%) were well below those noted using static image telepathology.[18,33,34]

Telepathology progress has typically been aligned with technologic advances. This evolution is nicely illustrated by the change of telepathology services that were offered by the US military. In 1993, the Armed Forces Institute of Pathology initiated a static imaging consult service in its pursuit of providing rapid expert consultation globally.[35] By 2001, dynamic telepathology was adopted by the US Department of Defense within the Army Telemedicine Program. In 2005, these systems were converted to a WSI platform. Since then, several companies have supplied competing products for digital imaging, providing users with an increasing range of scanning platforms and image viewers. Several commercial software solutions (eg, Corista, ePathAccess, Xifin) have started to build international networks, providing users and consulting groups with collaborative telepathology portals. These digital pathology networks provide virtual consultant consortiums with Web-enabled access to secure cloud services. With the growth of mobile health (mHealth) we are likely to witness greater use of telepathology using mobile devices (eg, tablets, cell phones, wearable glasses such as Google Glass).

TELEPATHOLOGY APPLICATIONS

Telepathology is currently most beneficial for providing pathology services to distant locations where the medical facilities lack on-site or easily accessible pathology services.[36] It is often logistically easier and cheaper to move an image around than it is to move a patient or pathologist. Telepathology can be used to expedite rapid consultation of remote cases where travel is not a viable option. It is also useful as a communication tool between general and sub-specialist pathologists.[5] Access to experts via telepathology, in which a teleconsultant remotely reviews digital images of challenging cases, has the potential to greatly improve patient care. In the appropriate setting, telepathology is therefore a cost-effective tool that ensures quick turnaround time, virtually eliminates expensive courier costs, improves resource utilization, permits load balancing, and creates added value.[37–39] **Table 2** highlights some of the advantages and disadvantages associated with telepathology applications.

Telepathology has been applied to all divisions of pathology, including surgical pathology, cytopathology, autopsy, and clinical pathology (especially hematopathology and microbiology).[40–43] Telepathology also has been used for sharing electron microscopic images,[44,45] and it has benefited veterinary medicine.[46] Telecytology, the practice of cytology at a distance, has been successful with both gynecologic specimens (eg, Pap tests) and nongynecological cases (eg, fine-needle aspirations).[47–54] Today, telecytology is mostly used for rapid on-site evaluation.[55] Diagnostic accuracy with telecytology is imperfect, and in early published studies ranged from 80% to 100%.[47,56] With improved technology (eg, robotic WSI scanners), diagnostic accuracy has improved. However, the interpretation of telecytology digital images is still hindered by the inability of images to accurately display cellular detail (eg, nuclear chromasia) and to change focus along the z-axis, especially in thick areas with overlapping cell groups.

Telepathology has been widely used for intraoperative consultation (eg, frozen section) at a remote location without a pathologist on-site and/or when traveling and/or when shipment of a specimen may be impracticable.[57–59] Most recently, telepathology has started to be used for making primary diagnoses, but this has occurred in countries (eg, Canada) outside the United States. Another area in which telepathology has been extensively used is to facilitate consultation between pathologists.[60,61] Patient-related material (eg, glass slides) may need to be referred for formal secondary review for a number of reasons; that is, expert opinion requested by the primary pathologist for a difficult case, per patient request, or as a result of a patient being referred to another institution for follow-up care. Traditionally, cases (glass slides) are physically sent via commercial

Table 2
Clinical advantages and disadvantages associated with telepathology applications

Advantages	Disadvantages
Primary Diagnosis	
• Facilitates rapid diagnosis • Cost-effective • Provides coverage for remote sites • Useful for remote frozen sections • Useful for immediate fine-needle aspiration evaluation • Potential to improve patient care • Load balancing	• Difficult to handle certain cases (eg, multiple simultaneous cases) • Deferral to glass slide may be needed • May take longer than glass slide review • Technology errors and downtime • System maintenance required • State limited licensure
Secondary Consultation	
• Access to expert opinions • Real-time consultation • Cheaper than courier services • Faster turnaround time • Original material retained at host institution • Avoids slide loss or damage • Portability of the telepathologist • Virtual collaboration (teleconferencing)	• Difficult to handle certain cases (eg, cases with multiple slides) • Technical failures • Image quality (especially for difficult cases) • Billing arrangements

courier services. Unfortunately, the risk is that shipped slides may get lost or broken.[62] This risk is virtually eliminated with telepathology, and is particularly helpful when making recut sections is unfeasible or when there are only limited slides available for review.

Telepathology and teleconferencing are ideal for educational purposes.[63] In addition to portability and the ease of sharing cases with multiple users, telepathology ensures consistency and longevity of imaged materials for educational purposes, and offers a mechanism to standardize teaching.[64] An increasing number of teaching programs (eg, medical schools, pathology residency training programs, cytotechnology schools) have created "virtual slide sets" to replace traditional slide boxes. Digital images, linked to case-related information, can be offered online for students anywhere, which can be viewed at any time.[65,66] An increasing number of professional societies and organizations are using WSI for conferencing, continuing medical education, scientific meetings, and proficiency testing.

TELECOMMUNICATION

Telecommunication is the transmission of messages over distances for the purpose of communication. Telepathology is becoming easier to implement in most laboratories, primarily because access to broadband telecommunications and wireless technology is more prevalent.[67] Telepathology systems can be linked to a local area

network or wide area network on the Internet via cables, an integrated services digitized network, satellite, or a Wi-Fi connection. The Internet provides universal, simplified, and affordable options for telepathology in most regions. Limitations imposed by the Internet include no guarantees on the quality of service, security and privacy concerns, and for some regions low bandwidth, which negatively impacts real-time applications.[68] Telepathology using wireless telecommunications and mobile phone cellular services has proven to be effective for clinical use.[69,70] Teleconferencing or desktop sharing software (eg, Skype, Lync, Team Viewer), which offers live (synchronous) online communication between distant users, has been used for some telepathology solutions.[71–73] Several online digital sharing services (eg, SecondSlide) have been established. When using a file hosting service (eg, DropBox, PathXchange) for cloud storage and/or file sharing, it is important to make sure that they meet privacy concerns for clinical use, such as the Health Insurance Portability and Accountability Act.

TELEPATHOLOGY MODES AND SYSTEMS

The various modes of telepathology (static, dynamic, WSI, hybrid) are compared in **Table 3**. Static telepathology involves the examination of precaptured still digital images (snapshots) that can be transmitted via e-mail or stored on a shared server. Dynamic telepathology involves the examination of live images or a sequence of images in real time

Table 3
Comparison of different telepathology methods

Telepathology Method	Image System	Remote Control	Images Per Case	Image Selection	Bandwidth Needed	Cost
Static	Still	No	Limited	Host	Low	Low
Dynamic	Live	Yes	Unlimited	Telepathologist	High	High
Whole-slide imaging	Still	Yes	Unlimited	Telepathologist	High	High
Hybrid	Still and Live	Yes	Unlimited	Telepathologist	High	High

using a live telecommunications link. In general, dynamic systems offer greater accuracy because the user can interpret images in real time without limited focus.[74] WSI involves digitization (scanning) of glass slides to produce high-resolution digital slides. Hybrid technology combines robotics with high-resolution imaging.[75–77]

There are several systems available for telepathology. These include gross workstations, microscope cameras, robotic microscopes, and whole-slide scanners. Gross workstations are used primarily to transmit macroscopic images of specimens for gross pathology. Telepathology can be performed using microscopic cameras in 3 ways: (1) static telepathology using a digital camera (or smartphone) attached to a microscope; (2) video microscopy using a video camera connected to a microscope; and (3) teleconferencing where software is used to share the desktop on which a microscopic image is displayed. Early studies using video technology were plagued by slow transmission and poor picture quality.[74,78–81] Robotic telepathology involves remote microscope robotic operation (eg, motorized stage, objectives, and focus). WSI has also been termed wide-field microscopy or "virtual" microscopy. Newer whole-slide scanners now offer remote robotic control to view slides in addition to WSI capabilities.

STATIC TELEPATHOLOGY

Static (store-and-forward) telepathology can be used to share digital images of just about anything in pathology, such as gross specimens, parasites, microbiology culture plates, histopathology, blood smears, and electrophoresis gels. These images may be shared with others via e-mail or stored on a shared server. The person sending the image and the pathologist receiving it do not need to do so simultaneously (ie, asynchronous telepathology).[82] In addition to still images, other types of information that can be transferred with this technique include audio, text, and video files. Static images can be viewed by a single telepathologist or simultaneously by multiple clients

during an online discussion.[83] The benefits of static telepathology are its relatively low cost, simple technology needed, vendor independence, and low maintenance. Moreover, the image files are small and hence easier to manage and store. However, there are several drawbacks, including no remote control access, sampling error, only limited fields of view are available for evaluation, and the host taking the images needs to have some expertise to select appropriate diagnostic fields.[84,85] Static telepathology is typically unsuitable for emergency consultations. Acquiring still images also is labor intensive.

ROBOTIC TELEPATHOLOGY

The first robotic telepathology system was invented and patented by Dr. R.S. Weinstein (Weinstein US Patent #5,216,596). The first patent application was submitted in 1987 and granted in 1993. This form of telepathology involves a robotically controlled microscope with a digital camera attached to the microscope linked to a networked computer. Robotic systems allow one to perform dynamic (real-time) telepathology. The telepathologist has software controls on his or her computer to remotely "drive" (ie, pan and zoom around a slide) and focus the microscope. Advantages of robotic telepathology include access to the entire slide, user control of the microscope and image with respect to fields (panning) and magnification, good image quality, and fast driving speed. In a review of 11 published studies from 1997 to 2007 using robotic telepathology for rendering remote frozen section diagnoses, the diagnostic accuracy ranged between 89% and 100%.[5] Some of the disadvantages include expensive technology, the need for integrated software for both host and recipient, high bandwidth requirements, and the need for ongoing technical support and maintenance.

WHOLE-SLIDE IMAGING

WSI telepathology offers another means to view an entirely digitized (scanned) slide. Whole-slide scanners typically include a slide loader, microscope with different objectives, digital camera, robotics, and software. Slide loaders range from trays that hold 1 to 4 slides to large racks or hotels that can stack up to 400 slides. For recently mounted slides (eg, frozen section slides with a movable coverslip), it is better to use horizontal loading rather than vertical placement. Slide scanning can be automated or done manually. Slides can be scanned using an objective lens magnification of ×20, ×40, or higher depending on the telepathology need. For routine surgical pathology work, ×20 should suffice; however, for hematopathology cases, ×40 may be preferred, and for telemicrobiology even higher magnification (eg, ×83 oil magnification). The focal plane (orthogonal disposition) also will need to be set before scanning. For cytology cases, z-stacking is often desirable. Although scanning at higher magnification takes longer and results in larger image files, the digital images are of better resolution and offer superior zoom capability. However, large files (eg, 150 GB without compression) require good computer microprocessors and adequate RAM to manipulate them.

WSI has been shown to be remarkably suitable for telepathology, because digital slides are of high resolution and permit access to an entire slide or set of slides at various magnifications.[86,87] Once the scanned slide is ready, viewing the digital image to render a diagnosis can be faster than using a robotic microscope, especially if performed on a computer with a high-speed network connection. The length of time required to prepare slides for scanning and conduct previsualization quality checks should be taken into account when using WSI for rapid telepathology, such as during frozen sections. In one study comparing the time requirements of robotic versus virtual slide telepathology for frozen sections, investigators found that slide preparation time for both modalities was comparable (average 10.33 minutes for robotic vs 12.26 minutes for virtual slides), but that slide interpretation time was far superior with digital slides (average 10.26 minutes for robotic vs 3.42 minutes for virtual slides).[5] Because of the ease related to sharing files and the interactive nature of viewing images, WSI is incredibly effective for education.[88]

At present, WSI telepathology equipment is still expensive for many laboratories. Added expense may be incurred with storage of large image files. With newer scanners, rapid scanning is possible. However, long scan times may result if high-resolution, multiplane images are desired or when digitizing slides with large, thick tissue sections. Scanning difficulties may arise as a result of cover slip misplacement or wet slides with too much mounting medium that stick with automatic slide feeders. Small tissue fragments, faint tissue, or material at the slide edge or even outside the coverslip may not get scanned. For cytopathology, WSI may be problematic without z-stacking. Anther disadvantage of WSI is related to the fact that with some scanners, slides may need to be scanned one at a time. Also, there is currently a lack of vendor interoperability, making it difficult to sometimes view proprietary image files with different viewers.

REFERENCES

1. Weinberg DS. How is telepathology being used to improve patient care? Clin Chem 1996;42:831–5.
2. Weinstein RS, Bhattacharyya AK, Graham AR, et al. Telepathology: a ten-year progress report. Hum Pathol 1997;28:1–7.
3. Kayser K, Szymas J, Weinstein R. Telepathology. Telecommunication, electronic education and publication in pathology. Berlin: Springer; 1999. p. 1–186.
4. Weinstein RS, Graham AR, Richter LC, et al. Overview of telepathology, virtual microscopy, and whole slide imaging: prospects for the future. Hum Pathol 2009;40:1057–69.
5. Evans AJ, Chetty R, Clarke BA, et al. Primary frozen section diagnosis by robotic microscopy and virtual slide telepathology: the University Health Network experience. Hum Pathol 2009;40:1070–81.
6. Evans AJ, Kiehl TR, Croul S. Frequently asked questions concerning the use of whole-slide imaging telepathology for neuropathology frozen sections. Semin Diagn Pathol 2010;27(3):160–6.
7. Agha Z, Weinstein RS, Dunn BE. Cost minimization analysis of telepathology. Am J Clin Pathol 1999;112:470–8.
8. Kayser K, Beyer M, Blum S, et al. Recent developments and present status of telepathology. Anal Cell Pathol 2000;21:101–6.
9. Weinstein RS, Descour MR, Liang C, et al. Telepathology overview: from concept to implementation. Hum Pathol 2001;32:1283–99.
10. Massone C, Brunasso AM, Campbell TM, et al. State of the art of teledermatopathology. Am J Dermatopathol 2008;30:446–50.
11. Graham AR, Bhattacharyya AK, Scott KM, et al. Virtual slide telepathology for an academic teaching hospital surgical pathology quality assurance program. Hum Pathol 2009;40:1129–36.
12. Lopez AM, Graham AR, Barker GP, et al. Virtual slide telepathology enables an innovative telehealth rapid breast care clinic. Hum Pathol 2009;40:1082–91.
13. Weinstein RS. Prospects for telepathology [editorial]. Hum Pathol 1986;17:433–4.
14. Weinstein RS, Descour MR, Liang C, et al. An array microscope for ultrarapid virtual slide processing

and telepathology. Design, fabrication, and validation study. Hum Pathol 2004;35:1303–14.

15. Williams S, Henricks WH, Becich MJ, et al. Telepathology for patient care: what am I getting myself into? Adv Anat Pathol 2010;17:130–49.

16. Kayser K, Szymas J, Weinstein RS. Telepathology and telemedicine: communication, electronic education and publication in e-health. Berlin: VSV Interdisciplinary Medical Publishing; 2005. p. 1–257.

17. Dunn BE, Choi H, Recla DL, et al. Robotic surgical telepathology between the Iron Mountain and Milwaukee Department of Veterans Affairs medical centers: a 12-year experience. Hum Pathol 2009;40:1092–9.

18. Halliday BE, Bhattacharyya AK, Graham AR, et al. Diagnostic accuracy of an international static-imaging telepathology consultation service. Hum Pathol 1997;28:17–21.

19. Nordrum I, Engum B, Rinde E, et al. Remote frozen section service: a telepathology project to northern Norway. Hum Pathol 1991;22:514–8.

20. Kaplan KJ, Burgess JR, Sandberg GD, et al. Use of robotic telepathology for frozen-section diagnosis: a retrospective trial of a telepathology system for intraoperative consultation. Mod Pathol 2002;15:1197–204.

21. O'Malley DP. Practical applications of telepathology using morphology-based anatomic pathology. Arch Pathol Lab Med 2008;132:743–4.

22. Pantanowitz L, Evans AJ, Hassell LA, et al. American Telemedicine Association clinical guidelines for telepathology. J Pathol Inform 2014;5:39.

23. Canadian Association of Pathologists Telepathology Guidelines Committee, Bernard C, Chandrakanth SA, et al. Guidelines from the Canadian Association of Pathologists for establishing a telepathology service for anatomic pathology using whole-slide imaging. J Pathol Inform 2014;28(5):15.

24. Lowe J. Telepathology: guideline from the Royal College of Pathologists. London. 2013. Available at: http://www.rcpath.org/Resources/RCPath/Migrated%20Resources/Documents/G/G026_Telepathology_Oct13.pdf. Accessed March 18, 2015.

25. Leung ST, Kaplan KJ. Medicolegal aspects of telepathology. Hum Pathol 2009;40:1137–42.

26. Güler NF, Ubeyli ED. Theory and applications of telemedicine. J Med Syst 2002;26:199–220.

27. Hoyt R, Sutton M, Yoshihashi A. Medical informatics. Practical guide for the healthcare professional. Pensacola (FL): University of West Florida Press; 2007. p. 197–206.

28. Fox BI. Telehealth. In: Felkey BG, Fox BI, Thrower MR, editors. Health care informatics: a skills-based resource. Washington, DC: American Pharmacists Association; 2006. p. 277–300.

29. Stanberry B. Telemedicine: barriers and opportunities in the 21st century. J Intern Med 2000;247:615–28.

30. Picot J. Meeting the need for educational standards in the practice of telemedicine and telehealth. J Telemed Telecare 2000;2(6 Suppl):S59–62.

31. Wells CA, Sowter C. Telepathology: a diagnostic tool for the millennium? J Pathol 2000;191:1–7.

32. Dunn BE, Almagro UA, Choi H, et al. Dynamic-robotic telepathology: Department of Veterans Affairs feasibility study. Hum Pathol 1997;28:8–12.

33. Weinstein RS, Bloom KJ, Rozek LS. Static and dynamic imaging in pathology. IEEE Proc Image Management Comm 1990;1:77–85.

34. Krupinski E, Weinstein RS, Bloom KJ, et al. Progress in telepathology: system implementation and testing. Advances in Path Lab Med 1993;6:63–87.

35. Mullick FG, Fontelo P, Pemble C. Telemedicine and telepathology at the Armed Forces Institute of Pathology: history and current mission. Telemed J 1996;2:187–93.

36. Ongürü O, Celasun B. Intra-hospital use of a telepathology system. Pathol Oncol Res 2000;6:197–201.

37. Ho J, Ahlers SM, Stratman C, et al. Can digital pathology result in cost savings? A financial projection for digital pathology implementation at a large integrated health care organization. J Pathol Inform 2014;5:33.

38. Henricks WH. Evaluation of whole slide imaging for routine surgical pathology: Looking through a broader scope. J Pathol Inform 2012;3:30.

39. Fine JL. 21st century workflow: a proposal. J Pathol Inform 2014;5:44.

40. Brebner EM, Brebner JA, Norman JN, et al. Intercontinental postmortem studies using interactive television. J Telemed Telecare 1997;3:48–52.

41. Fisher SI, Nandedkar MA, Williams BH, et al. Tolehematopathology in a clinical consultative practice. Hum Pathol 2001;32:1327–33.

42. McLaughlin WJ, Schifman RB, Ryan KJ, et al. Telemicrobiology: feasibility study. Telemed J 1998;4:11–7.

43. Suhanic W, Crandall I, Pennefather P. An informatics model for guiding assembly of telemicrobiology workstations for malaria collaborative diagnostics using commodity products and open-source software. Malar J 2009;8:164.

44. Schroeder JA. Ultrasructural telepathology: remote EM diagnostic via Internet. In: Kumar S, Dunn BE, editors. Telepathology, vol. 14. Berlin: Springer; 2009. p. 179–204.

45. Yamada A. Remote control of the scanning electron microscope. In: Kumar S, Dunn BE, editors. Telepathology, vol. 15. Berlin: Springer; 2009. p. 205–24.

46. Maiolino P, De Vico G. Telepathology in veterinary diagnostic cytology. In: Kumar S, Dunn BE, editors. Telepathology, vol. 6. Berlin: Springer; 2009. p. 63–70.

47. Pantanowitz L, Hornish M, Goulart RA. The impact of digital imaging in the field of cytopathology. Cytojournal 2009;6:6.

48. Lee ES, Kim IS, Choi JS, et al. Accuracy and reproducibility of telecytology diagnosis of cervical smears. A tool for quality assurance programs. Am J Clin Pathol 2003;119:356–60.

49. Raab SS, Zaleski MS, Thomas PA, et al. Telecytology: diagnostic accuracy in cervical-vaginal smears. Am J Clin Pathol 1996;105:599–603.

50. Schwarzmann P, Schenck U, Binder B, et al. Is today's telepathology equipment also appropriate for telecytology? A pilot study with pap and blood smears. Adv Clin Path 1998;2:176–8.

51. Ziol M, Vacher-Lavenu MC, Heudes D, et al. Expert consultation for cervical carcinoma smears. Reliability of selected-field videomicroscopy. Anal Quant Cytol Histol 1999;21:35–41.

52. Eichhorn JH, Buckner L, Buckner SB, et al. Internet-based gynecologic telecytology with remote automated image selection: results of a first-phase developmental trial. Am J Clin Pathol 2008;129:686–96.

53. Prayaga A. Telecytology: a retrospect and prospect. In: Kumar S, Dunn BE, editors. Telepathology, vol. 12. Berlin: Springer; 2009. p. 149–62.

54. Thrall M, Pantanowitz L, Khalbuss W. Telecytology: clinical applications, current challenges, and future benefits. J Pathol Inform 2011;2:51.

55. Kerr SE, Bellizzi AM, Stelow EB, et al. Initial assessment of fine-needle aspiration specimens by telepathology: validation for use in pathology resident-faculty consultations. Am J Clin Pathol 2008;130:409–13.

56. Allen EA, Ollayos CW, Tellado MV, et al. Characteristics of a telecytology consultation service. Hum Pathol 2001;32:1323–6.

57. Wellnitz U, Binder B, Fritz P, et al. Reliability of telepathology for frozen section service. Anal Cell Pathol 2000;21:213–22.

58. Winokur TS, McClellan S, Siegal GP, et al. A prospective trial of telepathology for intraoperative consultation (frozen sections). Hum Pathol 2000;31:781–5.

59. Liang WY, Hsu CY, Lai CR, et al. Low-cost telepathology system for intraoperative frozen-section consultation: our experience and review of the literature. Hum Pathol 2008;39:56–62.

60. Beltrami CA, Della Mea V. Second opinion consultation through the Internet. A three years experience. Adv Clin Path 1998;2:146–8.

61. Piccolo D, Soyer HP, Burgdorf W, et al. Concordance between telepathologic diagnosis and conventional histopathologic diagnosis: a multiobserver store-and-forward study on 20 skin specimens. Arch Dermatol 2002;138:53–8.

62. Rosen PP. Special report: perils, problems, and minimum requirements in shipping pathology slides. Am J Clin Pathol 1989;91:348–54.

63. Romer DJ, Suster S. Use of virtual microscopy for didactic live-audience presentation in anatomic pathology. Ann Diagn Pathol 2003;7:67–72.

64. Helin H, Lundin M, Lundin J, et al. Web-based virtual microscopy in teaching and standardizing Gleason grading. Hum Pathol 2005;36:381–6.

65. Bruch LA, De Young BR, Kreiter CD, et al. Competency assessment of residents in surgical pathology using virtual microscopy. Hum Pathol 2009;40:1122–8.

66. Dee FR. Virtual microscopy in pathology education. Hum Pathol 2009;40:1112–21.

67. Alfaro L, Roca MJ. Portable telepathology: methods and tools. Diagn Pathol 2008;3(Suppl 1):S19.

68. Dolla Mea V, Beltrami CA. Current experiences with Internet telepathology and possible evolution in the next generation of Internet services. Anal Cell Pathol 2000;21:127–34.

69. Frierson HF Jr, Galgano MT. Frozen-section diagnosis by wireless telepathology and ultra portable computer: use in pathology resident/faculty consultation. Hum Pathol 2007;38:1330–4.

70. Bellina L, Missoni E. Mobile cell-phones (M-phones) in telemicroscopy: increasing connectivity of isolated laboratories. Diagn Pathol 2009;4:19.

71. Marchevsky AM, Lau SK, Khanafshar E, et al. Internet teleconferencing method for telepathology consultations from lung and heart transplant patients. Hum Pathol 2002;33:410–4.

72. McKenna JK, Florell SR. Cost-effective dynamic telepathology in the Mohs surgery laboratory utilizing iChat AV videoconferencing software. Dermatol Surg 2007;33:62–8.

73. Klock C, Gomes Rde P. Web conferencing systems: Skype and MSN in telepathology. Diagn Pathol 2008;3(Suppl 1):S13.

74. Smith MB. Introduction to telepathology. In: Cowan DF, editor. Informatics for the clinical laboratory. A practical guide for the practicing pathologist, vol. 16. New York: Springer; 2005. p. 268–86.

75. Tsuchihashi Y, Mazaki T, Nakasato K, et al. The basic diagnostic approaches used in robotic still-image telepathology. J Telemed Telecare 1999;5(Suppl 1):S115–7.

76. Zhou J, Hogarth MA, Walters RF, et al. Hybrid system for telepathology. Hum Pathol 2000;31:829–33.

77. Della Mea V, Cataldi P, Pertoldi B, et al. Combining dynamic- and static-robotic techniques for real-time telepathology. In: Kumar S, Dunn BE, editors. Telepathology, vol. 8. Berlin: Springer; 2009. p. 79–89.

78. Callas PW, Leslie KO, Mattia AR, et al. Diagnostic accuracy of a rural live video telepathology system. Am J Surg Pathol 1997;21:812–9.

79. Baak JP, van Diest PJ, Meijer GA. Experience with a dynamic inexpensive video-conferencing system for frozen section telepathology. Anal Cell Pathol 2000;21:169–75.

80. Prasse KW, Mahaffey EA, Duncan JR, et al. Accuracy of interpretation of microscopic images of

cytologic, hematologic, and histologic specimens using a low-resolution desktop video conferencing system. Telemed J 1996;2:259–66.

81. Vazir MH, Loane MA, Wootton R. A pilot study of low-cost dynamic telepathology using the public telephone network. J Telemed Telecare 1998;4: 168–71.

82. Della Mea V. Prerecorded telemedicine. J Telemed Telecare 2005;11:276–84.

83. Brauchli K, Oberli H, Hurwitz N, et al. Diagnostic telepathology: long-term experience of a single institution. Virchows Arch 2004;444:403–9.

84. Della Mea V, Cataldi P, Boi S, et al. Image selection in static telepathology through the Internet. J Telemed Telecare 1998;4(Suppl 1):20–2.

85. Della Mea V, Cataldi P, Boi S, et al. Image sampling in static telepathology for frozen section diagnosis. J Clin Pathol 1999;52:761–5.

86. Wilbur DC, Madi K, Colvin RB, et al. Whole-slide imaging digital pathology as a platform for teleconsultation: a pilot study using paired subspecialist correlations. Arch Pathol Lab Med 2009;133:1949–53.

87. Furness P. A randomized controlled trial of the diagnostic accuracy of Internet-based telepathology compared with conventional microscopy. Histopathology 2007;50:266–73.

88. Góngora Jará H, Barcelo HA. Telepathology and continuous education: important tools for pathologists of developing countries. Diagn Pathol 2008; 3(Suppl 1):S24.

Mobile Technologies for the Surgical Pathologist

Douglas J. Hartman, MD

KEYWORDS

- Mobile technology • Education • Digital consultations • Mobile image analysis
- Barriers to implementation of mobile technology

ABSTRACT

Recent advances in hardware and computing power contained within mobile devices have made it possible to use these devices to improve and enhance pathologist workflow. This article discusses the possible uses ranging from basic functions to intermediate functions to advanced functions. Barriers to implementation are also discussed.

OVERVIEW

Recent advances in the hardware capabilities housed within cellular phones have led to the creation of so-called smartphones. These smartphones are being rapidly adopted and an emerging mobile health (mHealth) field has begun. This rapid growth represents an opportunity and a challenge for clinical laboratories.[1] Smartphones are cellular phones equipped with Internet functionality as well as having image capture capabilities through built-in cameras. Although smartphones are generally considered the predominant mobile device, tablet computers also run on the same operating systems (so-called mobile computing). For the purposes of this discussion, both smartphone technology and mobile computing are collectively referred to as mobile technologies. There are several mobile technologies now at the hands of the diagnostic surgical pathologist. These technologies can be grouped into 3 categories: (1) basic functions, (2) intermediate functions, and (3) advanced functions. Basic functions essentially represent electronic versions of paper documents or interfaces to clinical systems. Intermediate functions contain an interactive component (ie, calculators that take in data and provide an output or simplify a process). Advanced functions are in early development and have not yet been realized, but several possible directions are discussed. Each month new developments are introduced within this arena. By 2020, some experts have predicted that 25% of all patient encounters could be through mHealth.[2]

BASIC FUNCTIONS OF SMARTPHONE APPLICATIONS

FLASH CARDS

Several applications for pathology have been created for educational purposes. Some of this educational material is tailored toward United States Medical Licensing Examination (USMLE) Board pathology study materials, including Flash Cards for Robbins, Rubin's, Lange Medical, and McGraw-Hill (**Box 1**). Additionally, there is an application for Pathology Case Files from McGraw-Hill.

PUBLICATIONS

Some applications have been created for pathology publications. This is likely to increase in the coming years because it brings the educational material to the pockets/hands of the people who need the information. These advances mimic the increased consumer use of tablets/readers. Current pathology journals with mobile applications connected to published articles include *Journal of Pathology*, *American Journal of Clinical Pathology*, and *Cancer Cytopathology* (**Box 2**). The American Society for Clinical Pathology has also

---

Disclosure Statement: Author for one up-to-date on topic - Clinical Pathological Cases in Gastroenterology, otherwise no disclosures.
Department of Anatomic Pathology, University of Pittsburgh Medical Center, 200 Lothrop Street, A-607, Pittsburgh, PA 15213, USA
E-mail address: hartmandj@upmc.edu

Surgical Pathology 8 (2015) 233–238
http://dx.doi.org/10.1016/j.path.2015.02.007

Box 1
Electronic versions of traditionally paper-based resources

- Robbins Pathology Flash Cards
- Rubin's Pathology Flash Cards
- McGraw-Hill Flash Cards
- McGraw-Hill Pathology Case Files
- Lange Medical Flash Cards

published several e-books. More journals are likely to respond to this increased demand and offer their articles on a mobile platform.

NATIONAL MEETINGS/CONFERENCES

Some applications have been created to facilitate attendee experience at pathology conferences. These include PathVisions national meetings in 2012 and 2013, American Pathology Foundation meetings, and the American Society for Clinical Pathology national meeting (**Box 3**). These applications are intended to enhance the users' experience at the conference/meeting. They assist to digest/organize the numerous educational opportunities that are presented at national meetings.

LABORATORY INFORMATION SYSTEMS MOBILE APPLICATIONS

Several applications have been created to interface with pathology laboratory information systems and whole-slide imaging platforms. The most mature available whole-slide imaging product is the Aperio product, and a mobile application to view images on smartphones is available through the ePathViewer application. There is also a mobile application available for interface with PathX laboratory information system. Pathologists can use this application to view and sign out

Box 2
Journals/professional society meetings with mobile applications

- *Journal of Pathology*
- *American Journal of Clinical Pathology*
- *Cancer Cytopathology*
- American Society of Clinical Pathology e-books
- PathVisions Meeting (2012 and 2013)
- American Pathology Foundation
- American Society for Clinical Pathology national meeting

Box 3
Interfaces with machines/whole-slide imaging platforms

- SlidePath (Leica)
- PathX
- Mobile version of PathXchange
- InterPath (Aperio)
- ePathViewer (Aperio)

cases and follow their case queues; other clinicians also can view the current stage for pathology reports. Mobile applications to interact with the electronic medical record have recently been developed.[3,4] Within the University of Pittsburgh Medical Center Health System, we have piloted the use of a new mobile platform for accessing electronic health record systems.[4,5] This has received good reviews although it is still in the early phase of adoption.[4,5]

EDUCATION

There is great interest in increasing health education of the population with the use of mobile devices.[6–9] Some investigators, however, have implemented mobile-based teaching platforms for the education of future physicians. For instance, podcasting of medical lectures has become a popular activity in anatomy classes.[10–15] These devices offer resources at students' fingertips whenever they like to tap into resources. Mobile technology resources have also been developed to facilitate house staff and/or hospital staff education as well.[16–21]

INTERMEDIATE FUNCTIONS OF SMARTPHONE APPLICATIONS

Intermediate functions of smartphone applications can be seen in 3 subgroups: (1) electronic calculators (an application that returns a clinical recommendation based on user input), (2) differential diagnoses tools (differential diagnoses are proposed based on user input), and (3) digital consultations (streamlined process for more rapid processing of consultations).

ELECTRONIC CALCULATORS

In the era of evidence-based medicine, many clinical guidelines/algorithms have been developed for patient management. The complexity of these guidelines/algorithms reflects the increasingly specialized level of medical care now considered standard of care. This is particularly prevalent for cytology specimens. Sometimes the findings under the microscope are the sole determinant of clinical action whereas other times it is a combination of factors that determines the clinical management for a patient. Guidelines for the clinical management of patients with Papanicolaou smears have been around for a long time. Two smartphone applications can be used to input clinical data to determine the appropriate follow-up/next step in a patient's care—American Society for Colposcopy and Cervical Pathology (ASCCP) Mobile ($9.99, iTunes Store) and Pap Reader (free, iTunes Store). These applications accept input from user and return what the appropriate follow-up/next step should be. The inputs include cytology interpretation, human papillomavirus status, pregnancy status, and age. These steps are programmed based on the consensus guideline recommendations from the ASCCP. There are also applications for the interpretation/management of thyroid fine-needle aspiration results based on the 2009 American Thyroid Association guidelines (FNA Reader, free, iTunes Store).

Another such application, called HER2 Reader (free, iTunes Store), was produced by the American Society of Clinical Oncology and can be used to input HER2 immunohistochemistry (percentage of cells, circumferential membrane staining, and intensity) with a resulting interpretation. This same application can also calculate results of in situ hybridization when HER2 signals per cell and CEP17 signals per cell are supplied. This application can also provide an interpretation of estrogen receptor and progesterone receptor immunohistochemistry based on input of the percent of cells and the intensity.

TUMOR STAGING AND PEDIATRIC MEASUREMENTS

There are several tumor-staging guides (at least 11 within Apple's iTunes Store) based predominantly on the American Joint Committee on Cancer staging guidelines for carcinomas. Some are organ specific (just for lung or skin) whereas others are more general. The prices range between 0 to $4.99 for each application. PedsPath (free, iTunes Store) is a mobile application that allows "residents, fellows and attending physicians in the pediatric and perinatal pathology discipline to quickly look-up various measurement values applicable to live-born, stillborn, placenta and infants."

DIFFERENTIAL DIAGNOSIS TOOLS

Several applications have been created to help in generating a differential diagnosis. Two examples

of these are myDermPath (free, iTunes Store) and Oral Pathology Differential Diagnosis Generator ($119.99, iTunes Store). myDermPath application, developed by Drs R. Singh, T. Ferringer, and D. Elston, is "a user-friendly and interactive application for both learning and practice of dermatopathology." The Oral Pathology Differential Diagnosis accepts "category based user inputs" and returns a list of "non-ordered conditions" and "accessible full-articles from the U.S. National Library of Medicine" Of course, these diagnostic tools are not intended to replace an expert dermatopathologist or an oral pathologist.

IMAGE ACQUISITION

Mobile devices can be used for more than simple calculators or electronic resource libraries for surgical pathologists—they can be used for image acquisition from a microscope. Either by placing the camera against the ocular lens of a microscope or through the use of an inexpensive adapter, a smartphone can be used to acquire microscopic images.[22–24] The variety of smartphones described includes smartphones operating on Android, iPhone, and Windows mobile operating systems. The quality of camera contained within smartphones has shown a progressive improvement. In 2011, the standard camera on a smartphone was an 8-megapixel camera, which represented a drastic change from just 2 years prior.[25] The recent introduction of a 41-megapixel camera by Nokia is the largest megapixel camera available within a smartphone.[26]

CONSULTATION

An application called iDermpath (free, iTunes Store) has been developed for clients of Fleming Dermatopathology (a dermatopathology practice based in Milwaukee, Wisconsin). The application includes wireless access for clients to their pathology reports, including push notification when the new reports are completed. Both clinical requisitions and accompanying photographs can be submitted through the application. The application is Health Insurance Portability and Accountability Act (HIPAA) compliant and secure.

Some investigators have used mobile technology to provide medical expertise to underserved areas. Bellina and Missoni[27,28] have been using mobile technology to provide remote support for extensions in sub-Saharan Africa. The investigators report their experience with using built-in cameras not only to perform diagnostic work for underserved areas but also to provide educational training (particularly for women) so that underserved areas can have access to medical resources.[27,28]

POCKET PATHOLOGIST

Traditionally, consultations required packaging the original diagnostic glass slides (or a subset of them) and sending them through the mail or a shipping service to an external consultant. Given that the slides are important for medical/legal purposes, sending slides outside the original department can be problematic. Additionally, for a particular case, the sending pathologist must determine whether the case warrants a second opinion. The author and colleagues developed a tool for rapid consultation submission via an iPhone-based application, termed Pocket Pathologist (free, iTunes Store), that is connected to a digital consultation portal.[29] This tool allows a submitting pathologist to submit between 5 and 7 data points along with an image directly acquired by a smartphone camera from the microscope.[29] This is possible because there are several commercially available adapters that can be used to mount a smartphone to a microscope to obtain images.[29] Although the adapters designed for iPhones have less adjustment required during setup, there are adapters for non-iPhone smartphones and once the adjustment for an individual smartphone is performed the settings remain.[23] The images can either be acquired straight from the Pocket Pathologist application or they can be uploaded into the online submission form from the image gallery on the phone.[29] This process uses a secure server and is HIPAA compliant. Once uploaded, the case is sent to a center of excellence or designated pathologist via electronic mail notification. A consultation is completed and the submitting pathologist is notified via electronic mail that the digital consultation has been completed. If additional studies/images are needed, the Web-based application allows for communication between consultant and submitting pathologist.

MOBILE PHONE MICROSCOPE

One group has created a device using a 3-D printer that includes an LED light source powered by a watch battery coupled with a smartphone to replace the entire microscope setup.[30] The intended use for this is in resource-poor areas or outside the hospital environment. This represents a cheap alternative to a microscope along with the ability to tap into subspecialty expertise via the Internet. These features could help disseminate health care expertise to rural or underserved populations.

FUTURE DIRECTIONS/ADVANCED FUNCTIONS

Mobile technology's recent widespread adoption has led to a rapid expansion to the functional capabilities that can be performed with mobile devices. It is difficult to predict how future hardware and software advances will change the capabilities of these devices. The implementation of meaningful use is mandating patient engagement, and mobile technology represents a ready solution to for this requirement.[2]

HARDWARE

Hardware improvements are introduced with nearly each iteration of a device. In recent years, these improvements have been largely recognized within the camera hardware aspects. Improvements, such as better built-in video recording (largely driven by consumer demand), will likely make it easier to harness some of these functionalities for diagnostic pathology work. Although a single microscopic field may be of interest (because that is where the diagnostic question exists), a consultant may want to view an entire tissue contained on a slide or, at minimum, the surrounding tissues. Advanced video recording capabilities may facilitate the acquisition of a virtual whole-slide image, expanding the number of cases that may be amenable to digital consultation methods.

VIDEO

Additional changes within the video recording available on smartphones could potentially allow for a narrative by a submitting pathologist. By receiving a verbal description of a submitting pathologist's thought process, a consultant may be able to provide some further education along with diagnostic assistance on a difficult case. This technology could also be used to perform a 2-way verbal dialog between a submitting pathologist and consultant, creating an asynchronous interaction. Such interactions should improve the quality delivered by submitting pathologists as well as bring subspecialty expertise to the fingertips of submitting pathologists.

MOBILE IMAGE ANALYSIS

Mobile-based image analysis is still in its early stages. Although efforts, such as the Google Car, have been started to have computers interact with their environment, these systems are still heavily dependent on structured architecture (precise maps, specific heights for traffic lights, and so forth).[31] The development of image analysis software on standard computing platforms may represent a possible pathway to use image analysis on a mobile platform. Mobile devices have already been widely adopted for use, and the software needs to be developed to realize the gains of ready access and portable accessibility.

WHOLE-SLIDE IMAGING

Given the widespread availability of mobile devices, there is increased user demand to have the same functional capability within a mobile device that is present within desktop computing. Although the portability offered by mobile devices is highly desirable, the portability presents a new challenge for maintaining security measures. Although still early in implementation, the introduction of whole-slide imaging may be facilitated by the use of a mobile application that interacts with the whole-slide imaging program. Early navigation within whole-slide imaging applications has been largely mouse based, which creates a much different user experience from the traditional glass slide across a microscope stage.

WEARABLE TECHNOLOGY

Wearable mobile devices, such as glasses and watches, are now coming onto the market. There are several clinical applications that have been published using mobile technology to monitor chronic conditions, such as asthma, massive transfusion, and home care for pediatric patients after transplantation.[32–34] The use of glasses to capture images from a microscope may represent a streamlined and improved workflow for surgical pathologists. It is unclear how this functionality within the smartphones could be applied to surgical pathologists' workflow.

BARRIERS TO IMPLEMENTATION

Mobile devices have some inherent limitations—namely battery life, reception, and Internet connectivity—either through a 3G/4G network or a WiFi-enabled network connection. Each of these components is being improved on with the next iterations of the smartphones. Several operating systems exist within the mobile environment—Android, webOS, iOS, Symbian, Windows Mobile Professional, Windows Mobile Standard, Bada, and BlackBerry OS.[35] Although applications often are released around the same time for both iPhone and Android systems, the other operating systems may lag behind in development. The mobile device environment has seen major swings in the preferred device—for instance, BlackBerry devices were popular in the early 2000s but

have lost their place in the market. Certain components of the current image capture ability of smartphone cameras are locked by manufacturers, preventing developers from more fully exploiting the functionality of the cameras.[30] Although increased ability to modify components of image capture could be desirable, it also presents some challenges (companies need to support additional functions, and coordination between developers and manufacturers need to occur).[30] The current demand from the end user is a "bring your own device" mentality, which places the onus on the delivery system to be able to accommodate multiple mobile devices.[1] This is a labor-intensive task and likely to impede widespread adoption. Regulations, such as HIPAA, are changing to accommodate the rapid changes occurring in mobile security and technology.[2] Privacy and compatibility across devices have been cited as potential barriers to adoption of mHealth technology.[36]

SUMMARY

The recent advances in the hardware and computing power contained within mobile devices have made it possible to use these devices to improve and enhance pathologist workflow. The possible uses range from basic functions to intermediate functions to advanced functions. Basic functions include flash cards for USMLE and pathology board studies, published journal articles/e-books, and interfaces with clinical laboratory information systems. Intermediate functions include electronic calculators to decide about appropriate follow-up or next clinical management step, differential diagnosis tools for histologic findings, and digital consultation services. Advanced functions are still under development and are likely to be exciting new tools in the future.

REFERENCES

1. Available at: http://www.darkdaily.com/clinical-pathology-laboratories-ignore-the-rapid-growth-of-mobile-apps-in-healthcare-at-their-peril-921#axzz3C5DIJSKS. Accessed August 31, 2014.
2. Weinstein RS, Lopez AM, Joseph BA, et al. Telemedicine, telehealth, and mobile health applications that work: opportunities and barriers. Am J Med 2014; 127(3):183–7.
3. Kim Y, Kim SS, Kang S, et al. Development of mobile platform integrated with existing electronic medical records. Healthc Inform Res 2014;20(3):231–5.
4. Available at: http://upmctdc.com/Pages/convergence.aspx. Accessed August 31, 2014.

5. Available at: http://www.healthitoutcomes.com/doc/upmc-s-convergence-recognized-for-improving-ehr-access-0001. Accessed August 31, 2014.

6. Hartzler A, Wetter T. Engaging patients through mobile phones: demonstrator services, success factors and future opportunities in low and middle-income countries. Yearb Med Inform 2014;9(1):182–94.

7. Hallberg I, Taft C, Ranerup A, et al. Phases in development of an interactive mobile phone-based system to support self-management of hypertension. Integr Blood Press Control 2014;7:19–28.

8. Cho MJ, Sim JL, Hwang SY. Development of smartphone educational application for patients with coronary artery disease. Healthc Inform Res 2014;20(2):117–24.

9. Sharifi M, Dryden EM, Horan CM, et al. Leveraging text messaging and mobile technology to support pediatric obesity-related behavior change: a qualitative study using parent focus groups and interviews. J Med Internet Res 2013;15(12):e272.

10. Trelease RB. Diffusion of innovations: smartphones and wireless anatomy learning resources. Anat Sci Educ 2008;1(6):233–9.

11. Pickering JD. Anatomy drawing screencasts: enabling flexible learning for medical students. Anat Sci Educ 2014. [Epub ahead of print].

12. Jang HW, Kim KJ. Use of online clinical videos for clinical skills training for medical students: benefits and challenges. BMC Med Educ 2014;14:56.

13. Alegria DA, Boscardin C, Poncelet A, et al. Using tablets to support self-regulated learning in a longitudinal integrated clerkship. Med Educ Online 2014;19:23638.

14. Bahner DP, Adkins E, Patel N, et al. How we use social media to supplement a novel curriculum in medical education. Med Teach 2012;34(60):439–44.

15. Lewis TL, Burnett B, Tunstall RG, et al. Complementing anatomy education using three-dimensional anatomy mobile software applications on tablet computers. Clin Anat 2014;27(3):313–20.

16. Chu LF, Erlendson MJ, Sun JS, et al. Information technology and its role in anaesthesia training and continuing medical education. Best Pract Res Clin Anaesthesiol 2012;26(1):33–53.

17. Mather C, Cummings E. Mobile learning: a workforce development strategy for nurse supervisors. Stud Health Technol Inform 2014;204:98–103.

18. Hardyman W, Bullock A, Brown A, et al. Mobile technology supporting trainee doctor's workplace learning and patient care: an evaluation. BMC Med Educ 2013;13:6.

19. Sclafani J, Tirrell TF, Franko OI. Mobile tablet use among academic physicians and trainees. J Med Syst 2013;37(1):9903.

20. Korbage AC, Bedi HS. Mobile technology in radiology resident education. J Am Coll Radiol 2012;9(6):426–9.

21. Davis JS, Garcia GD, Wyckoff MM, et al. Use of mobile learning module improves skills in chest tube insertion. J Surg Res 2012;177(1):21–6.

22. Morrison AS, Gardner JM. Smart phone microscopic photography: a novel tool for physicians and trainees. Arch Pathol Lab Med 2014;138(8):1002.

23. Roy S, Pantanowitz L, Amin M, et al. Technical note: smartphone adapters for digital photomicrography. J Pathol Inform 2014;5:24.

24. Graff JP, Wu ML. The Nokia Lumia 1020 smartphone as a 41-Megapixel photomicroscope. Histopathology 2014;64:1044.

25. Available at: http://www.pcworld.com/article/2466500/how-the-smartphone-defeated-the-point-and-shoot-digital-camera.html. Accessed August 31, 2014.

26. Available at: http://www.nokia.com/us-en/phones/phone/lumia1020/. Accessed August 31, 2014.

27. Bellina L, Missoni E. Mobile cell-phones (M-Phones) in telemicroscopy: increasing connectivity of isolated laboratories. Diagn Pathol 2009;4:19.

28. Bellina L, Missoni E. Mobile diagnosis: bridging the sociocultural gaps and empowering women. Telemed J E Health 2011;17(9):750.

29. Hartman DJ, Parwani AV, Cable B, et al. Pocket pathologist: a mobile application for rapid diagnostic surgical pathology consultation. J Pathol Inform 2014;5:10.

30. Skandarajah A, Reber CD, Switz NA, et al. Quantitative imaging with a mobile phone microscope. PLoS One 2014;9(5):e96906.

31. Available at: http://en.wikipedia.org/wiki/Google_driverless_car. Accessed August 31, 2014.

32. Lv Y, Zhao H, Liang Z, et al. A mobile phone short message service improves perceived control of asthma: a randomized controlled trial. Telemed J E Health 2012;18(6):420–6.

33. Mina MJ, Winkler AM, Dente CJ. Let technology do the work: improving prediction of massive transfusion with the aid of a smartphone application. J Trauma Acute Care Surg 2013;75(4):669–75.

34. Facco F, Agazzi A, Manfredini L, et al. MoLab group. evaluation of a mobile clinical pathology laboratory developed for the home care of pediatric patients following transplantation of peripheral blood precursor cells. Clin Chem Lab Med 2013;51(8):1637–42.

35. Available at: http://en.wikipedia.org/wiki/Mobile_technology. Accessed August 31, 2014.

36. Mirza F, Norris T. Opportunities and barriers for mobile health in New Zealand. Stud Health Technol Inform 2007;129(Pt 1):102–6.

Selection and Implementation of New Information Systems

Keith J. Kaplan, MD[a],*, Luigi K.F. Rao, MD, MS[b]

KEYWORDS

- Laboratory information system • Implementation • Selection • Workflow

ABSTRACT

The single most important element to consider when evaluating clinical information systems for a practice is workflow. Workflow can be broadly defined as an orchestrated and repeatable pattern of business activity enabled by the systematic organization of resources into processes that transform materials, provide services, or process information.

OVERVIEW: SELECTION

BACKGROUND AND CONCEPTS

Do I really need a new system? How do I go about that process? Do I want to replace what I have? Is what I have good enough, so that all I need to do is surround it with additional capabilities?

How do you go about finding out which candidates are the correct systems for you? Do you want to go best of breed, or do you want to have a single vendor?

Regardless of your current practice—its members, partners, hospitals, and laboratories that comprise your practice—these questions are almost always the same.

Workflow can be broadly defined as an orchestrated and repeatable pattern of business activity enabled by the systematic organization of resources into processes that transform materials, provide services, or process information.[1]

The single most important element to consider when evaluating clinical information systems for your practice is workflow.[2] You want your anatomic pathology (AP) laboratory information system (LIS)

to fit your existing workflows or improve them but not redesign them to meet the requirements of the LIS. Software can be modified to meet your physical and virtual needs much easier than the converse. Many people make the mistake of evaluating the features of the software and all that they can and perhaps initially cannot do as areas for improvement and lose sight of how any of them fit into existing operations and desired workflows. Although many of the particular functions of the software may change or be modified as you customize the features, the particular workflows of your laboratory, perhaps on its third or fourth LIS system, are unlikely to change as often. Workflows within laboratories, ideally, are designed over time with particular goals or deliverables in mind and exist and persist to meet those goals after years of refinements. Although they may not seem ideal to an outsider, they may be completely practical and functional in an established laboratory to meet its specific needs with its patients, providers, technical staff, partner laboratories and/or hospitals, vendors, clients, and customers. An information system without your workflow in mind will not achieve the overall goals of any implementation—increased efficiency, increased productivity, and cost savings with measurable return on investment (ROI).

Practical matters, such as accessioning, gross processing, histology processing, workload assignment, case distribution, additional test ordering, case resulting, and result delivery, may seem like routine, mundane, basic requirements of any AP LIS; however, you may find particular vendors' thoughts on laboratory workflow may not fit yours. They may not appreciate assigning

---

Dr K.J. Kaplan is the Publisher for www.tissuepathology.com.

[a] PO Box 473431, Charlotte, NC 28247, USA; [b] Department of Pathology, Walter Reed National Military Medical Center, 8901 Rockville Pike, Bethesda, MD 20889, USA

* Corresponding author.

E-mail address: keithjkaplanmd@gmail.com

Surgical Pathology 8 (2015) 239–253

http://dx.doi.org/10.1016/j.path.2015.02.009

certain cases to certain pathologists perhaps at the time of accessioning based on client requirements rather than at case assembly as many laboratories have historically done. Conversely, you may not want cases assigned at accessioning but perhaps the following day when slides are cut and stained, the daily schedule is known, and the volume of cases, blocks, slides, and staffing are up to the minute.

Without getting too far ahead in the overall evaluation process, the most practical way to do this is to process a week's worth of specimens through a mock installation in tandem with your soon-to-be legacy system and see how one compares with the other, focusing not on "how" the system may necessarily perform a certain task but asking "why" does the system behave in this fashion. What rules, logic, recent enhancements/upgrades, or potential opportunities or issues upstream or downstream from that process may be affected for the next user in the process? For example, what may look like a nice shortcut or feature at accessioning may look attractive; if it creates potential for error at grossing, embedding, or with the immunohistochemistry stainer interface, you need to address the pain points early in the process to ensure workflow requirements are met for all users.

With that said, it cannot be assumed that a prospective LIS does something in a manner that is different from how you currently handle a portion of your workflow or that the new LIS, or at least that part of it, is inferior to your current system. Commercially available systems often represent an aggregate of workflow solutions that have been validated by current customers with enhancements provided in the form of upgrades to the current versioning of the application. Thus, much as new information is learned when conducting peer reviews of other laboratories and often new workflows are implemented based on experience elsewhere, the proposed solution in terms of a new LIS may offer some functionality that would be an improvement to your existing workflow but perhaps unable to perform due to current system limitations and workarounds put in place many years ago that have become routine workflow without anyone able to recall, "Why it is we do it this way?" other than the tried and true explanation, "That is the way we have always done it."

Vendors may make claims that their system supports your particular workflow or portion thereof that is of concern while perhaps not having done so before but would be willing to provide that specification as a customization to their existing system. In general, instead of implementing their current solution in your laboratory for a week, as previously discussed, to detail what level of customization to their source code is required to meet an important detail of your workflow, which is impractical, speak with current customers or references provided by the LIS vendor. Ideally you may know of or be provided a list of clients who use the software currently that are similar in scope and volume to your laboratory.

References are an economical source of valuable information, whether their experience has been overall positive or negative with the application. Most speak openly about a company, product, implementation, validation, testing, production, and ongoing service, support, and upgrades. Here you can uncover issues related to the performance of the company, the application, installation, or post go-live issues that another laboratory has experienced. Be prepared with a list of questions that address their experience today with a particular vendor and application. You may not need this list if you have a talkative reference, but it will help organize an important part of your due diligence in this process. Address workflow and any current or previous issues they had or uncovered that may be an issue for your operation. Also address any customizations that were or were not supported to address those concerns. Customization is a complex process that involves both the laboratory and the vendor to complete successfully. Hearing from another laboratory that it was or was not a pleasant experience may go a long way in your decision making. Be sure to address what resources they had internally to work with the vendor and what resource the vendor supplied to the project and balance those with your resources, or lack thereof, if you have the skills, support, and time to work with the vendor on developing.

SELECTION

Armed with a basic concept of how to approach system requirements within your laboratory's environment and workflow considerations and a decision made to explore and potentially select a new AP LIS, consider a request for information or request for proposal (RFI/RFP) from vendors to respond to for potential selection. Many companies, such as the College of American Pathologists and KLAS, regularly provide lists of commercially available LIS systems and ratings, respectively, to begin to research companies and products. Although much of the information is self-reported, both sources of information provide a common starting point for many to begin your own research.

A common starting point is to submit an RFI/RFP to vendors you think may be suitable based on install base, size and scope of clients, interface experience, previous experience, and customer feedback. This initial filter is important only in terms of considering how many companies you would like to potentially demonstrate their system for you, site visits to attend, and reference calls to make initially. You may want to choose from a wide range of small and large companies with any AP experience or limit the range. This commitment likely is long-term one for your laboratory, so be sure to address whether a particular product has been in use for several years at multiple locations and the likelihood it will continue to be so for years to come. What are the mission and vision for a company and its applications? Do they align with your core business model and practices?

The RFI/RFP may go a long way in terms of vendors selected for the next phase or eliminated from consideration based on their responses.

A couple of sample, high-level RFI/RFP approaches are provided in different forms to consider using as a road map for your own organization based on its specific needs and requirements. Some of these may not apply or be a short- or long-term consideration. At this phase, it may not hurt to ask about a company's thoughts on a particular specification should that need become necessary In a few months to years, perhaps during the time an implementation may be started or is finishing. The laboratory business is constantly changing and information technology (IT) needs to be fluid to respond to those changes and paramount to these are AP LIS performance issues even if they do seem like a "nice to have" but not a "must have" today.

Sample Request for Information or Request for Proposal #1

Technical environment

Hardware Describe the required hardware configuration, including descriptions of central processing unit(s), networking hardware, back-up devices, and uninterruptible power supply.

Describe the ability of the proposed system to support fail-safe data storage (redundancy, mirrored, and so forth).

Describe the requirements of system cabling for communication to the server and to the existing network.

Does the system employ 32-bit architecture?

What are the warranty periods provided for hardware?

Please outline service and maintenance costs for the system as proposed.

In an outreach environment, describe the connectivity of the proposed system.

Software Describe the operating systems under which the proposed system will operate (UNIX, DOS, Windows, Windows NT, and so forth).

Name and describe the database management program utilized by the system.

What programming language(s) was used to develop the system?

Describe the file purging/archiving methodology used by the proposed system.

List cost of license agreements, renewal, and upgrades.

Describe the length of time a software version is supported.

Please describe your system's database reporting tools.

Describe the security system used by the proposed system.

Describe your proposed disaster recovery plan to safeguard source code and ensure that the proposed system is recoverable in the event of a disaster at the headquarters of your facility.

Describe your proposed disaster recovery plan to ensure that data are safe and secure in the event of a disaster.

Network and interface issues Have you interfaced your LIS with other clinical information systems? (Provide names of interfaced systems.)

Describe the network topology of your outreach solution in conjunction with your LIS solution.

Describe the network topology of your outreach solution in conjunction with another vendor's LIS solution.

Can your outreach solution be a stand-alone application utilizing a different LIS?

Have you interfaced your outreach solution with other information systems (ie, the outreach solution needs to be able to accept orders from and send results to information systems that do not reside on the same local area network [LAN] or wide area network [WAN] as the laboratory)?

Does the proposed system comply with Health Level Seven International interface standards for importing and exporting data to and from other systems?

Have you interfaced your LIS with reference laboratories? (Provide names of interface reference laboratories.) Describe the interface functionality.

Does your LIS have the capability to provide a direct link to off-site locations for order entry and result retrieval? Describe this capability in detail.

What communication protocols are supported?

What speeds of network lines are required for proposed LIS to function on WAN?

What network infrastructure is needed to operate a true outreach operation (ie, the laboratory needs to accept orders from and send results to a nursing home that is not within the same LAN or WAN as the laboratory)?

SYSTEM IMPLEMENTATION AND TECHNICAL SUPPORT

Describe and attach your typical implementation plan. Describe the length of time your engineer will be on site during implementation and the exact scope of the work he/she will perform.

Describe the experience and qualifications of your installation team.

What kind of client communication and implementation planning is done prior to the installation?

Describe the training provided. Include a training outline.

Where is your technical support center located?

What are the methods for contacting technical support?

What are your hours of operation for technical support?

Describe the qualifications of your technical support staff.

Describe the organization and structure of your technical support services.

What percentage of your total employees is responsible for direct client support?

Describe the ongoing system support provided by the vendor.

Are software upgrades provided as part of the software support contract?

Describe your software upgrade process.

Are there "hot fixes" or "updates" between versions? Do these updates cost extra?

How often are new versions released?

How are customer requests for enhancements and customizations handled?

How many separate modifications were included in the last release?

How many separate modifications included in the last release requested by current users?

Describe the qualifications of your product development department.

What percentage of your total employees is responsible for product development?

Do you have a formal users' group?

Describe the company's policy regarding source code.

SYSTEM PROPOSAL

Provide a system proposal that includes

- Detailed listing of hardware provided
- Detailed listing of software provided
- Description of training provided, including location and time commitment
- Description and cost of ongoing support
- Cost of proposed system

Sample Request for Information or Request for Proposal #2

List of functional requirements

Assign one of the following availability codes to each item:

A—Feature is available off the shelf.

N—Feature is not available.

C—Feature is available with additional cost and custom programming.

- Detailed responses to and descriptions of each checklist item mentioned are required.
- Elaborate on any items that differentiate you from other vendors.
- Failure to complete or respond to all checklist items may result in dismissal of your RFI/RFP submission. If you do not have the functionality mentioned, please respond accordingly with "not available," "in development" or "in testing" or if you would propose doing so at additional cost and customization following the appropriate code (C).

Technical requirements
Describe hardware requirements (see previous example questions).
Describe software requirements (see previous example questions).
Describe network and interface issues (see previous example questions).

Interfacing	Security and auditing
Provide operational interfaces for the following applications: • Hospital information system (HIS) • Reference laboratory • Electronic medical record (EMR) • Billing system • Practice management system • Demographics system • Pathology module/software • Microbiology module/software • Radiology module/software • Other information system(s) Provide additional interfaces for multiple systems Provide all interfaces as an integral part of the application requiring no additional third-party software to implement or maintain the interface. Provide technical support for all active interfaces. Provide operational interfaces for the following applications (please provide a functional description of each interface available): HIS Reference laboratory EMR LIS Billing system Practice management system Demographics system Pathology module/software Microbiology module/software Radiology module/software Other information system Provide additional interfaces for multiple systems. Provide all interfaces as an integral part of the application requiring no additional third-party software to implement or maintain the interface. Provide technical support for all active interfaces.	Provide a multilevel security system that is separate from the LIS to ensure the confidentiality of patient-related information and to control access to outreach functions and features. Restrict access to specific areas of the application based on system function to be performed. Provide practice level security ensuring that associates of one practice cannot gain access to the patient records of another practice. Allow password protection at different levels (system administrator, phlebotomy, nursing, provider, and so forth). Allow a user of proper security clearance to modify the database parameters once the system is live, without requiring programming knowledge. Restrict access to configuration tables, profile indexes, and so forth to designated personnel via security controls. Maintain an automated system log of user sign-on activity. Maintain an audit trail for system entries, including user code, date, and time of each system transaction. Provide multilevel password security down to options within menus. Provide a multilevel security system that is separate from the LIS to ensure the confidentiality of patient-related information and to control access to outreach functions and features. Restrict access to specific areas of the application based on system function to be performed. Provide practice level security ensuring that associates of one practice cannot gain access to the patient records of another practice. Allow password protection at different levels (system administrator, phlebotomy, nursing, provider, and so forth). Allow a user of proper security clearance to modify the database parameters once the system is live, without requiring programming knowledge. Restrict access to configuration tables, profile indexes, and so forth to designated personnel via security controls. Maintain an automated system log of user sign-on activity. Maintain an audit trail for system entries including user code, date, and time of each system transaction. Provide multilevel password security down to options within menus.

Order entry

Allow multiple tests ordering for a single patient using a common demographic record.

Allow laboratory orders to be entered from any computer on or off the local network.

Allow the laboratory to develop and customize orderable items.

Allow simple test ordering: single header linked to a single test result field (eg, glucose).

Allow compound test ordering: single header linked to multiple test result fields (eg, complete blood cell count [CBC], lipid panel, and comprehensive metabolic panel).

Allow the user to order tests by entering test codes and/or by selecting from a test menu.

Automatically alerts users to previously ordered laboratory work.

Allow at the time of ordering a request that patient laboratory results be sent to more than one provider.

Allow the cancellation of orders for patients who do not show for appointment.

Provide medical necessity validation based on laboratory-defined valid diagnosis codes for each applicable test.

Allow the generation of Medicare-compliant Advanced Beneficiary Notice forms when test ordering fails medical necessity validation.

Allow entry of 4 diagnosis codes for each ordered test.

Provide automatic testing destination routing as specified in payor's contract.

Provide automatic label printing as orders are entered.

Allow laboratory-defined label configuration.

Describe the bar code formats your outreach solution accepts and prints.

Provide the specific sample requirements or sample tube types at the time of order entry.

Store diagnosis codes in registration function.

Support retrieval of patient records by partial (eg, first few letters of) patient last name.

Support sample storage and retrieval modules for the purpose of drug testing, add-on testing, and so forth.

Process orders for profiles that include multiple tests (eg, cardiac enzyme profile).

Allow a miscellaneous test code so previously undefined tests can be ordered and charged.

Ability to correct a field on a screen without having to re-enter entire order transaction.

Allow splitting one ordered test into more than one request (eg, group tests, pre-operative, and coagulation screen).

Automatically check for and warn of duplicate single test orders with profile orders.

Support cancellation of tests—logging accession number, test code, patient name, reason, date, time, and tech ID.

Provide simple method to order additional test requests on sample already received and processed in laboratory.

Allow cancellation of an order without canceling prior results.

Provide flexible, customizable sample ID formats.

Print sample collection labels for timed and routine collections.

Allow for multiple labels per test to print.

Print instructions/comments (eg, do not collect from right arm) on sample labels.

Print aliquot labels when more than one test is drawn in the same collection tube.

Provide that uncollected samples continue to appear on subsequent lists until canceled or collected.

Provide for easy free text entry of information, such as critical result notification, sample rejection, or culture sites.

Provide for intelligent prompting for accessioning (eg, when a wound culture is ordered, the system prompts the user for site/location).

Provide easy access to sample requirements for laboratory users.

Provide intelligent sample labeling—groups samples in chemistry together and prints on labels, while hematology tests print on separate label and microbiology prints separately. Allows for making the number of labels customizable for each test.

Provide intuitive user interface—easy to locate screens for accessioning, reporting queries, and so forth.

Provide for an easy, systematic, and logical method of adding, editing, or deleting tests in the test code dictionary.

When looking up a patient in the system, tests performed on that patient and test results are made available without additional steps.

Allow outreach clients to customize their own order entry screens to fit their practice's needs.

Allow outreach clients to customize colors and logos of the system for their practice only.

Result reporting

Provide ability to auto deliver results by the following methods:

Web delivered (ie, provider logs in to a Web site to retrieve results)

E-mail

Fax

Print

Electronic interface to client information system (EMR, HIS, medical practice management software, and so forth)

Accept images, graphics, and linked documents from a host LIS via interface to display on reports.

Provide ability to designate HTML or PDF format of reports.

Maintain patient result history indefinitely.

Provide ability to purge results after a specific amount of time if desired.

Provide ability to graph historical results on a report.

Provide scheduler for automatic result delivery.

Allow redelivery of results.

Automatically maintain a record of reports delivered by each reporting modality (fax, printer, and e-mail, and so forth). Provide easy access to these results at any time.

Allow patient test to be incomplete for at least 8 weeks in the system.

Print daily detailed master log of all work performed in laboratory for audit purposes.

Display abnormal or critical results uniquely from other results.

Allow for cumulative result reporting. Please explain.

Describe the procedure for correcting test results that have been resulted. After correcting, are the corrections able to be altered?

Print list of received but untested samples due to insufficient quantity.

Allow for a comment to be placed on the sample accordingly.

Includes features that allow batch reporting.

Allow features for customizable patient report formats.

Display patient results in an easy to view format for all patients of a provider or location.

Provide ability to batch print and batch acknowledge receipt of results.

Provide the date/time reported on reports transmitted by fax, laser printer, and e-mail.

Provide a permanent log of all test results that have been edited.

Workstations work independently of each other. Multiple functions can occur simultaneously without one party having to exit the system.

Provide flexible reporting formats.

Provide the ability to access all patients of a particular client by name, date, or date range.

Allow look-up of patient and patient results by client number.

Rules-based logic

Ability for rules-based logic where laboratory personnel can define criteria in "if-then" statements.

Ability for rules program to evaluate all rule entries for tests, not just the first one, so that complex or "cascading" rules may easily be designed, where several rules can be invoked based on one scenario.

Provide rules-based report routing.

Provide the ability to create rules to assist in decision support.

Must have ability to flag results based on criteria other than standard reference ranges to include testing location, drawing location, ordering provider, patient age, and priority of order.

Charge rule capability.

Provide ability to customize order entry rules.

Allow rules to be enabled by practice (ie, one practice has certain rules enabled and another practice does not).

Sample status and tracking

Provide the ability to track patient samples throughout the testing process.

Provide identification (ID) of the individual who ordered the test, collected the sample, and released the test results, including the date and time of these occurrences so that this information is accessible throughout the process.

Support user-defined priorities.

Support a way to identify the phlebotomist (doctor, nurse, and so forth) in system for samples not drawn by laboratory personnel.

Include data for tracing order (dates, times, tech ID, and results) from order entry to final reporting in master log.

Provide index to master log by accession number.

Provide customizable sample storage tracking, including ID of freezers, refrigerators, and so forth.

Allow sample storage/retrieval by use of a barcode scanner (ie, the requisition is scanned into the system and the system tells the laboratory where the sample is stored in the laboratory).

Management and administration

Provide ability to create completion reports by date.

Provide ability to create billing summary reports by date.

Provide ability to create reports of failed medical necessity checks.

Provide ability to create canceled test reports that include test name and reason for cancellation.

Provide for a customizable overdue report that would indicate tests, such as urine cultures, that become overdue at 4 days while blood cultures become overdue at 7 days and CBC overdue at 4 hours.

Provide ability to create turnaround time reports by date.

Provide a summary report for test usage over a user-definable period of time.

Provide physician utilization report (eg, number of tests requested by a physician).

Provide ability to print a list of draws that need to be performed.

Patient records

Provide ability to easily generate historical patient reports.

Allow patient database search based on

Patient name

Patient account number

Patient Social Security number

Allow the user to search previous patient results for specific tests and easily view historical results of that test.

Allow the user to graph patient results by test to identify possible trends.

Allow historical results for multiple tests to be graphed on one normalized graph.

Describe how the system handles storage of old results. Is archiving/purging necessary?

Allow the user to review specific patient's results without paging through the entire list of patient results.

Data mining

Provide user-friendly report generator with graphic user interface as an integral part of the outreach application.

Provide ability to create reports from any computer.

Provide ability to create a billing report.

Provide ability to create a report showing all tests completed during a date range.

Provide ability to create a report for order exceptions.

Provide ability to generate patient lists (with certain demographic data) that meet specific result criteria for public health reporting.

Provide ability to create reports on standing or recurring orders.

Provide ability to write queries using logic in great detail within the application.

Support the use of commercially available tools for report generation.

Provide ability to save commonly performed searches.

Provide ability to schedule automatic, unattended runs of data reports.

Provide ability to create reports to mine patient data for specific practices within the application.

Provide online help screens to assist novice users in all applications.

After responses to the RFI/RFP (Table 1) customized from the options and others, you may want to include for your laboratory get cost quotations for the system according to your requirements. Be sure to look at initial implementation costs as well as costs for the following 1-, 3-, and 5-year periods for total cost of ownership with ongoing support and maintenance as well as depreciation on the hardware for the total cost of the system to gain a full measure of ROI. Again, at this point, telephone reference checks are an economical way to talk with your peers about the system you are considering.[3]

Once you have narrowed down the possible list of candidate systems to choose from, it is time for vendor demonstrations. Demonstrations are extremely important. If you are going to have 2 or 3 vendors come in, have them come in at the same time or as close to it possible. You have an opportunity to go from one vendor to the other,

Table 1
Sample request for information or request for proposal #3

Enterprise Features	Required/Desired Optional	Score
Multisite capability?		
Sign-out via Web interface? (No need for VPN, Citrix, or terminal server?)		
Clinical pathology system included		
Build our own interfaces to clients, EMRs, instruments, etc., without vendor fees or involvement?		
Subtotal		
Scalability		
Can system accommodate current volumes?		
Can system accommodate 100% increase to current volumes?		
Database supports mirroring/replication failover?		
Experience configuring and supporting mirrored/replicated environments?		
Subtotal		
System set-up and accession		
Build our own part types?		
Field to store office chart number?		
Mini vs maxi accessioning capability?		
Custom data entry screens by site? Specimen type?		
Enter both AP and clinical data?		
Configurable workflows?		
Custom report generation without vendor assistance?		
Subtotal		
Histology production		
Dynamic notification of special stain and recut orders? E-mail notification?		
Automated logs? Print on defined schedule?		
Subtotal		
Outreach tools		
Interface to practice management systems?		
Result interfaces for common EMRs and hospital systems?		
Autofax/fax on demand?		
Fax chutes by location, client, physician?		
Real-time numeric and graphic client data tracking volume, etc.?		
Custom client productivity reports?		
Subtotal		
Interface capabilities		
Interfaces to Aperio?		
Interfaces to stainer(s)?		
Interfaces to slide and cassette printers?		
Support for scanned supporting documentation (Reqs, Ins, send-out reports, etc.?)		
Import slide images remotely via Citrix or terminal server?		
Subtotal		
Paperless solutions		

(continued on next page)

Table 1
(continued)

Enterprise Features	Required/Desired Optional	Score
Ability to scan documents in?		
Bar coding?		
RFID?		
Launch case automatically on screen with gross description/ preliminary transcription, attached scan of req, prompted by slide bar code/RFID detection?		
Subtotal		
Transcription productivity		
Quick text templates?		
Medical spell check?		
Synoptic reports (CAP-approved cancer reporting)?		
Means to designate cancer registry reports?		
WYSIWYG throughout report generation?		
Subtotal		
Sign-out		
Ability to easily navigate from module to module without need to exit one or the other?		
Do quick searches?		
Check on history?		
Ability to know if a pathologist has referred the case to another pathologist?		
Transmit e-mail to pathologist that case is transcribed (for rush or other critical cases)?		
One-click sign out? (Cases automatically move to the next in line after sign out.)		
Subtotal		
Vendor qualifications		
Other software products that could be integrated with these products are available.		
Active user group exists for each product.		
User group influences release of the product (eg, controls x% of enhancements to the product).		
Reference sites provided for each product		
Published evaluations of software provided		
Proof of success in similar organization provided		
Willing to demonstrate products: at customer site; at vendor site		
Proposed contract provided		
Sample plans provided (eg, implementation, training)		
Software license agreements provided (eg, software maintenance, support)		
Subtotal		
Warranty/support		
Documentation updated for any fixes		
Procedures for vendor-initiated fixes provided		
On-site expertise available at no or low cost		

(continued on next page)

Table 1
(continued)

Enterprise Features	Required/Desired Optional	Score
Customer can modify software without impacting warranty or support		
Updates, enhancements, and new releases covered under maintenance agreements		
Failure to install an update, enhancement, or new release impacts the warranty/support/maintenance after		
30 d or Less		
31–60 d		
61–90 d		
91+ d		
Warranty/support/maintenance is provided for modifications specifically requested by the customer.		
Subtotal		
Total score		

Abbreviations: Reqs, requisitions; RFID, radio frequency identification; VPN, virtual private network; WYSIWYG, what you see is what you get.

see something at the first vendor, then go to the second vendor and see if that vendor has it as well. Also, if you spread demonstrations out over time, people are going to forget what they saw. Be sure to include as many shareholders/stakeholders in the process as possible. This is a critical time for someone in accessioning or billing or for a pathologist to question something seen, or more importantly not seen, or that the company was not able to address clearly, to raise concerns about workflow functionality.

Understand your vendor's business strategy. Where are they going? What market are they after? If you are a midsize reference laboratory, for example, and the vendor's primary target market is large academic teaching hospitals, you need to consider the consequences. Also, what do you need to do to install and keep the system running? If you cannot have a medical technologist who is fairly up on IT components and can write the expert rules, and you have to hire 3 programmers to do that, that is something you have to understand.

This visit is also important for understanding the basic architecture of the system and what operating system the system runs on, which are important in the context of other laboratory software applications for functionality as well as those of any corporate partners, hospitals, or clients.

Be cognizant of site visit(s) and users' opinions of the system from due diligence through contracting, implementation, validation, testing, go-live, post–go-live support, and maintenance/upgrades since go-live. Be sure that knowledgeable IT, technical, and professional personnel are available to discuss the pros and cons with you openly. The vendor should not be present at these discussions to allow the client to be completely transparent with their opinions about the company and product. Make a concerted effort to follow specimens from collection to sign-out to see all components of the system. If billing or result interfaces are required or desired, be sure to inquire what systems their LIS interfaces with and their experiences. A site with multiple users/customers who express serious doubts about the company and/or product may be a red flag. Although no system can be everything to everyone, a current user who expresses nothing but frustration with the company and/or the product and regrets either implementing a solution or migrating from a previous solution needs to be addressed in your due diligence. It may be that a customer's expectations were not met based on functionality that did not exist or it may be that a customer was misled by the vendor, as discussed previously. This needs to be sorted out.

Although vendors have different strengths and weaknesses, the aggregate—the area under the end of the curve in integral calculus—for most of the leading vendors is about the same. What is different is how we/they do certain things.[3]

It is also worthwhile to make the time and necessary budget to visit a vendor's headquarters during this process and meet with leadership and see how the customer service center operates and what the corporate culture is like. Now is the time to know if it has a full-functional 24/7 help desk within the headquarters or whether it out-sources that service and how that is managed. One question we like to ask at the headquarter visit of the chief executive officer or chief operating of-ficer is, "What are 3 items you are working on now?" or "What 3 major functionalities do you see on the short-term horizon of importance to clinical laboratories?" Meet the people who are going to be installing and supporting your system. You are going to be business associates and col-leagues for potentially the next 7 to 10 years.

Scenarios to provide each vendor may be help-ful so that you can compare how one system does a specific function to another. For example, have 10 to 15 scenarios for them to demonstrate, such as assigning specific cases to specific pa-thologists based on client requests, processing reflex testing, preordering special stain requests, and running a report for client services on vol-umes of orders/tests received as a month-to-month comparison for business analytics. Ensure that the demonstrations and site visits are the current version and not "mocked up" with func-tionality that does not exist in a production envi-ronment or a database that is unrealistic for clinical use with missing patient identifiers or generic specimen sources, types, or procedures. Try to have the team get some hands-on expo-sure, to the extent possible, during demonstra-tions and perhaps on the site visit(s) interact with the system enough to get a flavor of working with the system. You and your laboratory will be seeing this wallpaper on their computer screens for some time.

Folks who are part of the due diligence process need to record and share their thoughts at every stage of the process in the event it is later dis-covered that part of the RFI/RFP, responses, demonstration, or site visit was incomplete, and that they need to go back to and ensure the spec-ification or functionality was discussed as to whether the system has the capability or not and how it is currently used in a similar clinical environment, if at all.

When multiple vendors are on site at the same time, you have a chance to revisit these vendors, confirm things, and fill in the gaps. If you see a demonstration of one component from one vendor and 2 hours later see the same demonstration from another vendor and see something they are doing that is totally different, go back and ask the first vendor, "Show me how you could do that same function."[3]

Lastly, make a decision and stick to it. You are entering into a long-term relationship most likely, so time is required to make the right decision but the decision-making process should not take longer than it will to implement and validate the system for use, in general. Begin the process of contracting with 4 major principles in mind[3]:

1. The worst time to negotiate a contract is during contract negotiations. You have lost leverage if you have told the vendor they are your choice over all the others.
2. There are standard contracts that are pre-sented. These are a good baseline but the final version may not resemble the original boiler-plate version you were initially presented. Often there is good infrastructure there with which to work that you can build on.
3. The contract has to cover the entire system. If you are acquiring hardware, software, imple-mentation services, support, database training, user training, and more, the contract should cover it all.
4. The contract has to be fair and protect the inter-ests of both parties. Without going into an exhaustive review of types of contracts and stip-ulations within contracts, the reader should recognize legal counsel should be sought for assistance in contract matters of this complexity.

Have a negotiation team prior to contracting. If you want the first year of on-site support to be included beginning at go-live, be sure to include this in negotiations or better yet within the RFI/RFP as a requirement. This is important (discussed later). The vendor may agree to include support but it may affect the price inclusive at implementa-tion rather than an optional line item in the con-tract. Both sides need to be flexible and not adversarial. Again, the intent is a long-term rela-tionship that requires the terms of the relationship are clearly delineated on the front end. Being treated poorly before you are a client during this process may present some additional information as to whether you want to associate your business with theirs.

A contract checklist should include, but may not be limited to, the following items[3]:

1. System specifications
2. Operational characteristics, including perfor-mance criteria, reliability and availability criteria, and backup and recovery
3. Acceptance testing criteria. Make installment payments for capital expenses and implemen-tation based on milestones the vendor has to achieve to be remunerated. For example, you may want to propose 20% of purchase price due at signing, 20% due at database configuration, 15% due at validation, 15%

due at testing, 10% due at go-live, and 20% due at 60 or 90 days post–go-live to resolve any bugs that are identified.

4. Terms and conditions of the license. How much are additional licenses and how few can be purchased at 1 time?

5. Payment terms (discussed previously)

6. Source code availability and user programming provisions and constraints. If the vendor goes out of business, you have the right to find some fallback procedure, whether it is access to source code or the ability to hire a third party to maintain the system for you.

7. Warranties

8. Inclusion of RFI/RFP responses. It is important that they respond to the RFI/RFP in a manner that reflects they meet a particular requirement that was demonstrated and that the production version satisfies the response and demonstration.

9. Confidentiality of data

10. Provisions for additional locations

11. Rights to future applications

12. Manuals and other documentation

13. Legal conditions and remedies. Consult an attorney.

If all goes right, you will have selected the best system to meet your needs within your workflows, to add efficiencies, productivity, and data mining capabilities for both clinical and operational business considerations with a measurable ROI. And in 7 to 10 years' time you may want to do it all over again!

SYSTEM IMPLEMENTATION

Now that the critical aspects of selection of a new information system are covered, focus shifts to implementing this designated system. Although your institution-specific considerations will drive many of the significant decisions surrounding whether to use your chosen vendor's standard functionality or configure for your own environment, the general principles highlighted cover many possible scenarios. And although the discussion remains focused on AP, the overarching themes of the criticality of workflow considerations, a team-centric approach, and multiple iterations of testing remain the same in meeting the needs of implementing a clinical pathology or digital imaging system (among other potential applications).

It would be remiss to not mention the implications of the widespread adoption of electronic health records on the LIS arena,[4] particularly as EHR vendors begin to encroach into space that historically was the lone domain of LIS companies. These developments have often compelled LIS managers and their teams to take on a more involved role, and such involvement needs to be considered because personnel time commitments and expectations rapidly change in this type of scenario. Such considerations are particularly worth dedicating thought and time to if your practice and associated IT support are small in size and/or perhaps larger with more resources and personnel but geographically spread across a large swath of area. Should your technical group be limited in either number, time, and/or adaptability, utilizing a contractor, either wrapped within the original contract with your vendor or as a third-party consultant, may be worthwhile, especially if it offers expertise and seasoned experience as a broker for both sides (of course not losing sight of this temporary but not insignificant expense). Regardless of which approach is taken, a project manager ultimately responsible for the implementation's success should be designated to guide the team through the overall process to completion.

PREPARATION PHASE

In the preparation phase, it is essential to ensure that you and your working environment have made any necessary upgrades to hardware (including computer workstations, servers, printers, and ports) required to take on the new information system. Along the same vein, ensuring that your bandwidth capacity can withstand the demands of the new network requirements is also of prime importance, especially in the context of your institutional security parameters.

Your data conversion and contingency plans are of paramount significance because they will cover which data are carried forward, how the data elements are moved, and by which means legacy data will be accessible while migrated to your new system. Depending on your institution's requirements, you may not feel the need for comprehensive coverage but expect to ask for total 100% conversion of prior data as your default starting point.

Before getting to day zero when you will turn on the new system for full real use, it is imperative to request and establish a testing environment in addition to your live production environment. This allows you and your team to properly go through unit and integrated testing, working through any bugs and problems that arise, in a separate arena that will not disrupt the current clinical service work utilizing the live system.

SYSTEM CONFIGURATION, IMPLEMENTATION TESTING, AND VALIDATION

After you have established dual-environment arrangements, your team's next milestone is to arrange for your system to be configured with existing laboratory instrumentation as well as software interfaces with your EHR, clinical LIS, and outreach and reference sites. Once your system has been configured, the new setup can be tested and validated. The importance of this next order of business in establishing and completing a test plan cannot be understated—it can be the sole criterion on which your project is deemed a rousing success or an utter failure. Once a test plan is in place, complete with test procedures for each function that was approved and laid out in the system design deliberations as well as any interfaces that are modified or new, the ideal testing set should involve the system's new hardware and software configurations, working within anticipated security requirements and current clinical workflows.

Prior to go-live, validation of the system and its new functionality should take place wherein the gamut of anticipated potential clinical scenarios are put together and tested for both the ordering/input component of the transaction and the results/output transmittal side of the equation. Final, end to-end integration testing incorporating order entry, result delivery, background financial processes, and associated interface crossing with test patients and their tracer specimens is needed to ensure that all the components of the system are present and verified to be in correct working order.

TRAINING

Training involves a multitiered approached in which your team's project manager, the system manager(s), superuser(s), and designated trainer(s) are given initial instruction on the system, often at one of your selected vendor's training sites (with associated travel costs typically and presumptively built into your contract). This will allow for more extensive "train the trainer" preparation from the vendor directly and set your team leaders to become established to the point where they will be able to lead local training sessions for your end users. Be sure to inquire with the vendor about online modules or other remote training offerings that may obviate the time and financial burdens associated with training time. Whether distance training or not, be prepared to dedicate time slots for your laboratory's personnel to undergo this requisite commitment and have appropriate staffing coverage.

GO-LIVE

A few pragmatic items to mention before proceeding with your system's go-live revolve around communication and minimizing distractions. For the former, it is prudent to inform your client base (providers, outreach facilities, and the like) that you will be switching to a new system and that, although you do not anticipate any problems during the change, there may arise unforeseen hiccups during the transition. With regard to the latter, setting aside the go-live date for just your new system and avoiding any overlap with high-resource utilization periods, such as EHR installations, bringing on board new laboratory analyzers, or possible accreditation or inspection windows, is a preferred approach if such events are within your institution's control.

When the time has come to flip the switch on your new system, rest assured that you and your team's preparation and due diligence have set up for success. Granted there are postimplementation considerations surrounding issues of system maintenance or the inevitable workflow idiosyncrasy that is unique to your laboratory setting that the vendor's solution does not meet that will need to be addressed (and of course tested). But once you have reached this point, you can breathe easy—it will only be a few years before the refresh cycle comes full circle and you need to consider if and when to update your system again. Should you decide to do so, you will be better off having done it before and undoubtedly be better equipped with the lessons learned from the previous installation. We hope this article has helped you in modernizing one of the most important pieces of your laboratory's daily work.

REFERENCES

1. Anonymous. Available at: https://www.ftb.ca.gov/aboutFTB/Projects/ITSP/BPM_Glossary.pdf. Accessed June 23, 2014.
2. Sinard JH. Practical pathology informatics: demystifying informatics for the practicing anatomic pathologist. London: Springer-Verlag; 2006. p. 380.
3. Winsten D, Weiner H. Landing a new lis. Northfield: CAP Today; 2007. Available at: http://www.cap.org/apps//cap.portal?_nfpb=true%26cntvwrPtlt_actionOverride=%2Fportlets%2FcontentViewer%2Fshow%26_windowLabel=cntvwrPtlt%26cntvwrPtlt%7BactionForm.contentReference%7D=cap_today%2Ffeature_stories%2F0507NewLIS.html%26_state=maximized%26_pageLabel=cntvwr. Accessed July 15, 2014.
4. Sinard JH, Powell SZ, Karcher DS. Pathology training in informatics: evolving to meet a growing need. Arch Pathol Lab Med 2014;138(4):505–11.

Health Information Systems

S. Joseph Sirintrapun, MD[a],[*], David R. Artz, MD[b]

KEYWORDS

- Laboratory information system • Health information systems • Electronic medical record
- Electronic health record • Computerized provider order entry • Decision support

ABSTRACT

This article provides surgical pathologists an overview of health information systems (HISs): what they are, what they do, and how such systems relate to the practice of surgical pathology. Much of this article is dedicated to the electronic medical record. Information, in how it is captured, transmitted, and conveyed, drives the effectiveness of such electronic medical record functionalities. So critical is information from pathology in integrated clinical care that surgical pathologists are becoming gatekeepers of not only tissue but also information. Better understanding of HISs can empower surgical pathologists to become stakeholders who have an impact on the future direction of quality integrated clinical care.

PART 1–A. HEALTH INFORMATION SYSTEMS—SETTINGS AND FUNCTIONS

Hospitals and health care organizations are complex systems comprising innumerable intricate operations and processes. Factoring advances in technology and medical knowledge, this complexity is further compounded. With such complexity, there is generation of immense amounts of information. Health information systems (HISs) are computing systems that capture, store, manage, or transmit this vast amount of information as it pertains to the health of individuals, clinical care, or the activities of health-related organizations. **Fig. 1** provides an overview of various HISs, which can be divided into 4 categories: (1) foundational systems, (2) financial systems, (3) departmental systems, and (4) electronic medical records (EMRs).

Foundational systems handle the managerial aspects for health care organizations and include the master patient index (MPI) and computing systems, which inform other HISs about admission, discharge, and transfer (ADT) activities. The transmitted message from an ADT system includes demographic information, such as name, date of birth, and gender. The MPI serves to index this information, like name, date of birth, gender, race, and social security number, ensuring that all registered patients are represented once without duplicate identities. The MPI also ensures consistent demographic information across all HISs within a health care organization.

Financial systems handle the accounting aspects for a health-related organization and include billing systems, which handle hospital charges. The general ledger is another accounting system that serves as the backbone for financial and nonfinancial data. There are also financial systems that handle financial and strategic decision support (DS).

Departmental systems are computing systems that are specific to departmental needs and operations. The most visible system to surgical pathologists is the anatomic pathology laboratory information system (AP-LIS). The AP-LIS supports a vast array of operations and functionality for the anatomic pathology laboratory. As a counterpart, the clinical laboratory has the clinical laboratory information system, which frequently is not interoperable with the AP-LIS. Radiology has the radiology information system (RIS), which deals with patient lists, patient tracking, orders, workflows, and results entry with reporting. Serving in conjunction with the RIS in radiology is the picture archiving and communication system, which manages the

Disclosures: The authors have nothing to disclose.
[a] Department of Pathology, Memorial Sloan Kettering Cancer Center, 1275 York Avenue, New York, NY 10065, USA; [b] Memorial Sloan Kettering Cancer Center, 633 3rd Avenue, New York, NY 10017, USA
* Corresponding author.
E-mail address: sirintrs@mskcc.org

Surgical Pathology 8 (2015) 255–268
http://dx.doi.org/10.1016/j.path.2015.02.014

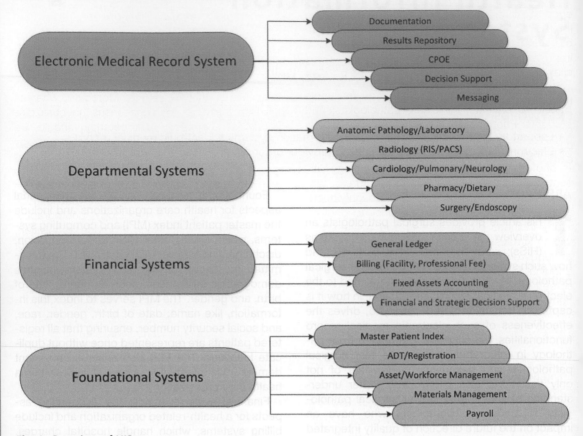

Fig. 1. Overview of HISs.

large repository of radiologic images. Cardiology also has its own version, separate from that in radiology, which handles cardiology images, such as echocardiograms and cardiac catheterization procedures. There are departmental systems for departments that perform specialized testing (ie, ECGs in cardiology, pulmonary function tests for pulmonology, and electromyograms for neurology). Some institutions may bring various imaging modalities together in a separate system, called a vendor neutral archive. Departmental systems exist for pharmacy and dietary departments to streamline workflows by handling medication and dietary orders, coordination administration, and distribution.

Clinical laboratories and financial management departments were the first to adopt HISs. Other types of HISs sprouted to reflect the operational and functional needs of their respective departments. As a consequence of this subspecialization, however, HISs developed independently in silos and with their own individual database infrastructure. This occurred with the AP-LIS and the clinical laboratory information system, and the consequence was a lack of interoperable HISs

that do not interface or interact with each other seamlessly. There are other reasons for this lack of interoperability, such as lack of standardization for interoperability. Vendors of departmental HISs had incentive to create dependency of health care organizations and not come together to create interoperable standards with other competing vendors. This ethos continued until recently where forces advocating for interoperability had become strong enough to influence policy.

The realization for the breakdown of silos and having a more interoperable HISs was not a recent idea, but began as early as 1991. Then, the Institute of Medicine (IOM) set forth a vision and issued a strong call for nationwide implementation of computer-based patient records.[1] The IOM acknowledged that physician groups, hospitals, and other health care organizations operated as silos, often providing care without the benefit of complete information about a patient's condition, medical history, services provided in other settings, or medications prescribed by other clinicians.[2] The IOM called for interoperability through automation and linking of information on services provided to patients in ambulatory and institutional settings (eg, encounters, procedures, and ancillary tests). This interoperability would in turn provide a rich source of information for quality measurement and improvement purposes to enable quality integrated clinical care.[2]

Because of reports like those issued by the IOM, there has been recent widespread adoption of EMRs. Most importantly, federal incentive programs have targeted EMRs to redesign the health care system to create quality integrated clinical care. The EMR is discussed later.

Key Points

- There are 4 categories of HISs
  - Foundational systems
  - Financial systems
  - Departmental systems
  - EMR
- Pressure for HIS interoperability is not new, but only recently with aid of federal incentive programs, has there been push for redesign of the health care system to create quality integrated clinical care.
- This has led to widespread adoption of EMRs.

PART 1–B. HEALTH INFORMATION SYSTEMS—ARCHETYPAL ARCHITECTURES

Interoperability by HISs occurs by 2 archetypal architectures: (1) integrated systems and (2) interfaced systems. Integrated systems are those in which data are housed in the same database and used by various HISs (ie, departmental, financial, and foundational). Interfaced systems are those where HISs are separate applications and data are housed in their own databases. Data are communicated between each separate system through an interface engine usually using a Health Level Seven International 7 (HL7) protocol. Most of the U.S. healthcare organizations are on some iteration of Version 2 for HL7; otherwise specified as HL7 Version 2.x (V2). The significance of HL7 Version 2.x (V2) will be addressed later. Valid arguments exist for both archetypal architectures in terms of advantages and disadvantages.

With integrated systems, information flow is theoretically more seamless because of the foundation of one database. Imagine an integrated system for anatomic pathology, clinical laboratory, and molecular pathology in reporting a hypothetical bone marrow core specimen. Currently such an optimized integrated system does not exist. Under an optimized integrated system however, a pathology report on a bone marrow core can be generated from the AP-LIS with seamless incorporation of a complete blood count (CBC) and/or aspirate result from the clinical laboratory information system. Once the ancillary molecular test results return, an addendum can be tagged into the report, all transactions happening hypothetically under one application without need for different logins, copy-paste actions, or correcting formatting issues.

There is a general sense, however, that integrated systems are not optimized for operational and functional needs of departments. Large vendors are better positioned to create integrated systems but by their size are believed less focused or receptive to the operational and functional needs of each individual department. Large vendors also are thought less nimble to handle nuanced changes that enhance applications. Moreover, because these integrated systems are built on one database, small changes in one application can have unforeseen downstream consequences to the other integrated applications. Along the same lines, integrated systems are more vulnerable to disruption. Corruptions to the database, downtimes, or upgrades affect all applications because they are not able to function independently. The theoretic simplification that occurs because disparate systems run on the same database is a selling point of integrated systems.

With interfaced systems, departments can keep their own departmental HIS, which often addresses the operational and functional needs of respective department more optimally. The term, *best of breed*, derives from the description of such departmental systems. Most of the nuances and customizations demanded by departments may be handled more effectively with a best of breed system. Best of breed systems usually stem from smaller more nimble vendors with incentives for self-preservation to make the most optimized system in their domain. Often such vendors are more receptive and better able to handle changes to their products.

Interfaced systems are heavily dependent on well-implemented communication and routing. This is the reason why more testing is required under such archetypal architecture. In practice, even under the best interfaced system, interoperability is never really fully achieved. With the same scenario under an interfaced system, having an integrated report for the same bone marrow core becomes more difficult. A pathology report on a bone marrow core is generated from an AP-LIS, but there is no seamless incorporation of CBC and/or aspirate result from the clinical laboratory information system. Tagging a molecular addendum poses a similar challenge. The sign-out process mandates separate logins and, once results are obtained, mechanisms for transferring the results to the AP-LIS are usually copy-paste. Without seamless automation for results transfer, errors can occur. The overall sign-out process becomes disruptive because of the different logins, copy-paste actions, and correcting of formatting issues.

In practice, most organizational clinical computing systems are combinations of integrated and interfaced systems, with varying degrees of each. In an ideal world, an integrated system should be optimized for the operational and functional needs of departments. Likewise, an interfaced system should have the seamless modes of interfacing between various applications.

Key Points

- Two archetypal architectures
  - Integrated systems
    - Advantages: one database, more interoperabilty
    - Disadvantages: arguably less customized functionality, more vulnerability of disruption due to interdependency, changes/upgrades more difficult due to interdependency (entire enterprise affected)
  - Interfaced systems
    - Advantages: arguably more customized functionality, less vulnerability to disruptions, changes/upgrades can be staggered and are more manageable (only portions of the enterprise affected)
    - Disadvantages: multiple databases, less interoperability, interface engine dependent

---

PART 2. ELECTRONIC MEDICAL RECORD SYSTEMS AS A FOUNDATIONAL TOOL

The Committee on Quality of Health Care in America in 2001 called for health care organizations to aim for health care that is safe, effective, timely, efficient, equitable, and patient centered. This would require greater access to shared information, expanding communication channels, and overcoming sociotechnical challenges. This also spelled a key role for information technology. Only through support from carefully and consciously designed information systems would health care be enabled to meet these aims.[2] The solution was the EMR, which acts as a foundational tool by helping users better integrate, distribute, organize, interpret, and react to health information and knowledge. **Table 1** lists the advantages and disadvantages of the EMR.

There will be much discussion of the value added by EMRs; however, a few of the disadvantages should be highlighted. EMRs can be expensive. There often seems to be a level of technical familiarity as prerequisite in using EMRs. There are costs in training because EMRs are not necessarily designed to be intuitive for less computer savvy individuals. Workflow disruptions are also notable, particularly with electronic notes, which have had many reported downsides. Data entry for documentation via clicking, typing, and scrolling may take some users longer than scribbling on paper.[3]

The advantages of an EMR in terms of its functionalities seem to override the obstacles. A well-designed and functioning EMR further enables users to utilize this health information and knowledge to influence policy and decision-making, action, individual and public health outcomes, and research. The functionalities of the EMR are listed in **Box 1** and discussed in sequence.[4]

ADMINISTRATIVE PROCESSES

Depending on the health care organization, foundational and financial systems can occur as separate HISs interfaced with the EMR. With such interface types of architecture, extensive testing is required to ensure that the care that occurred along with the documentation noted in the EMR coincides and matches correctly with the billing

---

Table 1
Advantages and disadvantages of the electronic medical record

Advantages	Disadvantages
- Integrative virtual work environment	- Costly
- Accessibility and availability	- Training
○ Portable	- User resistance
○ Multiple user view	- Workflow disruption (ie, electronic note entry and documentation)
- Messaging and alerts	
- Patient care safety	
○ Legibility	- Inadequate results display
○ Audit trails	
- Error reduction	- Technical issues (ie, network, interface)
○ Computerized order entry	
○ Computerized Decision Support	
- Information capture and management	
○ Quality improvement	
○ Research	

Box 1
Functionalities for the electronic medical record

- Administrative processes
- Centralization of health information and knowledge
- Results management
- Messaging (electronic communication and connectivity)
- Computerized Provider Order Entry
- Decision Support
- Patient support
- Data capture, reporting, and population health management

---

codes and list of patients and providers in the foundational and financial systems. EMRs have evolved to incorporate the functionalities of foundational and financial systems in an integrated manner. This integration of foundational and financial HISs to manage documentation for regulatory, compliance, quality assurance, and billing ends up being the back end of modern EMRs.[5]

CENTRALIZATION OF HEALTH INFORMATION AND KNOWLEDGE

The front end of the EMR is the most visible system to clinicians and patients. It is this front end that is ubiquitous in numerous clinical settings (listed in **Table 2**).

The EMR serves as an integrative work environment, centralizing health information for display and presentation. Much like the paper chart, health information is acquired, collected, collated,

---

Table 2
Electronic medical record settings

- Ambulatory clinic
- Outpatient surgical center
- Emergency room
- Operating room
- Skilled nursing facility
- Long-term acute care facility
- Home

- Inpatient
  - Acute care
  - Psychiatry
  - Rehabilitation service
  - ICU
    - Trauma/surgical
    - Pulmonology
    - Cardiology
    - Neurology/neurosurgery
    - Neonatal

---

and stored from other information systems like the AP-LIS. But beyond a paper chart, the EMR is accessible, portable, and available—factors that have been the source of physician satisfaction with such an information system. The EMR has enhanced the practice of surgical pathology. EMRs overcome the issues of accessibility and portability of paper charts, such as physical filing and retrieving of information and misplacement. No longer is there a need to request a paper chart or call or e-mail for clinical correlation. Health information is available during all 24 hours and multiple users can access a single patient record on demand, which is a difficult task with a paper chart.

RESULTS MANAGEMENT

For surgical pathology, results management translates into how surgical pathology reports are presented in the EMR. Surgical pathology reports are reconstructed visually in the EMR through HL7 Version 2.x (V2) messaging and rendered in unformatted text. This translation results in style and formatting loss in the rendered EMR report. EMR reports are not able to handle bold, italics, colors, tables, figures, or pictures. The HL7 Version 2.x (V2) messaging standard rendering reports in an EMR works best for laboratory reports, which are shorter and less textual than surgical pathology reports. The HL7 Version 2.x (V2) messaging standard was not intended to display surgical pathology reports in an intuitive layout. Surgical pathology reports are considerably longer; consider tumor resections with long synoptic checklists. The beautiful reports generated by genitourinary and molecular diagnostic laboratories are not readily reconstructed in the same manner in institutional EMRs. Pathologists, who aligned their data through an aligned column format in Microsoft Word, are often surprised that the information displayed in the EMR does not maintain alignments well. An even more dangerous example is with certain symbols like "~", where the words that follow the symbol can be deleted. Thus statements like "~no carcinoma identified" become "carcinoma identified." Pathologists should be aware of the representation of their reports in the EMR and not just from the AP-LIS. In addition it is the responsibility under Clinical Laboratory Improvement Amendments (CLIA) of a laboratory to know how the results are displayed in the EMR and, if there are multiple institutional EMRs, that results are consistent. Pathologists should be aware of where the results of their generated reports are mapped in the EMR and if there are possibilities for hidden results under any permutation.[5]

Having surgical pathology reports that are human readable and easier to comprehend rapidly proves increasingly difficult with the onset of advanced molecular testing with next-generation sequencing (NGS). NGS is inherently complicated and intuitive layouts presumably require figures, graphs, tables, charts, and so forth, in contrast to unstructured paragraphs of text. Even worse, NGS, unlike the cancer checklists for reporting, has no established guidelines for reporting NGS information. To enhance reporting capabilities in the EMR, some institutions have implemented a PDF interface to overcome the limitations of HL7 Version 2.x (V2) reconstructed reports. The report in PDF format is good for complex reporting because it enables intuitive layouts with capabilities of including bold and colors and the ability to recreate figures, graphs, tables, charts, and so forth. Not only does this avert misinterpretation through formatting and transmission errors but also it becomes a form of passive clinical decision support (discussed later).

Implementing a PDF interface from an AP-LIS requires partnerships from information technology teams from other HISs within the institution, notably the interface engine and the EMR. Many EMRs do not have the functionality to display PDFs or do not have the functionality readily available. Moreover, institutions with data warehouses might resist the idea because PDFs only display and render information that is not easily data mineable. To circumvent such concerns, processes should be ensured to all parties that data streams are maintained if current information mining processes are in place. **Fig. 2** is one example of an institution's information workflow, which has enabled PDF functionality. When the Microsoft Word Document is created from the sign-out in the AP-LIS, this triggers creation of a PDF version

that sits on an accessible institutional server. The HL7 Version 2.x (V2) message that is created after the sign-out of the report then contains a pointer field, which triggers the EMR to retrieve the PDF document for display into the EMR. The institutional data warehouse, in this example, captures information through parsing the HL7 Version 2.x (V2) message and thus the feeder data stream is maintained. As value added for clinical care, a polished PDF report is rendered for display in the EMR.

The PDF interface represents the first stage in enhanced reporting and arguably passive decision support. It can act as the enhanced reporting solution within the confines of HL7 Version 2.x (V2). The next stage in reporting may come through the concept of clinical document architecture (CDA). The current iterations of HL7 Version 2.x (V2) do not encompass CDA. Rather CDA is a component of HL7 Version 3 (V3) which is the next generation of HL7 messaging. CDA was intended for transmission standards to take into account the structural components of clinical documents, in particular the clinical visit note, which is highly textual. Clinical visit notes are not just accumulated lines of text but also documents with structural components, such as the physical examination, review of systems, and assessment and plan section. Surgical pathology reports, also highly textual, can be considered analogous to clinical visit notes with structural components like the final diagnosis section, gross description section, addendum section, and so forth. CDA provides organizational context for how reports are structured and positioned and standardizes the appearance of documents in the EMR.[6] The advantage over a PDF interface is that with CDA capability, the data stream or report rendered EMR becomes more structured and more amenable to processing and data mining unlike

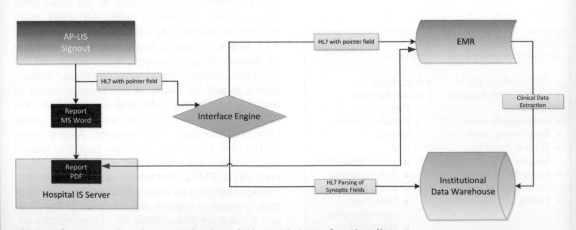

Fig. 2. Information flow for an Institution which enabled PDF functionality.

the unstructured PDF. Fortunately, CDA functionality is likely to appear in all US commercial EMRs because this functionality is included in the requirements for meaningful use under the United States HITECH Act. Whether this implementation of CDA occurs through adoption of HL7 Version 3 (V3) remains unclear however due mainly to the hesitancy of EMR vendors to adopt towards HL7 Version 3 (V3) standards.

The reasons for EMR vendors not adopting HL7 Version 3 (V3) standards are multifactorial. Because EMR vendors of today are large and widely implemented, the competition incentive to evolve toward better messaging standards is absent. Such vendor systems also create a higher reliance and interdependency. Because all components of such vendor systems are interdependent, developments and improvements have unintended consequences throughout the system, making even incremental developments harder to implement. In short, systems become too big to improve and disruptive or even revolutionary changes are even harder to incorporate. There are also prohibitive costs in terms of infrastructure changes to the EMR for adoption of an HL7 Version 3 (V3) standard. HL7 Version 3 (V3) is not backwards compatible with HL7 Version 2.x (V2). This was by design because the intent of HL7 Version 3 (V3) was to be completely revolutionary and not to be hamstrung by the legacy constraints of HL7 Version 2.x (V2). Further compounding is the fact that HL7 Version 3 (V3) is highly complex and experience for implementation is still immature. In other words, there are growing pains with adopting something new like the HL7 Version 3 (V3), pains that EMR vendors are reluctant to take on unless further pressured. Because of the difficulties with adoption of HL7 Version 3 (V3) by EMR vendors, the implementation of CDA may occur through modalities like Fast Healthcare Interoperability Resources (FHIR). The discussion of FHIR is beyond the scope of this article, however a simplified view of FHIR is of a hybrid messaging solution. FHIR can act as a standalone messaging standard and encompass many of the beneficial functionalities of HL7 Version 3 (V3), like CDA. The advantage over HL7 Version 3 (V3) is that FHIR can be used in partnership with current HL7 Version 2.x (V2) standards.

Surgical pathology reports are in need of more dynamic capabilities for managing updates. Updates on reports often come in the form of addendums. The pathology specimen is signed out as the initial report, and then ancillary testing is performed with results usually tagged at the end of the initial report. This is sufficient for a 1-time study, like an immunohistochemical predictive/ prognostic panel performed on, for example, a breast specimen. But if there are multiple tests performed on multiple parts of a specimen, tagging addendums to the end of a report makes the report layout less intuitive. NGS poses this dilemma because NGS can be run on multiple tumor sites listed as different parts within a specimen. Ideally, tagging an addendum to its associated part is the most intuitive layout; however, this requires parts to be separated as components of the final diagnosis section, which is a functionality that most AP-LIS vendors lack.

With genomic reporting, AP-LISs are simply not ready because there are too many unresolved issues. Information, such as the performance characteristics of an assay or whether an assay is single analyte versus multiparametric, is difficult to convey. There are questions in reporting mutations or in negative results and regarding whether sequence information, such as location, sequencing depth, sequencing quality, and regions interrogated, should be stored. Current communication interfacing standards with HL7 Version 2.x (V2) do not support data formatting and metadata for genomic information, such that only dumbed-down genomic results are reportable.

For now, the PDF interface represents the best mechanism to perform enhanced pathology reporting with CDA to occur sometime in the future. This somewhat overcomes the current limitations that current communication interfacing standards have imposed with conveying information in a graphical or interactive manner. Perhaps the optimal solution to enhanced reporting will come from an application program interface (API), which utilizes hyperlinks in an HTML Web-based manner for distribution of information to and from an EMR. The advantage is that information and reports can be updated dynamically, thus creating truly interactive reports. There also will be the ability to deliver report metadata, limitations for interpretation, and level of evidence for interpretation through background and references on demand.

Key Points

- Surgical pathology reports are reconstructed visually in an EMR through HL7 Version 2.x (V2) messaging and rendered in unformatted text.

- HL7 Version 2.x (V2) messaging standard was not intended to display surgical pathology reports in an intuitive layout.

- Responsibility under CLIA resides with the laboratory to know how the results are displayed in the EMR and, if there are multiple institutional EMRs, that results are consistent.

- HL7 Version 2.x (V2) messaging proves more inadequate for NGS reporting with possible solutions including a PDF interface, further development of CDA, or evolution toward a more interactive HTML-based API.

- Updates of reports, as with ancillary testing with NGS, are future issues because tagging addenda to the ends of reports is not ideal

MESSAGING (ELECTRONIC COMMUNICATION AND CONNECTIVITY)

It is no longer sufficient to just render a pathology report in an EMR and assume that all of the clinical team is aware and receiving the information adequately, particularly when there are updates on reports. Clinical care, now that it is more integrated, mandates various clinical teams and personnel receiving updated information about multiple patients. Managing when, who, and where the reports with any updates are routed is paramount. This poses a difficult challenge in how EMRs handle transmitted information of reports with updates, notably addenda.

Often the associated submitting provider for a pathology specimen is not the person the updated information in the addenda is intended for. Some EMRs lack functionality to alert the appropriate provider for such updates. If a breast lumpectomy specimen is signed out, the submitting surgeon is fine with knowing the final pathology with resection margin status. If NGS is requested by an oncologist on the same specimen, however, and then there is a handover in care to another oncologist provider, routing the results of an NGS addenda to the new oncology provider is considerably difficult. Catastrophic errors can occur if results are not relayed appropriately, with certain crucial members of a clinical team unaware of actionable test results.

EMRs are getting better with managing changing providers and distribution of information, but alerting mechanisms via the EMR for updated pathology reports is still a work in progress. Some EMRs are able to do group providers involved in care such that alerts for results go to the entire group to enhance electronic communication with the clinical team. Idealized EMRs would track chain of custody of care, but alternative mechanisms include messaging capabilities for providers, such as an inbox, orders to approve, results to acknowledge, and forwarding mechanisms, such as faxes, printing, and transmission to other systems. Unfortunately some EMRs in use today lack such robust forwarding

capabilities, and, even if present, mechanisms are not well established to determine the appropriate provider to forward results to.

Key Points

- It is insufficient to just render a pathology report in the EMR without knowing how the results are received adequately.

- Managing when, who, and where the reports, with any updates, are routed is paramount.

- Results routing is a future challenge for how EMRs handle transmitted information of reports with updates, notably addenda.

- Idealized EMRs would track chain of custody of care, but alternative mechanisms include messaging capabilities for providers, such as an inbox, orders to approve, results to acknowledge, and forwarding mechanisms, such as faxes, printing, and transmission to other systems.

COMPUTERIZED PROVIDER ORDER ENTRY

Computerized provider order entry (CPOE) is a process that allows an ordering provider to use a computer to directly enter medications, procedures, orders, consultations, and tests, notably radiology and laboratory. Orders are entered in the EMR, and the system then transmits this order over a network via HL7.

From a quality and safety perspective, CPOE has shown a reduction in medical errors. In a study by Bates and colleagues,[7] medical ordering errors were cut by more than half. CPOE reduces errors through (1) eliminating misinterpretation through illegible handwriting or transcription; (2) readily identifying the ordering provider; (3) minimizing inappropriate, unnecessary, or redundant tests; and (4) ensuring that sufficient information is included with orders and improves compliance with medical staff policies. **Fig. 3** shows an example of a CPOE menu for ordering an NGS panel on a surgical pathology tumor specimen. In addition to eliminating misinterpretation through illegible handwriting on paper requisitions, the order provider is readily identifiable, and the system does not allow for duplicate orders if an order is already placed. In addition, the order cannot be processed until sufficient information is placed into certain menu items.

The AP-LISs of today unfortunately lack interface capability for CPOE with EMRs. Moreover, hospital systems are not designed or have not developed workflow to handle the components of

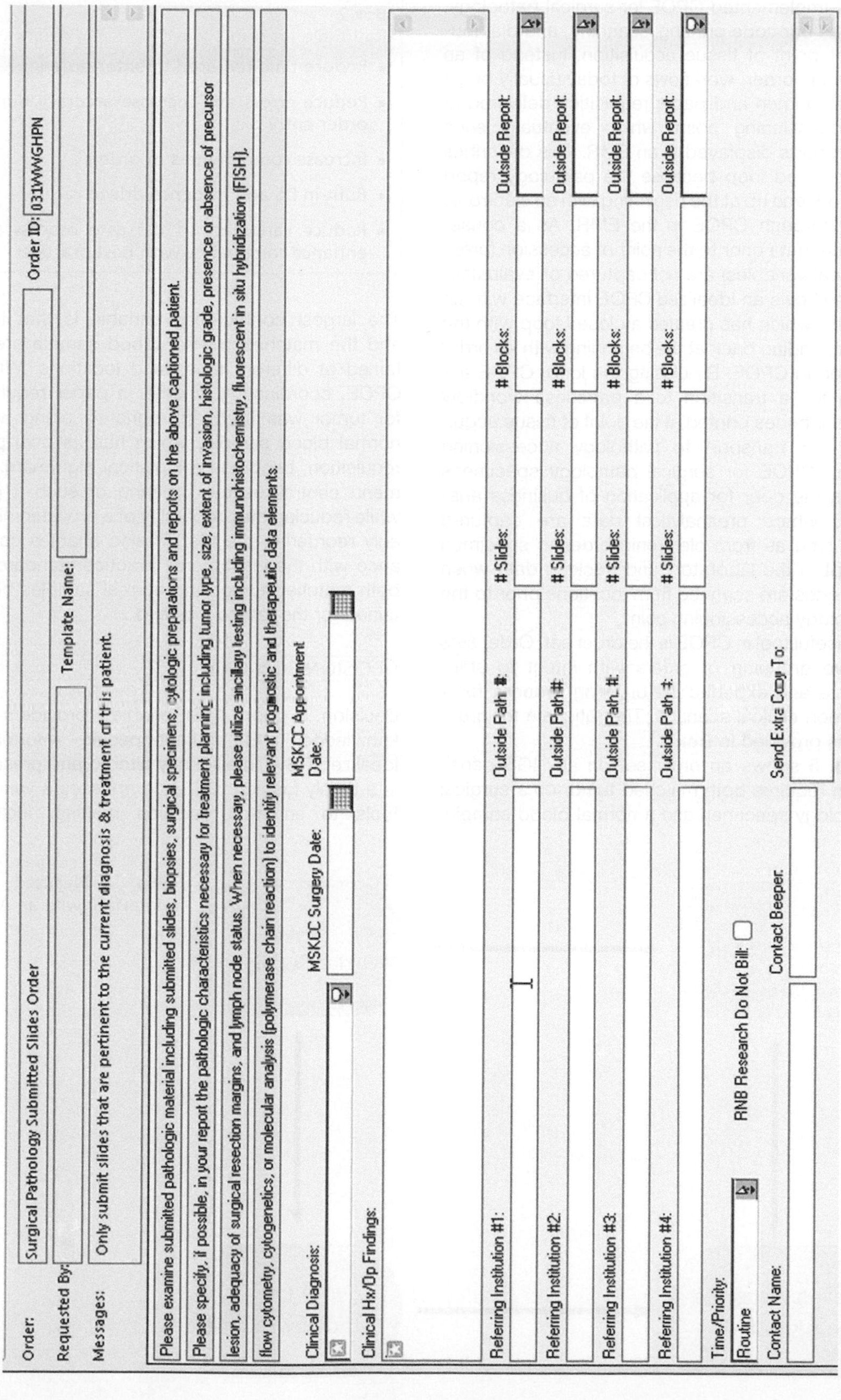

Order: Surgical Pathology Submitted Slides Order | Order ID: 031WWGHPN

Requested By:

Template Name:

Messages: Only submit slides that are pertinent to the current diagnosis & treatment of this patient.

Please examine submitted pathologic material including submitted slides, biopsies, surgical specimens, cytologic preparations and reports on the above captioned patient.

Please specify, if possible, in your report the pathologic characteristics necessary for treatment planning including tumor type, size, extent of invasion, histologic grade, presence or absence of precursor

lesion, adequacy of surgical resection margins, and lymph node status. When necessary, please utilize ancillary testing including immunohistochemistry, fluorescent in situ hybridization (FISH),

flow cytometry, cytogenetics, or molecular analysis (polymerase chain reaction) to identify relevant prognostic and therapeutic data elements.

Clinical Diagnosis: | MSKCC Surgery Date: | MSKCC Appointment Date:

Clinical Hx/Op Findings:

Referring Institution #1: | Outside Path #: | # Slides: | # Blocks: | Outside Report:

Referring Institution #2: | Outside Path # | # Slides: | # Blocks: | Outside Report:

Referring Institution #3: | Outside Path. #: | # Slides: | # Blocks: | Outside Report:

Referring Institution #4: | Outside Path #: | # Slides: | # Blocks: | Outside Report:

Time/Priority: | RNB Research Do Not Bill: ☐

Routine

Contact Name: | Contact Beeper: | Send Extra Copy To:

Fig. 3. Screenshot of a CPOE menu for ordering an NGS panel on a surgical pathology tumor specimen.

a well-implemented CPOE for surgical pathology, such as bar code printing, scanning, and distribution at point of tissue acquisition. Instead of an electronic order, workflows of today usually begin with specimen and paper requisition delivered at an accessioning point, which eventually ends with reports displayed in an EMR. This describes an unclosed loop because the pathology report does not end up at the beginning with an electronic order through CPOE in the EMR. As a consequence, data prior to the point of accession (preanalytical variables) are not captured or evaluated. **Fig. 4** shows an idealized CPOE interface with an AP-LIS, which has created a closed loop with the report, ending back at the beginning with an order entered in CPOE. By closing the loop, CPOE enables for a transition to a paperless workflow with bar codes printed at the point of tissue acquisition for transport to pathology accessioning points. CPOE for surgical pathology specimens opens the door for application of business analytics, where preanalytical data are captured such time as from electronic order to specimen receipt in the laboratory and tracking data when bar codes are scanned from locations prior to the pathology accessioning point.

A useful tool in CPOE is the order set. Order sets involve grouping of orders with intent to standardize and expedite the ordering process for a common clinical scenario. The rationale for order sets is provided in **Box 2**.[8]

Fig. 5 shows an order set on an NGS panel, which requires both matched tumor on a surgical pathology specimen and a normal blood sample.

Box 2
Rationale for order sets
• Reduce time required to enter orders
• Reduce errors and increase accuracy during order entry
• Increase completeness of orders
• Built-in DS and evidence-driven care
• Reduce variability in the care process and enhance compliance with best practices

The largest confounding variable is that tumor and the matched normal blood sample are obtained at different times and locations. Without CPOE, coordinating whether a paper requisition for tumor was filled appropriately along with a normal blood sample, which has its own paper requisition, becomes a logistical nightmare. This menu centralizes the ordering of such a panel while reducing the probability of a provider mistakenly reordering the test. It also enables compliance with the institutional practice standard that both matched tumor and normal samples be obtained for the test to proceed.

DECISION SUPPORT

Decision support (DS) enables providers with knowledge and patient-specific information. Idealized DS is intelligently filtered and presented in a timely fashion. DS encompasses a variety of tools to enhance decision making, including

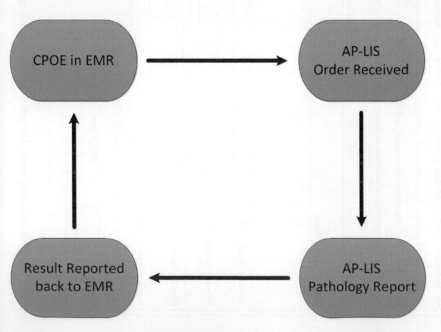

Fig. 4. Idealized CPOE interface with an AP-LIS.

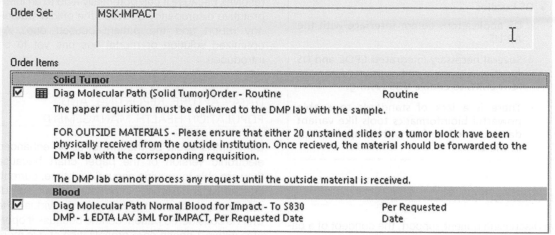

Order Set: MSK-IMPACT

Order Items

Solid Tumor

☑ Diag Molecular Path (Solid Tumor)Order - Routine   Routine

The paper requisition must be delivered to the DMP lab with the sample.

FOR OUTSIDE MATERIALS - Please ensure that either 20 unstained slides or a tumor block have been physically received from the outside institution. Once recieved, the material should be forwarded to the DMP lab with the corrseponding requisition.

The DMP lab cannot process any request until the outside material is received.

Blood

☑ Diag Molecular Path Normal Blood for Impact - To S830   Per Requested
DMP - 1 EDTA LAV 3ML for IMPACT, Per Requested Date   Date

Fig. 5. Screenshot of a NGS order set at MSKCC.

computerized alerts and reminders to providers, clinical guidelines, condition-specific order sets, documentation templates, diagnostic support, and contextually relevant reference information.[9] As discussed previously with reporting of NGS results, a focused PDF report and summary can be a passive version of DS. Many institutions already have implemented a PDF interface as a component of their clinical reporting of NGS to integrate back in EMRs.[10]

DS is becoming necessary to address the growing information overload clinicians face and to provide a platform for integrating evidence-based knowledge into care delivery. A majority of DS applications operate as components of comprehensive EMRs. DS is also becoming the reason for implementing EMRs to fulfill government mandates for meaningful use.

DS is often coupled with CPOE, where electronic orders can be linked to clinical guidelines, contextually relevant reference information educational content, and rules engines to check orders (duplicates) and to generate alerts. The condition-specific order set seen in **Fig. 5** is also a form of DS. The implementation of such menus improves physician ordering patterns by locking down variations in ordering habits. In **Fig. 5**, order for an NGS panel cannot be processed unless both tumor and normal samples are checked and requested.

DS is not without its hurdles. Ideally, DS applications interface with the AP-LIS; however, most AP-LIS vendors have not yet developed such interfacing functionality. DS also, if poorly designed, creates inefficiency with interruptions, such as too many pop-ups, warnings, hurdles, and alerts to initiating an order, otherwise known as "alert fatigue." DS is seen as a necessary component of NGS testing and reporting because DS systems can use panomic data to guide treatment selection and precision medicine.[11] Currently there are several necessary integrated CPOE and DS functionalities that are not supported by current EMRs to enable NGS testing. There is no seamless mechanism to have records for consent and counseling conveyed to an NGS laboratory. For germline genetic testing, there is no mechanism to ensure no unnecessary expensive repeat testing, such as referring to a preexisting test result or having a lifetime duplicate test check rule. Complex tests, such as NGS, do require assistance. Clinicians should not be held to a level of sophistication of knowing when ordering fluorescence in situ hybridization (FISH), karyotyping, or NGS is appropriate under all sorts of scenarios. Another large hurdle is the lack of standards to enable powerful bioinformatics tools like variant databases to interface with DS applications in the EMR.[10]

Key Points

- DS enables providers with knowledge and patient-specific information and ideally DS is intelligently filtered and timely presented.

- DS is becoming necessary to address the growing information overload clinicians face and to provide a platform for integrating evidence-based knowledge into care delivery.

- Clinicians should not be held to a level of sophistication of knowing when ordering FISH, karyotyping, or NGS is appropriate under all sorts of scenarios.

- DS hurdles
  - DS applications do not interface with the AP-LIS.
  - Several necessary integrated CPOE and DS functionalities are not supported by current EMRs to enable NGS testing.
  - There is a lack of standards to enable powerful bioinformatics tools like variant databases to interface with DS applications in the EMR.

PATIENT SUPPORT

In discussing patient support, the concept of a patient portal is introduced. A patient portal is a secure online Web site that gives patients convenient 24-hour access to personal health information from anywhere with an Internet connection. EMRs of today are implementing patient portals to enhance patient-provider communication, empower patients, support care between visits, and, most importantly, improve patient outcomes. Patient portals are seen as a solution to meet the expectations of stage 1 of meaningful use in engaging patients in their own health care.[12] Many patient portals display laboratory results, but surgical pathology reports raise another set of issues.

From the surgical pathologist perspective, when and how pathology reports are displayed in a patient portal become issues. If a patient has a resection for a tumor, what is the appropriate time for the report to be displayed in the portal? If the report is displayed too soon, the patient may not see the provider in time for a discussion about issues about prognosis. How the report is displayed is also important. Would a patient be able to interpret a pathology report written for clinicians, or will that lead to more questions fielded by clinicians or potentially even pathologists.

As implementation of patient portals becomes more widespread, should a more patient-focused report with appropriate language and terminology be done and would this create more issues than it resolves because it can potentially lead to an interpretative discrepancy between the official pathology report and the patient-focused one? An optimized solution or model has has yet to be introduced.

DATA CAPTURE, REPORTING, AND POPULATION HEALTH MANAGEMENT

Early EMRs could be thought of as an enhanced electronic version of the paper chart because they are able to provide secure, real-time, current, interactive, and portable information on an individual. Because of this focus on the individual, the EMR is considered patient centric because it operates within 1 health care organization and is more focused on episodes/encounters and immediate health care, like clinical information collected from a provider's office.[5]

Another term that is used interchangeably, although mistakenly, is electronic health record (EHR). EMRs and EHRs have similar functionality because they both work as enhanced electronic versions of paper charts. EHRs are more longitudinal, encompassing the entirety of a patient's episodes/encounters and across health care organizations. Unlike EMRs, EHRs can encompass more than just the one health care organization that originally collected and compiled the information. They are built to share information with other health care providers, such as laboratories and specialists, so they contain information from all the clinicians involved in the patient's care. In theory, the EHR enables the ability to easily share medical information among stakeholders and to have a patient's information follow that person through the various modalities of care engaged by that individual. Information can move with the patient—to a specialist, a hospital, a nursing home, the next state, or even across the country. This allows for comparison of various records of an individual and allows for extraction of data from records across different individuals. This mobility of information enables EHRs to go beyond the health and immediate patient-centric health care, toward the goal of bettering population health. The heart of a well-implemented HER is sophisticated data capture, which is amenable to computer processing.[13]

An immense wealth of data is contained in the databases of EMRs/EHRs; consider clinical notes and reports from laboratory, pathology, and radiology. Countless other types of data elements are captured by the EMR/EHR, such as clinic visit dates, blood pressure readings, and vaccinations. Such data can be tracked over time and used to

---

Key Points

- Patient portals are seen as a solution to meet the expectations of stage 1 of meaningful use in engaging patients in their own health care.

- There are many issues that arise and are unresolved with the advent of patient portals.

- Pathologists should be active in the management of results in patient portals.

check on how patients are doing and to identify which patients due for screenings or checkups. Through this monitoring of captured data, EMRs/EHRs, in concept, improve overall quality of care within the health organization. With even more advanced queries and monitoring of EMR/EHR database and the mobility of the extracted data from different records, information can be used for audits, research, outcomes assessment, research, and surveillance. The ability to use this information in more meaningful ways to elucidate insight and knowledge is a key goal of EHRs.

With this promise for better overall health care for individuals and population health, there are obstacles that require solutions before the full potential of EHRs is achieved in the setting of improving health care of individuals and of population health. EMRs, despite containing immense wealth in data, have most of the data captured unstructured and not easily amenable to computer processing. This is usually not an issue with data elements, like clinical visit dates, blood pressures, and laboratory data, which are often short, numeric, and less textual. For data elements contained in textual documents, such as clinical notes and pathology reports, however, the accumulated lines of text in some EMRs provide little structure or context to create parsing algorithms to mine and extract the data. An example is capturing data from a family history section of a clinical note for familial correlations of disease processes. The family history is sometimes reported as accumulated lines of text that offer no structure or context to a computer. Graphical representation with family trees hypothetically is a better mechanism for data capture; however, this functionality is far from universal.

The narrative text-based format of sections like the family history may change in the future with meaningful use by mandating that EMRs capture data better through more structured mechanisms. CDA, as discussed previously, may be a step forward and holds promise for such structured capture. For now, however, templates can lock down the structure of certain data elements of a document. Synoptic reporting of cancer specimens has been widely implemented and easily utilized and applied. Because of the consistency and structure of the information, these synoptic cancer templates have structured lines of text in a manner amenable to computer processing. Templates for many EMR clinic notes have received mixed reactions, with the downside a limitation on flexibility in applying the template to nuanced situations. This basically forces documentation into frameworks without the ability to tailor for clinical exceptions.

Referring to **Fig. 2**, an institution that possesses a data warehouse has created mechanisms for clinical data extraction from the EMR database to provide clinical correlations while also enabling parsing algorithms to capture data from synoptic templates in cancer pathology reports from the transmitted HL7 Version 2.x (V2) message. In this way, the institution is able to create a streamlined automated information flow, which coordinates the association between clinical data, such as clinical trials and treatment, with the cancer reporting elements into the institutional data warehouse.

As mechanisms improve for capturing data, EHRs will also continue to evolve better transmission mechanisms to public health databases focused on reportable diseases to better population health. This reporting to public health agencies for more global surveillance of disease is also mandated under meaningful use. Consider the reporting of infectious diseases for outbreak surveillance as well as tumor cases for cancer registries. Such tasks were difficult in the days of paper records, but now, using captured data elements in EHRs, transferring directly to cloud-based public health data centers with their own information systems is more seamless.

Key Points

- Information sharing is the ultimate key goal of EHRs with the hope of improving the quality of health in the population.

- Mobility of the extracted data from different records can enable information to be used for audits, research, outcomes assessment, research, and surveillance.

- Extracted and shared information can be evaluated toward more meaningful ways to elucidate insight and knowledge.

- Cancer synoptic reporting helps enable better and more automated data sharing for public databases, such as cancer registries.

SUMMARY

Pathologists have become gatekeepers of tissue and information. Pathologists must acknowledge their role in quality integrated clinical care and engage information system teams outside of the departmental AP-LIS. EMRs/EHRs are developing functionalities for which pathologists should be stakeholders to provide valuable pathology domain knowledge. This requires moving out of the traditional siloed mind-set and collaborating with clinical colleagues, administrative teams, and vendors as part of institutional information system teams to coordinate efficient flows for information.

REFERENCES

1. Dick RS, Steen EB, Detmer DE, editors. The computer-based patient record: an essential technology for health care, revised edition. Washington, DC: The National Academies Press; 1997.
2. Institute of Medicine (IOM). Crossing the quality chasm: a new health system for the 21st century. Washington, DC: The National Academies Press; 2001.
3. Mamykina L, Vawdrey DK, Stetson PD, et al. Clinical documentation: composition or synthesis? J Am Med Inform Assoc 2012;19(6):1025–31.
4. Institute of Medicine (IOM) Committee on Data Standards for Patient Safety. Key capabilities of an electronic health record system: letter report. Washington, DC: The National Academies Press; 2003.
5. Pantanowitz L, Tuthill JM, Balis UG. Pathology informatics: theory & practice. Chicago, IL: American Society of Clinical Pathologists Press; 2012.
6. Dolin RH, Alschuler L, Beebe C, et al. The HL7 clinical document architecture. J Am Med Inform Assoc 2001;8(6):552–69.
7. Bates DW, Leape LL, Cullen DJ, et al. Effect of computerized physician order entry and a team intervention on prevention of serious medication errors. JAMA 1998;280(15):1311–6.
8. Payne TH, Hoey PJ, Nichol P, et al. Preparation and use of preconstructed orders, order sets, and order menus in a computerized provider order entry system. J Am Med Inform Assoc 2003;10(4):322–9.
9. HealthIT.gov. Clinical Decision Support (CDS). Available at: http://www.healthit.gov/policy-researchers-implementers/clinical-decision-support-cds. Accessed July 8, 2014.
10. Tarczy-Hornoch P, Amendola L, Aronson SJ, et al. A survey of informatics approaches to whole-exome and whole-genome clinical reporting in the electronic health record. Genet Med 2013;15(10):824–32.
11. Yu P, Artz D, Warner J. Electronic health records (EHRs): supporting ASCO's vision of cancer care. Am Soc Clin Oncol Educ Book 2014;225–31.
12. HealthIT.gov. What is a patient portal? Available at: http://www.healthit.gov/providers-professionals/faqs/what-patient-portal. Accessed July 8, 2014.
13. HealthIT.gov. Health Information Exchange (HIE). Available at: http://www.healthit.gov/providers-professionals/health-information-exchange/what-hie. Accessed July 8, 2014.

Translational Bioinformatics and Clinical Research (Biomedical) Informatics

S. Joseph Sirintrapun, MD[a],*, Ahmet Zehir, PhD[b], Aijazuddin Syed, MS[b], JianJiong Gao, PhD[b], Nikolaus Schultz, PhD[b], Donavan T. Cheng, PhD[b]

KEYWORDS

- Translational informatics • Bioinformatics • Clinical research informatics • Biomedical informatics
- The Cancer Genome Atlas • TCGA • cBioPortal • Cancer genomics

ABSTRACT

Translational bioinformatics and clinical research (biomedical) informatics are the primary domains related to informatics activities that support translational research. Translational bioinformatics focuses on computational techniques in genetics, molecular biology, and systems biology. Clinical research (biomedical) informatics involves the use of informatics in discovery and management of new knowledge relating to health and disease. This article details 3 projects that are hybrid applications of translational bioinformatics and clinical research (biomedical) informatics: The Cancer Genome Atlas, the cBioPortal for Cancer Genomics, and the Memorial Sloan Kettering Cancer Center clinical variants and results database, all designed to facilitate insights into cancer biology and clinical/therapeutic correlations.

OVERVIEW OF TRANSLATIONAL BIOINFORMATICS AND CLINICAL RESEARCH (BIOMEDICAL) INFORMATICS

Translational bioinformatics and clinical research (biomedical) informatics are the primary domains related to informatics activities that support translational research. Although arguably distinct, clinical research (biomedical) informatics and translational bioinformatics are often used interchangeably. Translational bioinformatics focuses more specifically on the computational techniques in the areas of genetics, molecular biology, and systems biology.[1,2] By contrast, clinical research (biomedical) informatics involves the use of informatics in the discovery and management of new knowledge relating to health and disease.

Clinical research (biomedical) informatics uses computational techniques related to secondary research use of clinical information for understanding disease processes. These computational techniques span a wide set of interdisciplinary fields and encompass resources, devices, and methods that optimize the acquisition, storage, retrieval, transformation, and communication of clinical information.[1,2]

Driving both translational bioinformatics and clinical research (biomedical) informatics is the management and refinement of data: how data are captured, transmitted, processed, and conveyed into information in order to generate meaningful knowledge. How data are captured for translational bioinformatics begins after tissue acquisition and tissue processing, and uses advanced molecular techniques for data generation. How data are captured for clinical research (biomedical) informatics starts with data compiled from health information systems (discussed in an article elsewhere in this issue).

Disclosures: None.
[a] Department of Pathology, Memorial Sloan Kettering Cancer Center, 1275 York Avenue, New York, NY 10065, USA; [b] Memorial Sloan Kettering Cancer Center, 417 East 68th Street, New York, NY 10065, USA
* Corresponding author.
E-mail address: sirintrs@mskcc.org

Surgical Pathology 8 (2015) 269–288
http://dx.doi.org/10.1016/j.path.2015.02.015

One application of clinical research (biomedical) informatics is managing information related to clinical trials. Another application is linking large-scale DNA data banks with electronic medical record systems for discovery of genotype-phenotype associations.[3] Informatics of biospecimens and biorepositories also falls under the scope of clinical research (biomedical) informatics and is discussed briefly.

With biospecimens and biorepositories, there are immense infrastructural needs from information technology. Biospecimens and biorepositories must have associated quality clinical and pathology information with the specimens, which means efforts to determine which data elements to capture and easy mechanisms to associate and annotate samples. Optimal information systems can update whether studies have institutional review board approval using samples and associated clinical data elements. Moreover, there should be security maintenance and processes in place for de-identification of protected health information. Tools for de-identification could include an honest broker system, which maintains linkages between samples and clinical data elements through a third-party mediator.

Information systems for biospecimens and biorepositories should encompass operational logistics, such as inventory tracking, sample processing, storage, and distribution management. Sophisticated information systems have barcoding systems to facilitate such operational logistics. Crucial are functionalities to document how specimens are acquired and collected. Other functionalities include refrigeration and location, specimen distribution, and usage and control user accessibility. Biospecimens and biorepositories are costly investments and there are pressures for such information systems to enable cost recovery measures.[4]

Creating an optimal information systems infrastructure for biospecimens and biorepositories has proved daunting. The cancer Biomedical Informatics Grid (caBIG) initiative began in 2004 to create an interoperable academic/commercial biomedical information system, built on community-driven, precompetitive open source standards for data exchange and interoperability in the cancer research enterprise. This initiative held hopes for widespread dissemination throughout the cancer community. The guiding principles of caBIG of open access, open development, and open source were appealing. The ideal vision for caBIG was to make large and diverse cancer research data sets sustainably available for analysis, integration, and mining. In doing so, caBIG would become the platform by which cancer researchers would access data and biospecimens across institutions to perform genomic analysis and to find and analyze clinical data. The caBIG initiative never achieved its ideal vision for multiple lengthy reasons which will not be discussed and, sadly, the caBIG initiative was retired.[5]

ILLUSTRATIVE EXAMPLES OF TRANSLATIONAL BIOINFORMATICS AND CLINICAL RESEARCH (BIOMEDICAL) INFORMATICS

This article details 3 projects that are hybrid applications of translational bioinformatics and clinical research (biomedical) informatics. The first is TCGA, the second is the cBioPortal for Cancer Genomics, the third is the MSKCC CVR system database; all were designed to facilitate insights into cancer biology and clinical/therapeutic correlations.

PART 1. THE CANCER GENOME ATLAS

TCGA is a comprehensive and coordinated multi-institutional effort to create a detailed catalog, or atlas, of genetic mutations in cancer using advanced genome sequencing and translational bioinformatics associated with specific types of tumors to improve the prevention, diagnosis, and treatment of cancer. Its mission was to accelerate the understanding of the molecular basis of cancer through the application of genome analysis and characterization technologies.

TCGA began in 2006 as a pilot project funded by the National Cancer Institute (NCI) and National Human Genome Research Institute, both parts of the National Institutes of Health. Initially, TCGA focused on characterization of only 3 types of cancers but since has grown to at least 30 tumor types and many more subtypes.[6,7] The cancers were selected by TCGA because of their poor prognosis and overall public health impact. The power of the project is the quality of tissue acquisition. TCGA samples are consistent in their processing with extensive quality controls (QCs) in place. TCGA research network encompasses centers for genome characterization, protein characterization, and genomic data analysis centers, which enable the process for genomic discovery. TCGA network comprises scientists, bioinformaticians, bioethicists, doctors, nurses, and cancer advocates. The data generated includes gene expression, protein expression, DNA copy number alterations (CNAs), epigenomics (noninherited DNA modifications), and microRNAs (miRNAs), which are short RNAs that control gene expression. Genome sequencing centers perform exome (coding gene region) sequencing on all cases, with some cases selected for whole-genome (coding and noncoding gene region) sequencing. Genomic data analysis centers, through developed tools, analyze the vast amount of data generated in TCGA. This project has collected an unprecedented number of high-quality human cancer samples and matching normal controls to identify important genomic changes in the development of cancer.

The data are accessible for prepublication by (1) the Cancer Genomics Hub (https://cghub.ucsc.edu/), a database that houses lower-level sequence data and alignments, or (2) TCGA Data Portal (https://tcga-data.nci.nih.gov/tcga/tcgaHome2.jsp [**Fig. 1**]), where all other data, including some clinical information, are deposited. TCGA Data Portal hosts data sets that are queryable and include exome (variant analysis), single-nucleotide polymorphism (SNP), methylation, mRNA, miRNA, and de-identified patient clinical information from both tumor and matching normal samples (**Fig. 2**).[7] The data can also be accessed by several tools and portals developed by the genomic data analysis centers, including the Broad Firehose (http://gdac.broadinstitute.org/), Regulome Explorer

(http://explorer.cancerregulome.org/), TumorPortal (http://cancergenome.broadinstitute.org/), University of California Santa Cruz Cancer Genomics Browser (https://genome-cancer.ucsc.edu/), Integrative Genomics Viewer (IGV) via the "Load from Server" option (http://www.broadinstitute.org/igv/), and cBioPortal for Cancer Genomics (http://cbioportal.org/) (discussed later).

PART 2. CBIOPORTAL FOR CANCER GENOMICS

Large-scale cancer genomics projects, such as TCGA, generate overwhelming amounts of cancer genomics data from multiple different technical platforms, which increases the challenges of performing data integration, exploration, and analytics, especially for scientists without a computational background. There have been issues with making the large raw data sets more easily accessible and integrating the clinical information in a meaningful manner.[8–10]

The cBioPortal for Cancer Genomics (http://cbioportal.org [**Fig. 3**])[2] was specifically designed

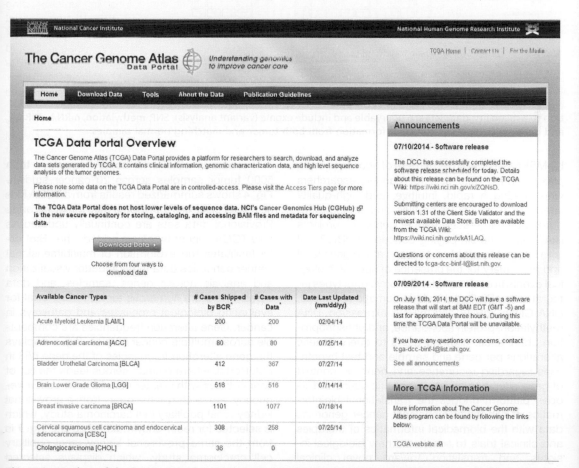

Fig. 1. Screenshot of the home page for TCGA Data Portal (https://tcga-data.nci.nih.gov/tcga/tcgaHome2.jsp).

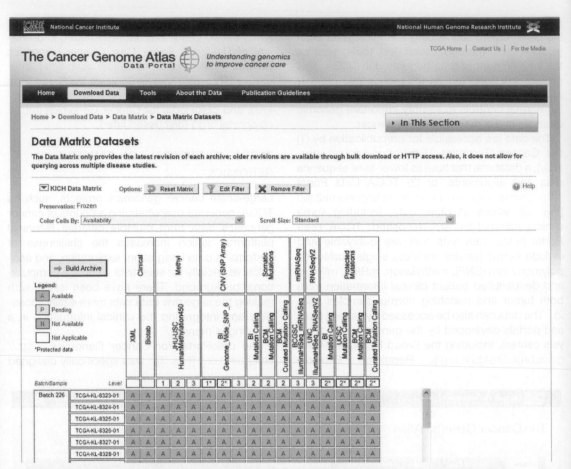

Fig. 2. Screenshot of a Web page in TCGA Data Portal for hosted data matrix/matrices of tumor samples. In addition to availability, data sets are queryable and include exome (variant analysis), SNP, methylation, mRNA, miRNA, and de-identified patient clinical information from both tumor and matching normal samples.

by MSKCC to lower the barriers of access to complex genomic data sets for cancer researchers who needed a rapid, intuitive, and high-quality interface to molecular profiles and clinical attributes from large-scale cancer genomics projects like TCGA. The simplifying concept of cBioPortal is to integrate multiple data types at the gene level and then query for the presence of specific biological events in each sample. Genomic data types integrated in cBioPortal include somatic mutations, DNA CNAs, mRNA and miRNA expression, DNA methylation, protein abundance, and phosphoprotein abundance, allowing users to query genetic alterations per gene and sample and test hypotheses regarding recurrence and genomic context of gene alteration events in specific cancers. This open platform bridges the translational bioinformatics of rich multidimensional cancer genomics data with the biomedical informatics of therapies and clinical trials to accelerate new biological insights and translation toward novel clinical applications.[8–10]

The data in cBioPortal come from more than 5000 tumor samples across 20 cancer studies. **Fig. 4** shows summarized results from a TCGA kidney renal clear cell carcinoma study in cBioPortal. Provisional data sets are continually updated as new TCGA cancer types are added. The cBioPortal facilitates the exploration of multidimensional cancer genomics data through better visualization and analysis across genes, samples, and data types. There are numerous tools in cBioPortal for evaluating biological processes and pathways in cancer. Gene alteration frequencies are comparable across multiple cancer studies. **Fig. 5** displays the gene alteration frequencies of the gene p53 in cBioPortal, where ovarian serous leads the list of cancer types with greater than 90% alteration frequency. **Fig. 6** shows the query from a provisional kidney renal papillary cell carcinoma study, which is selected for recurrently mutated genes. **Fig. 7** is from the same provisional kidney renal papillary cell carcinoma study, which displays selected genes from genomic regions with CNAs.

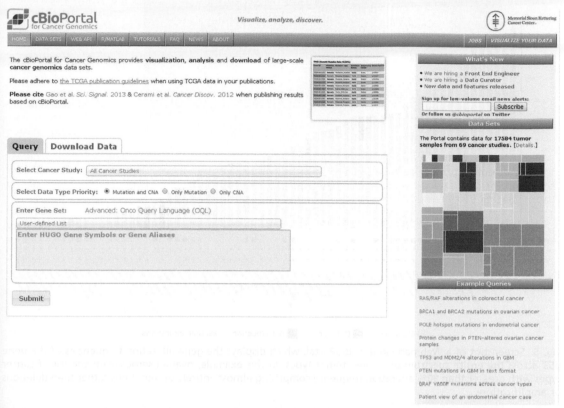

Fig. 3. Screenshot of the home page for the cBioPortal for Cancer Genomics (http://cbioportal.org).

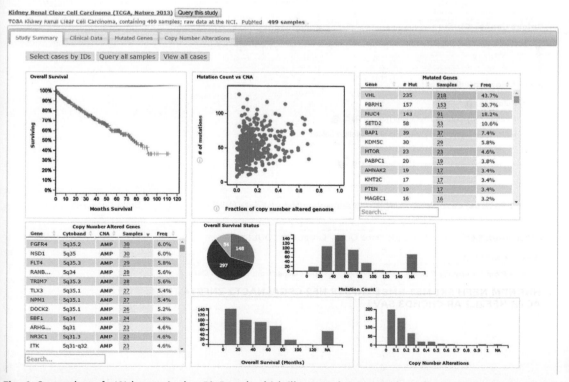

Fig. 4. Screenshot of a Web page in the cBioPortal, which illustrates how research studies are integrated and summarized visually. This Web page shows summarized results from a TCGA kidney renal clear cell carcinoma study correlating molecular information (ie, mutation count and CNAs) with clinical outcome data (ie, overall survival).

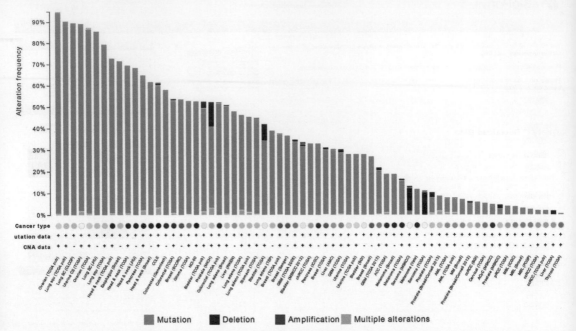

Fig. 5. Screenshot of a Web page in the cBioPortal, which displays the gene alteration frequencies of the gene p53 across the entire spectrum of studied tumor types. In this example, ovarian serous leads the list of cancer types with greater than 90% alteration frequency comprising almost entirely of mutations rather than deletions or amplifications.

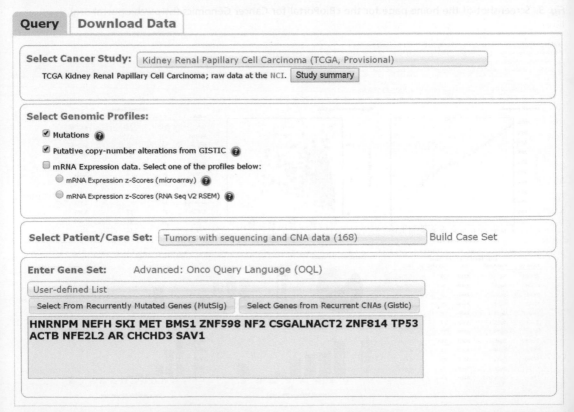

Fig. 6. Screenshot of a Web page in the cBioPortal illustrating the power of discovering recurrently mutated genes by tumor type. This example shows a query from a provisional kidney renal papillary cell carcinoma study, which is selected for recurrently mutated genes, such as MET.

Recurrent Copy Number Alterations (Gistic)

Click on a gene to select it Filter by Gene:

Amp Del	Chr	Cytoband	#	Genes	Q Value
	9	9p21.3	4	CDKN2A CDKN2B C9ORF53 CDKN2B-AS1	5.0e-18
	19	19p13.2	1	INSR	4.3e-17
	1	1p36.31	0		7.36e-6
	2	2q37.3	0		8.10e-5
	11	11q24.2	0		1.63e-3
	11	11q22.3	0		3.02e-3
	2	2q32.1	1	FSIP2	4.09e-3
	3	3p22.1	1	ULK4	1.21e-2
	19	19q13.42	0		1.53e-2
	14	14q11.2	0		2.21e-2
	17	17q25.2	0		2.47e-2
	14	14q32.2	0		3.65e-2
	5	5q35.2	0		3.77e-2
	16	16q24.1	0		7.99e-2
	7	7q22.1	0		8.55e-2
	6	6q22.31	1	NKAIN2	8.60e-2
	3	3q22.3	13	FOXL2 PIK3CB MRAS ARMC8 FAIM less BPESC1 CEP70 ESYT3 NME9 PRR23B PRR23C C3ORF72	0.11

Showing 1 to 26 of 26 entries

Select Genes

Fig. 7. Screenshot of a Web page in the cBioPortal illustrating the power of discovering selected genes from genomic regions with CNAs. This example is from the same provisional kidney renal papillary cell carcinoma study illustrated in **Fig. 6** and, for all described CNAs, the corresponding genes located in those regions are listed.

Additional CNA details are viewable in cBioPortal through launching a Web start version of IGV. **Fig. 8** is the IGV showing the segmented copy number data of the provisional kidney renal clear cell carcinoma study with copy status of all queried genes.[8–10]

The OncoPrint of cBioPortal provides a concise and compact graphical summary of genomic alterations in genes involved in the selected cancer type. **Fig. 9** is the OncoPrint from the provisional kidney renal clear cell carcinoma study and shows that gene alterations in von Hippel-Lindau (VHL) comprise 54% of the cases but with the added insight that several of these cases show co-occurrence of alterations in genes PBRM1, SETD2, and BAP1. **Fig. 10** shows a mutation diagram for the PIK3CA gene from the same provisional kidney renal clear cell carcinoma study. Mutations and individual samples with PIK3CA mutations, as well as each mutation's number of occurrences in the Catalogue of Somatic Mutations in Cancer (COSMIC), are listed and annotated on PIK3CA protein domains.[8–10]

Information on co-occurrence (gene events occurring together) or mutual exclusivity (gene events not occurring together) is discoverable in cBioPortal. **Fig. 11** displays the statistics for co-occurrence and mutual exclusivity for genes from the provisional kidney renal clear cell carcinoma study. Through correlation plots, users have several different ways of visualizing discrete genetic events (CNAs or mutations) and continuous events, such as data regarding mRNA or protein abundance, or DNA methylation. **Fig. 12** shows the correlation plot between SETD2 mRNA expression and VHL mRNA expression, from the same provisional kidney renal clear cell carcinoma study. As shown in the OncoPrint in **Fig. 9**, a considerable number of cases show both mutations in SETD2 and VHL.[8–10]

The cBioPortal has the functionality for interactive analysis and visualization of altered networks. The networks consist of pathways and interactions from the Human Protein Reference Database,[11] Reactome,[12] NCI Pathway Interaction Database,[13] and the MSKCC Cancer Cell Map (http://cancer.cellmap.org), as derived from the open source Pathway Commons Project.[14] **Fig. 13** is the network view of altered gene nodes, such as VHL derived from the provisional kidney renal clear cell carcinoma study.[8–10]

The biomedical informatics component of cBioPortal can display overall survival analysis and disease-free survival rates, if survival data are

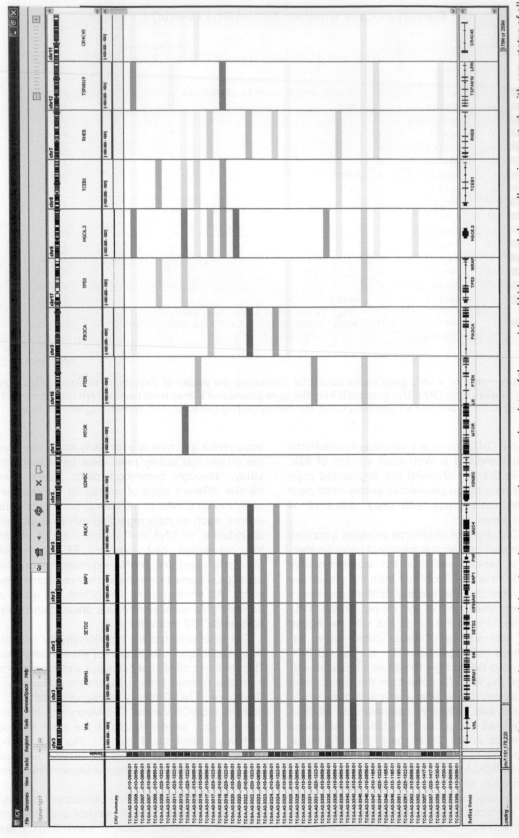

Fig. 8. Screenshot of the IGV in the cBioPortal showing the segmented copy number data of the provisional kidney renal clear cell carcinoma study with copy status of all queried genes.

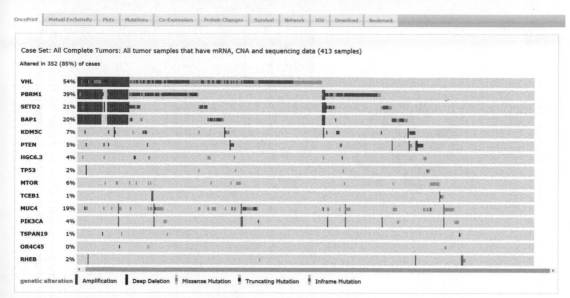

Fig. 9. Screenshot of an OncoPrint in the cBioPortal illustrating its power as a concise and compact graphical summary of genomic alterations in genes involved in the selected cancer type. This example is from the a provisional kidney renal clear cell carcinoma study and shows that gene alterations in VHL comprise 54% of the cases but with the added insight that several of these cases show co-occurrence of alterations in genes PBRM1, SETD2, and BAP1.

available. Overall survival and disease-free survival differences are computed between tumor samples that have at least one alteration in one of the query genes and tumor samples that do not. The results are displayed as Kaplan-Meier plots with *P* values from a log-rank test. **Fig. 14** shows the Kaplan-Meier plots focused on BAP1 from the provisional kidney renal clear cell carcinoma study and demonstrates a statistically significant difference in survival of cases with alterations of the BAP1 gene versus cases without alterations of the BAP1 gene.[8–10]

cBioPortal is currently being transitioned into a tool for the visualization genomic and clinical information of individual tumors (or even patients with multiple tumors), with the goal of its eventual use as a decision support system that can be used in patient treatment. Because tumor samples often have few driver mutations in a sea of background mutations, one key challenge is to identify the most likely driver events found in a tumor sample. cBioPortal does this by using prior information about genes and prior occurrence of specific mutations (eg, via the COSMIC database). cBioPortal also summarizes the key clinical annotation about a tumor sample, including basic demographic data of the patient, as well as stage and grade information about the tumor. For tumor samples from TCGA, links to the Cancer Digital Slide Archive are available, which allow fast and convenient

viewing of histopathologic slides of all TCGA tumors. Furthermore, de-identified pathology reports can be viewed in PDF format for all TCGA samples. In the future, cBioPortal can be more tightly integrated with other clinical information systems in a hospital.

PART 3. MEMORIAL SLOAN KETTERING CANCER CENTER—CLINICAL VARIANTS AND RESULTS DATABASE

The volume of genetic variants identified by clinical NGS assays poses a challenge in terms of variant visualization, classification, pathologist review, and sign-out. Guidelines from regulatory agencies, such as the College of American Pathologists or New York State Department of Health, impose additional requirements on tracking changes made during the sign-out process (passing or failing variant calls, editing of variant annotations, and so forth). From a longer-term perspective, a systematic organization of variant information and associated clinical and analysis metadata are essential to enable retrospective data mining and clinical phenotype correlative studies for biomarker discovery. To address these concerns the clinical bioinformatics group at MSKCC developed an in-house solution, called the CVR system, to organize and efficiently manage variants called by clinical NGS assays. The back-end CVR

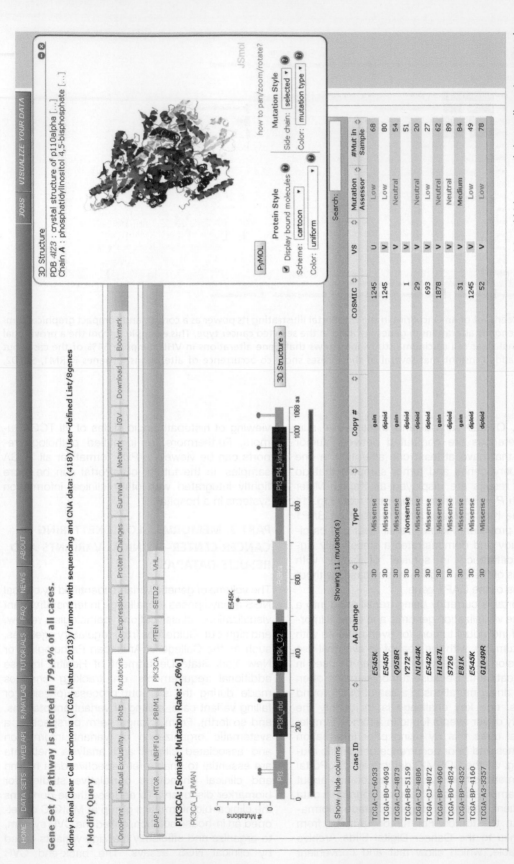

Fig. 10. Screenshot of a mutation diagram in the cBioPortal. This example illustrates the PIK3CA gene from the same provisional kidney renal clear cell carcinoma study illustrated in **Fig. 9**. Mutations and individual samples with PIK3CA mutations, as well as each mutation's number of occurrences in COSMIC, are listed and annotated on PIK3CA protein domains.

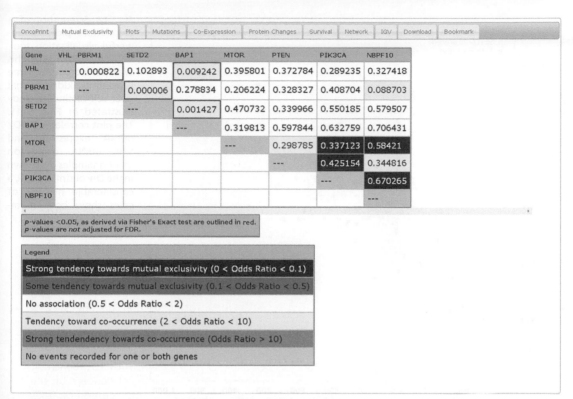

| OncoPrint | Mutual Exclusivity | Plots | Mutations | Co-Expression | Protein Changes | Survival | Network | IGV | Download | Bookmark |

Gene	VHL	PBRM1	SETD2	BAP1	MTOR	PTEN	PIK3CA	NBPF10
VHL	---	0.000822	0.102893	0.009242	0.395801	0.372784	0.289235	0.327418
PBRM1		---	0.000006	0.278834	0.206224	0.328327	0.408704	0.088703
SETD2			---	0.001427	0.470732	0.339966	0.550185	0.579507
BAP1				---	0.319813	0.597844	0.632759	0.706431
MTOR					---	0.298785	0.337123	0.58421
PTEN						---	0.425154	0.344816
PIK3CA							---	0.670265
NBPF10								---

p-values <0.05, as derived via Fisher's Exact test are outlined in red.
p-values are *not* adjusted for FDR.

Legend

Strong tendency towards mutual exclusivity (0 < Odds Ratio < 0.1)

Some tendency towards mutual exclusivity (0.1 < Odds Ratio < 0.5)

No association (0.5 < Odds Ratio < 2)

Tendency toward co-occurrence (2 < Odds Ratio < 10)

Strong tendendcy towards co-occurrence (Odds Ratio > 10)

No events recorded for one or both genes

Fig. 11. Screenshot of a data matrix/matrices in the cBioPortal displaying the statistics for both co-occurrence and mutual exclusivity for genes. Through correlation plots, users have several different ways of visualizing discrete genetic events (CNAs or mutations) and continuous events, such as data regarding mRNA or protein abundance, or DNA methylation. This example is from the same provisional kidney renal clear cell carcinoma study illustrated in Figs. 9 and 10.

database is paired with an intuitive Web interface to streamline variant classification through manual review and sign-out.

The CVR system sits at the end of a clinical sequencing pipeline (shown in **Fig. 15**). The Clinical Laboratory Improvement Amendments–approved NGS tests at MSKCC are mainly targeted sequencing panels that vary in terms of assay technology (hybridization capture vs amplicon polymerase chain reaction), sequencing platform (Illumina vs Ion Torrent), scale (high throughput vs benchtop sequencer), and analysis pipeline. The CVR system is designed to be agnostic for the variables (listed previously) and accepts as its input a variant call format (VCF) or tab-delimited text file with a prespecified format. Metadata from a wet laboratory and analysis parts of the pipeline are managed by different laboratory information systems respectively: various procedures in the wet laboratory process are documented and tracked using an NGS-specialized laboratory information management system (LIMS), whereas metadata regarding sequencing

QC and various analysis metrics are tracked using an in-house developed data management system (DMS). These metadata may be used to place variant calls into context during sign-out, and the CVR system uses API Web service calls to retrieve these metadata from the LIMS and DMS, for presentation in the sign-out Web interface.

Use cases for the clinical variants and results system

The development of the CVR system was motivated by the following use cases.

Development of a data warehousing solution

As NGS testing scales up in a clinical laboratory, the results of different runs of various tests may be stored in an ad hoc manner in scattered locations, complicating data backup and subsequent information retrieval. The authors desire a central storage system where all molecular pathology diagnostic test results can be systematically housed and looked up in subsequent queries.

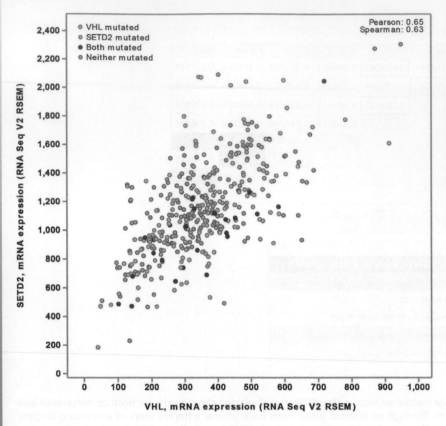

Fig. 12. Screenshot of a correlation plot, a powerful visualization tool, in the cBioPortal. This example is from the same provisional kidney renal clear cell carcinoma study illustrated in **Figs. 9–11**. The plot correlates SETD2 mRNA expression and VHL mRNA expression among samples. As shown in the OncoPrint in **Fig. 9**, a considerable number of cases show both mutations in SETD2 and VHL.

Improving how change history is tracked

Pathologists may reject variant calls based on experience and prior knowledge or even edit the cDNA and amino acid annotations for a given mutation to be compliant with Human Genome Variation Society (HGVS) standards. These changes should be memorialized in a database, so there is accountability for differences between variants called by the pipeline and variants that are entered into a patient's pathology report.

Facilitating the sign-out process

Depending on the size of the targeted sequencing panel, whether a patient matched normal is used, or filters set in the data analysis pipeline, NGS tests may return on the order of tens to thousands of variants. Reviewing each variant during sign-out by browsing for the appropriate alignment file and manually entering variant coordinates is a time-consuming process that cannot be scaled to large volumes. An automated solution for quick visualization of genomic data and variant calls is needed for facilitating sign-out of NGS test results.

Providing a start-to-finish dashboard view of laboratory operations

Many steps in the NGS pipeline (sample QC, wet laboratory workflow, and analysis steps) can affect the quality of the final variant calling output. To streamline and optimize processes and turnaround time, laboratory directors should have access to a laboratory operations dashboard, which integrates collected metadata from various parts of the pipeline (LIMS and DMS) and is capable of correlating various metrics against pipeline output (CVR).

Implementation

Database schema

The underlying schema of the MSKCC CVR database is based on the central idea that a set of variant calls is the product of an analysis pipeline configuration applied to the sequencing output for a given sample. Changes to either the pipeline configuration or sequencing result for a sample can alter the variant calling output, and it is essential to capture metadata on the pipeline, sample,

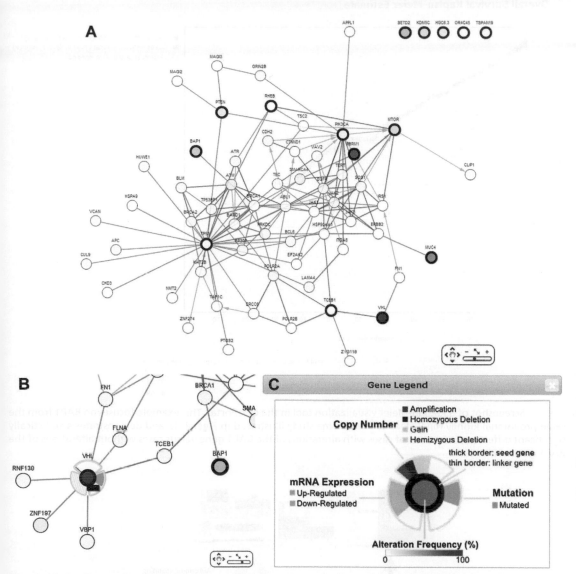

Fig. 13. Illustrates a network visualization tool of altered gene nodes in the cBioPortal. This example is from the same provisional kidney renal clear cell carcinoma study illustrated in **Figs. 9–12.** (*A*) The generalized network view of altered gene nodes. (*B*) Focuses on the VHL altered gene node and some interconnected gene nodes (ie, TCEB1). The BAP1 gene node is also within the proximity although not in direct connection with VHL. (*C*) Mouseover screenshot over the VHL altered gene node illustrating highly granular data, such as frequency of mutation, CNA, and mRNA expression.

and variant result levels to ensure provenance (**Fig. 16**). Examples of analysis pipeline metadata include time and date information, file system locations, pipeline versions, pipeline configurations, identifiers for bioinformatics analysts kicking off the pipeline, and so forth. Most of these metadata are already tracked by the DMS system, so the CVR system merely stores a DMS entity identification (ID), which it can use to retrieve the full set of metadata associated with the pipeline run from the DMS, using a Web service call if necessary. The CVR recognizes that a single patient may have multiple samples sequenced in various batches, which may differ in terms of sample type (ie, primary vs metastasis vs normal vs liquid biopsy), processing method (ie, formalin-fixed paraffin-embedded vs fresh vs frozen), or even purpose of inclusion within the sequenced batch (ie, clinical sequencing vs clinical validation vs translational research). Similar to the analysis

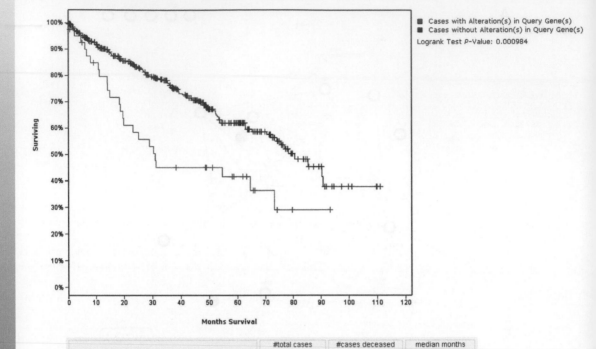

Fig. 14. Screenshot of a Kaplan-Meier visualization tool in the cBioPortal. This example focuses on BAP1 from the same provisional kidney renal clear cell carcinoma study illustrated in **Figs. 9–13** and demonstrates a statistically significant difference in survival of cases with alterations of the BAP1 gene versus cases without alterations of the BAP1 gene.

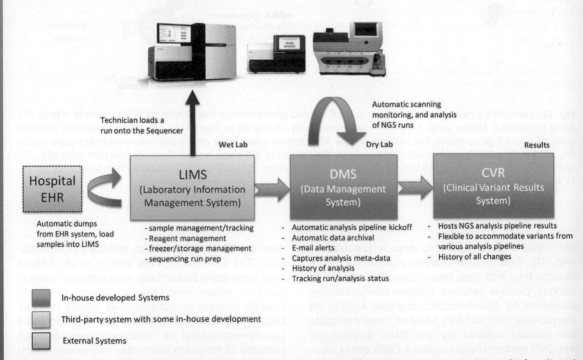

Fig. 15. Schematic of the clinical sequencing pipeline at MSKCC. The CVR system sits at the end of a clinical sequencing pipeline.

MSK Clinical Variant Results Database

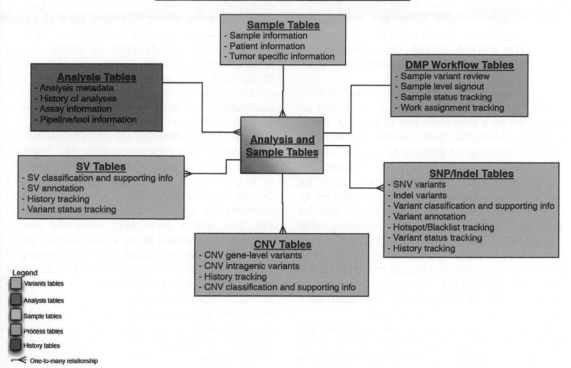

Sample Tables
- Sample information
- Patient information
- Tumor specific information

Analysis Tables
- Analysis metadata
- History of analyses
- Assay information
- Pipeline/tool information

DMP Workflow Tables
- Sample variant review
- Sample level signout
- Sample status tracking
- Work assignment tracking

Analysis and Sample Tables

SV Tables
- SV classification and supporting info
- SV annotation
- History tracking
- Variant status tracking

SNP/Indel Tables
- SNV variants
- Indel variants
- Variant classification and supporting info
- Variant annotation
- Hotspot/Blacklist tracking
- Variant status tracking
- History tracking

CNV Tables
- CNV gene-level variants
- CNV intragenic variants
- History tracking
- CNV classification and supporting info

Legend
- Variants tables
- Analysis tables
- Sample tables
- Process tables
- History tables
- One-to-many relationship

Fig. 16. Relational schematic underlying the MSKCC CVR database.

pipeline metadata, most of the sample and patient information can be retrieved from the wet laboratory LIMS via a Web service call, so the CVR stores an LIMS entity ID instead of replicating most of this information. The atomic data unit within the CVR can thus be thought of as a DMS entity–LIMS entity data unit pair, which allows flexibility for situations where the same sample is put through various iterations of analysis or if the same analysis pipeline is repeatedly applied to multiple samples.

The CVR entity data unit (analysis pipeline sample pair) is linked to data tables describing various classes of mutation events (eg, point mutations [single nucleotide variations], indels, CNAs [whole-gene and partial/intragenic events], and structural rearrangements [translocations, tandem duplications, and inversions]). Similar to a reference SNP identifier (rsID) in the Single Nucleotide Polymorphism Database (dbSNP), or a COSMIC ID, each mutation observed is given a distinct CVR variant ID to facilitate queries of mutation prevalence (ie, the most commonly observed mutation in a given tumor type). The schema is flexible to accommodate both somatic and germline variants, but germline mutations are deliberately stored in a separate set of data tables, which

can be access regulated depending on the level of patient consent.

Each set of data tables is provisioned by corresponding history tables, which maintain a detailed history of changes to table content, along with the ID of the user responsible for the changes. Data tables may be reverted to a previous version to undo changes, if necessary. In particular, individual variants may be deemed low-confidence or false-positive results (artifacts) over the course of manual review and sign-out. These variants are not deleted from the data tables but rather annotated with different flags under variant status: pending, rejected, and signed out. User IDs responsible for changes are not only tracked for accounting purposes but also managed, so that only certain users within specified user groups have modification privileges. The codebase for various modules regulating the CVR system is complex—the back-end for the database interactions is written in Python, and SQLAlchemy is used to abstract the underlying server technology.

Web portal

The Python Web development framework, Flask, is used for Web application development. The interface is supplemented with several JavaScript libraries to facilitate better usability and is hosted through an Apache server. A Web interface allows users to view variants using the IGV directly through hyperlinks, update clinical and diagnostic information, and automatically generate clinical reports reflecting assessments made during sign-out.

Fig. 17 shows the index page of the CVR Web portal that a pathologist sees when logging on and selecting a diagnostic test to sign out. In this example, Memorial Sloan Kettering–Integrated Mutation Profiling of Actionable Cancer Targets (MSK-IMPACT) is chosen, a hybridization capture-based targeted sequencing panel for 341 cancer-related genes. Different batches, or clinical runs, are listed as rows and can be expanded to display all sequenced samples within a given batch. Samples are colored based on their status: blue for pending (awaiting sign-out), yellow for sign-out complete but clinical report not generated, and green for sign-out complete and clinical report submitted to the pathology electronic health records database (ie, Cerner CoPath).

On selecting a particular sample, a pathologist is brought to a new tab in the Web portal, where salient patient and sample information is displayed up front (**Fig. 18**), including patient first and last names, whether a matched normal was used for somatic mutation calling, medical record number,

sample accession number, and gender and depth of sequencing coverage for the sample (usually >500× for MSK-IMPACT). Fields, such as tumor type, sample type (primary vs metastasis), and tumor purity (ie, usually 20% or higher—a QC requirement for testing), are editable at the point of sign-out; they are populated with suggested content based on information imported from other databases, but pathologists are required to check, confirm, and/or edit these fields at sign-out.

The mutations detected are listed below the patient and sample information (**Fig. 19**). Pathologists are able to filter and search for mutations in a given gene of interest by typing into a Google-style search field. The listed mutation locations are a set of hyperlinks to IGV session XML files, which, on clicking, direct the user to the specific mutated locus in the sample alignment file (BAM file) using IGV. Mouseovers of the Human Genome Organisation (HUGO) gene symbols listed in the table bring up additional information from other cancer genome annotation resources, such as My Cancer Genome. The table also contains coverage and sequencing statistics for each variant call, including sequencing depth at the location of the variant, number of mutant reads, and mutant allele frequency in both the tumor and comparator normal. Pathologists are able to edit cDNA and amino acid annotations to

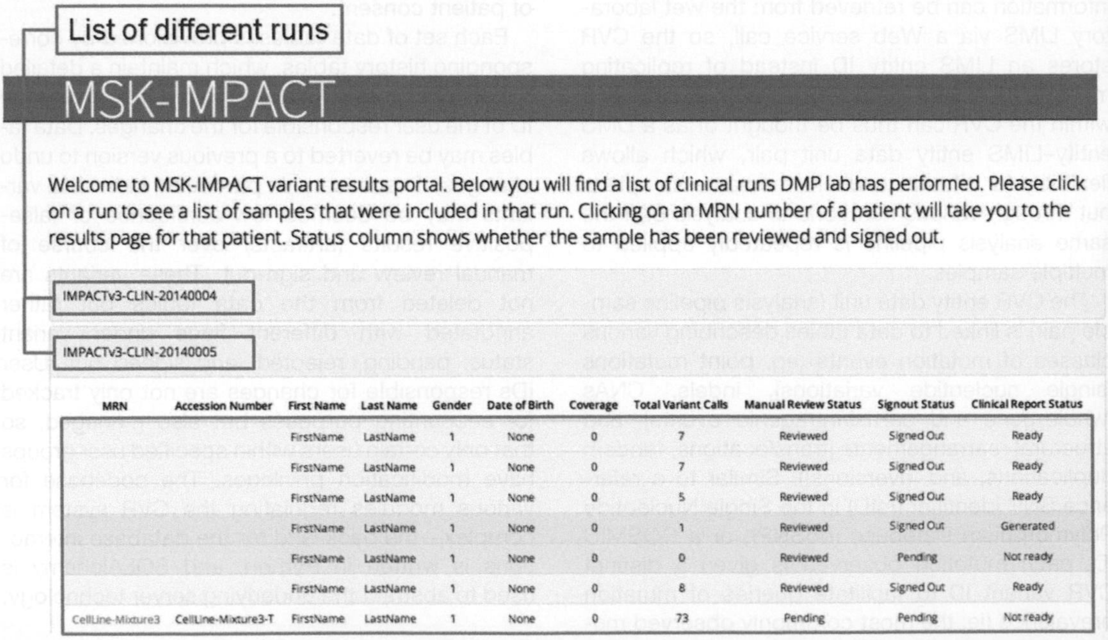

Fig. 17. Screenshot of the index page of the CVR Web portal, which represents the pathologist workspace environment for interpretation of the clinical sequencing pipeline at MSKCC that a pathologist sees when logging on and selecting a diagnostic test to sign out. This example shows the MSK-IMPACT test, a hybridization capture-based targeted sequencing panel for 341 cancer-related genes.

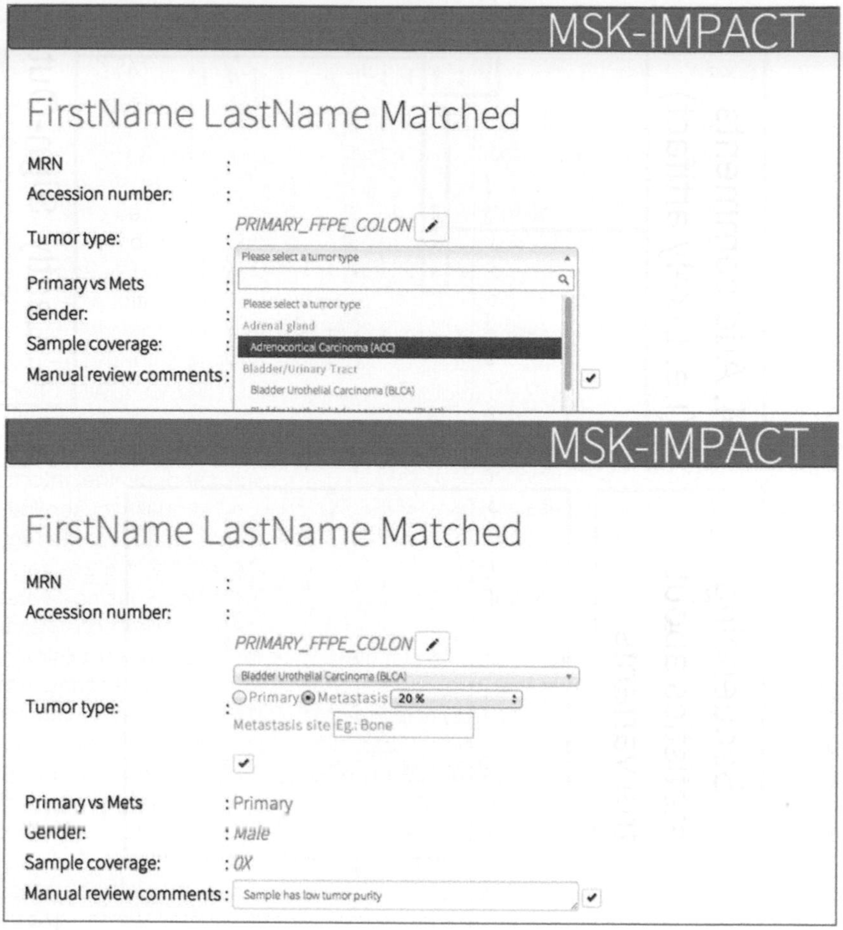

Fig. 18. Screenshot of subsequent tab from the index page in the CVR Web portal, on selecting a particular sample. The salient patient and sample information is displayed up front.

ensure compliance with HGVS standards by clicking on an "edit" button and "drop" variants that they consider low confidence or artifacts (**Fig. 20**). In addition, pathologists can memorialize their rationale for editing or dropping variants as free text comments using the portal interface, by typing into the "comments" field and clicking "save."

Analytics

Applications pulling data from the LIMS, DMS, and CVR databases allow laboratory directors to monitor various aspects of laboratory operations. For instance, because the sample, analysis pipeline, and mutation results are consolidated in their respective databases, directors can ask which solid tumor service or disease management team has been ordering the most number of diagnostic tests on a month-to-month basis (**Fig. 21**). Users

can also perform high-level analytics to identify correlations between wet laboratory QC metrics (input DNA yield, tumor purity, library concentration, and so forth) and variant calling output, which may help identify thresholds or criteria on these metrics, below which a sample is sent to alternative means of diagnostic testing.

Extension to molecular diagnostic assays in general

The CVR database was initially designed as a warehouse for results of clinical NGS assays, but its underlying database schema is flexible enough to be extended to storing the results of non-NGS–based molecular diagnostic tests (eg, Sanger sequencing, fluorescence in situ hybridization, and short or tandem repeat assays). Depending on the assay output, additional variant tables may need to be created to handle the different

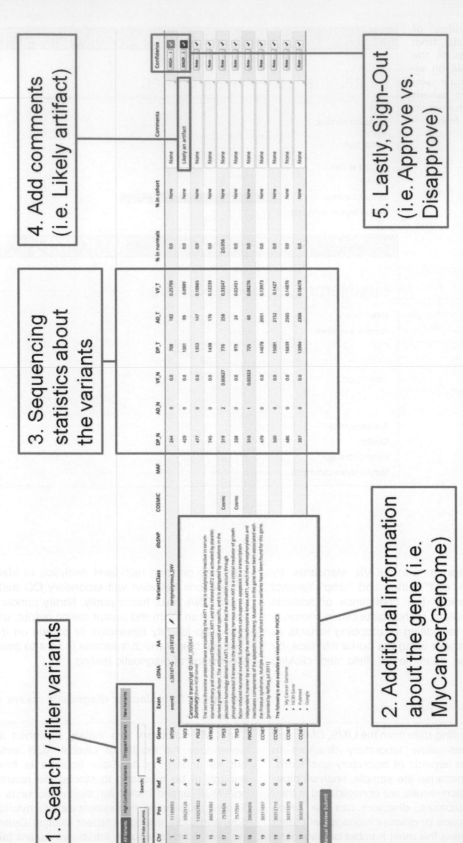

Fig. 19. Additional screenshots of the CVR Web portal environment. The mutations detected are listed below the patient and sample information and the pathologist is able to filter and search for mutations in a given gene of interest by typing into a Google-style search field. The listed mutation locations are a set of hyperlinks to IGV session XML files, which, on clicking, direct the user to the specific mutated locus in the sample alignment file (BAM file) using IGV.

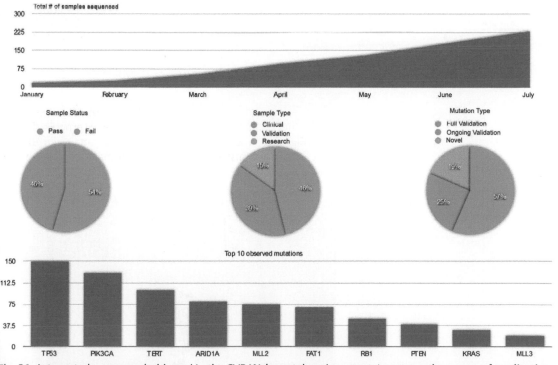

Annotation for APC - (NM_000038) variant ×

Please make sure the new annotations you've entered are HGVS compliant.

Position	112157607
Variant Class	stopgain_SNV
cDNA annotation	c.1327G>T
Amino acid annotation	p.E443X
Reference allele	G
Alternate allele	T

Submit   Cancel

Variant editing dialog box gives user control over every aspect of the variant in case an edit is required

Fig. 20. Annotate/edit function in the CVR Web portal environment. Pathologists are able to edit cDNA and amino acid annotations to ensure compliance with HGVS standards by clicking on an "edit" button and "drop" variants that they consider "low confidence" or artifacts.

classes of mutations called. Finally, to include non-NGS diagnostic assays under the same umbrella of DMSs developed for NGS tests, it is likely that the LIMS and DMS systems would also need to be extended to manage non-NGS tests. This may be more challenging for the DMS system than for the LIMS, because the LIMS is assay agnostic and certain assays may be run with vendor-proprietary software that is not amenable to integration with an in-house developed analysis pipeline management system. In such cases, workarounds (ie, considering vendor software systems as a black box) may be necessary.

Fig. 21. Integrated summary dashboard in the CVR Web portal environment. Leverages the power of applications pulling data from the LIMS, DMS, and CVR databases to allow laboratory directors to monitor various aspects of laboratory operations and query for answers to administrative/operational questions, such as which solid tumor service or disease management team has been ordering the most number of diagnostic tests, on a month-to-month basis.

REFERENCES

1. Clinical research informatics. Available at: http://www.amia.org/applications-informatics/clinical-research-informatics. Accessed July 9, 2014.
2. Pantanowitz L, Tuthill JM, Balis UG. Pathology informatics: theory & practice. Chicago, IL: American Society of Clinical Pathologists Press; 2012.
3. Ritchie MD, Denny JC, Crawford DC, et al. Robust replication of genotype-phenotype associations across multiple diseases in an electronic medical record. Am J Hum Genet 2010;86(4):560–72.
4. Dash RC, Robb JA, Booker DL, et al. Biospecimens and biorepositories for the community pathologist. Arch Pathol Lab Med 2012;136(6):668–78.
5. Digital capabilities to accelerate research. Available at: https://cabig.nci.nih.gov/. Accessed August 1, 2014.
6. Wikipedia. The Cancer genome atlas. Available at: http://en.wikipedia.org/wiki/The_Cancer_Genome_Atlas#cite_note-2. Accessed July 9, 2014.
7. Atlas, T.C.G. Program overview. Available at: http://cancergenome.nih.gov/abouttcga/overview. Accessed July 9, 2014.
8. cBioPortal. Available from: http://www.cbioportal.org/public-portal/. Accessed August 1, 2014.
9. Cerami E, Gao J, Dogrusoz U, et al. The cBio cancer genomics portal: an open platform for exploring multidimensional cancer genomics data. Cancer Discov 2012;2(5):401–4.
10. Gao J, Aksoy BA, Dogrusoz U, et al. Integrative analysis of complex cancer genomics and clinical profiles using the cBioPortal. Sci Signal 2013;6(269):pl1.
11. Keshava Prasad TS, Goel R, Kandasamy K, et al. Human Protein Reference Database–2009 update. Nucleic Acids Res 2009;37(Database issue):D767–72.
12. Matthews L, Gopinath G, Gillespie M, et al. Reactome knowledgebase of human biological pathways and processes. Nucleic Acids Res 2009;37(Database issue):D619–22.
13. Schaefer CF, Anthony K, Krupa S, et al. PID: the Pathway Interaction Database. Nucleic Acids Res 2009;37(Database issue):D674–9.
14. Cerami EG, Gross BE, Demir E, et al. Pathway Commons, a web resource for biological pathway data. Nucleic Acids Res 2011;39(Database issue):D685–90.

Training in Informatics
Teaching Informatics in Surgical Pathology

Lewis Allen Hassell, MD*, Kenneth E. Blick, PhD

KEYWORDS

• Informatics • Surgical pathology • Milestones • Problem-based learning • Competency

ABSTRACT

This article presents an overview of the curriculum deemed essential for trainees in pathology, with mapping to the Milestones competency statements. The means by which these competencies desired for pathology graduates, and ultimately practitioners, can best be achieved is discussed. The value of case (problem)-based learning in this realm, in particular the kind of integrative experience associated with hands-on projects, to both cement knowledge gained in the lecture hall or online and to expand competency is emphasized.

OVERVIEW

What, me worry?
—Alfred E. Neuman

The ability to stand calm and "keep your head when all about you are losing theirs" ("If," Rudyard Kipling) can come from 1 of 2 sources: (1) the confidence born of solid preparation, study, drill, and experience under stress or (2) the nonchalance derived from some combination of ignorance and apathy, oft epitomized by the hero of *Mad* magazine (quoted previously). For practicing pathologists today, and for the soon-to-be practitioners of that art and craft, the latter approach to the issues surrounding the informatics field is a recipe for more than comic-book disaster. But the challenge has been centered on how to form the foundation of knowledge and integrate the kind of drill and experience within the protected environs of a training program that can formulate the former

kind of calm. The prior articles in this volume and an extensive literature on this topic have made the case for the essential skills of pathology informatics (PI), and most practices currently have at least one and often many staff members using these to some degree or another. This article aims to describe a less-than-haphazard or nonchalant approach to acquiring and instilling those essential information technology (IT) skills and knowledge within the context of existing learning models and training programs. This approach entails a review of learning and teaching approaches in the existing graduate medical education setting (residencies and to a lesser degree fellowships) and the post-graduate environment.

THE WHAT—CURRICULUM CONTENT

Residency education generally, and pathology specifically, has migrated from a time-based apprenticeship model validated by a highly knowledge-based examination to an approach strongly emphasizing specific demonstrated competencies.[1] This follows a trend toward competency emphasis across medical education generally but most strongly manifests in graduate medical training.[2,3] Pathology has not been a laggard in this move and, accordingly, used the opportunity to flesh out learning and skill needs in an array of areas beyond conventional medical knowledge of diseases and morphologies to include the growing areas of molecular diagnostics, genomics, laboratory management, and informatics. The detailed and comprehensive exposition of the learning objectives and skill areas in informatics was developed soon after the Accreditation Council for Graduate Medical

Department of Pathology, University of Oklahoma Health Sciences Center, BMSB 451, 940 Stanton L Young Boulevard, Oklahoma City, OK 73104, USA
* Corresponding author.
E-mail address: Lewis-hassell@ouhsc.edu

Surgical Pathology 8 (2015) 289–300
http://dx.doi.org/10.1016/j.path.2015.02.008

Education (ACGME) introduced its 6 competency areas by Henricks and colleagues[4] working in collaboration with the Association for Pathology Informatics (API). Significantly, their approach carefully divided the knowledge areas essential to pathologists along with the applications of that understanding in common use from the informatics proficiencies or skill sets to be sought or demonstrated by the learners.

The Pathology Milestones Project codified this effort on a broad scale into an array of competency statements and descriptors that capture different levels of competency within each area. Looking at the Milestones superficially, it might be concluded that only 1 category (Systems-Based Practice [SBP] competency 7—Informatics: Explains, Discusses, Classifies, and Applies Clinical Informatics) is pertinent to the topic of this article.[5] But in reality, a more comprehensive and inclusive definition, such as might be drawn from a review of model curricula of informatics, reveals that a host of other competency statements within the Milestones document also has direct bearing on informatics knowledge and skills (Table 1).

This question of what PI is and, therefore, what may need to be taught to enable practitioners to be proficient in it's essential uses is a nontrivial one—although neither is it a particularly foreign debate. Pathology has always fostered camps of *lumpers* and *splitters*, who look at their fields of investigation differently, broadly and narrowly, respectively (see, for example, Tischler[6]) Seen broadly, PI encompasses an extensive knowledge and skill base that enables effectively collecting, storing, managing, maintaining, retrieving, analyzing, interpreting, and creating data pertinent to the care of patients who come under the care of a laboratory or a caregiver using a laboratory. The required skill set may include the management of the metadata of the laboratory itself, the medical literature, or other data sets pertinent to 1 or more of the these activities. A more narrow definition is that proposed by Gabril and Yousef[7] of "using highly advanced technologies to improve patient diagnosis or management," which they largely distilled down to the use of current advanced tools in imaging and image transmission along with data mining. Although the authors acknowledge that a majority of "advanced practitioners" of PI will be using and managing those tools, the reality is that the broad definition means that every pathologist must have certain PI skills and knowledge to be effective. It is also the more broad definition that has formed the foundation of several recent solid textbooks in PI. Table 2 summarizes the core curriculum content for residency-level training.

This curriculum content has recently been integrated into a tool for use by training programs, the result of joint work of the Association of Pathology Chairs (APC), College of American Pathologists (CAP), and API. This project and tool, Pathology Informatics Essentials for Residents (PIER), meshes well with the Milestone SBP7 and provides a graduated progression corresponding to the competency levels desired from residents during each year of training (Fig. 1). This program does not, however, attempt to address the broad needs (captured in Table 1) in the many other Milestones with PI components, perhaps with the recognition that a core understanding has many spin-off effects applied to other areas of training.

Looking further at postresidency-level training, either in a formal fellowship or a continuing medical education context, Table 3 outlines recommended added content.[8] Training experience at this level, however, becomes more project driven and experiential, leading to a portfolio of competencies based on successful performance and endeavor in solving informatics-based problems.

THE HOW—METHOD(S) OF TEACHING/LEARNING PATHOLOGY INFORMATICS

Unlike much of the training in anatomic pathology, which is individual patient case based and more easily organized around ongoing clinical materials, acquiring skills in PI cannot be readily compartmentalized into a single rotation of a few weeks (Box 1). Although the content and knowledge have been organized for transmission via texts[9,10] or lectures on an intermittent or even condensed basis and presented in a case-study format using more or less real situations, these approaches often fall short of producing the level of competency required in the SBP7 and other competencies listed in Table 1. Nevertheless, such efforts help build IT vocabulary and create the foundation from which more applied skills can be developed. The PIER approach also recognizes that although some content can be encapsulated into time blocks, the higher-level applications can best be acquired using a variety of approaches, including journals, texts, mentors, and project-based experiences.

Several model programs have published their approach to laying this foundation. For example, Dr Pantanowitz's group has applied the crowdsourcing power of a wiki to maintain the core content in their informatics block.[11] This approach builds on their prior efforts via a "virtual rotation"[12] and on efforts in other aspects of medical training where expertise may be otherwise difficult to access. Students can also benefit from these shared responsibilities.[13] This method of teaching/learning seems highly effective as witnessed by outcomes showing significantly higher levels of student IT performance based on assessments after implementation. This success is due in large part to the greater level of student engagement in the learning process. The old adage, "see, do, teach," is followed to a much greater degree as the students interact with the existing material and critique and refine it to make the content more meaningful on a personal basis.

PI is also a core competency area in the Laboratory Management University offering created by the American Pathology Foundation and the American Society for Clinical Pathology, launched in 2013.[14] This curriculum uses a blended learning model of online and live sessions coupled with a virtual community and offers numerous courses in each of the core management competency areas, including IT. The offerings are taught and developed by leaders in the field and geared to both the resident-level and also a new-in-practice leadership audience. This curriculum content is also being mapped to the Milestones (R. Weiss, personal communication, 2014) for use in developing other tools to assist program directors. The authors' experience in using these tools in resident education has been that the courses provide a solid foundation for discussion of a variety of topics, including PI; these discussions prompt potential topics for further competency development through chartered projects or other associated learning activities. Also, the authors have often coupled the discussions with evaluation of real and simulated case studies and have observed that trainees learn surgical pathology through both real time and historical cases; this same pattern adapts well to the learning PI.

The doing component of learning that fully demonstrates competency is never fully accomplished by didactic methods, updating a wiki, discussing a business-style case study, and/or self-paced learning from a textbook or virtual rotation. The authors have observed, however, that resident engagement in longitudinal projects seems highly valuable in cementing the skills needed to achieve the level of performance competency required. Table 4 lists a sampling of resident-led longitudinal learning projects, some of which resulted in publications; many of these have significant informatics components. These kinds of doing projects, however, seldom fit nicely into a 2- to 4-week elective, or informatics block, in the resident schedule. So how do programs and learners find the time to allow this kind of experience when so much of their other clinical material–based learning is neatly divided into time-based blocks? Different programs use different strategies to accomplish this, although informal surveys indicate that few programs require or significantly (ie, structurally) facilitate these kinds of hands-on resident projects. At the University of Oklahoma, such projects typically occur during a senior integrated rotation covering 3 months, during which they assume a variety of high-level duties. This timing, however, often does not allow the luxury of seeing the follow-up stage of project implementation. To counter this problem, programs may pair residents of different years. Another program has proposed chartering long-term projects early in training and using a time bank of resident elective time to offer short-term coverage for needed activities when a resident is engaged in a clinically demanding rotation (Massachusetts General Hospital forum on clinical informatics, 2014, personal communication).

Fellowship-level training in PI pertinent to surgical/anatomic pathology builds on the resident experience foundation that has been developed. Several models have been used, but many seem to draw on the diversity of individual fellow experiences to enrich the whole, contemporaneously as well as through revival of prior projects in the form of case studies.[9,15,16] These various structured fellowship programs have addressed the varying anticipated practice needs of their fellows by offering flexibility to adapt their experiences and the period or duration of fellowship training differently depending on the desired career path. This type of flexible structuring, although advantageous to trainees seeking a broad portfolio, opens potential for shorter-term training in focused areas and may help existing practitioners or fellows in other pathology disciplines acquire PI skills.[16] Additionally, the educational methods used in these programs, including operational projects, research time, core didactic sessions, clinical conference attendance, and special retreats focused on decision-making and management and governance issues, nicely capture the spectrum of modalities thought most useful in the acquisition of PI skills.

For pathologists beyond an active training stage of their career, the acquisition of PI skills is harder to gauge for a variety of reasons. On the one hand, need is the mother of invention and a motivated learner, seeking to solve a vexing problem, is a more efficient learner given appropriate resources. On the other hand, the kind of effective instruction that may make this learning less painful is often not available for subject matter like PI. Consultation on mobile surgical pathology materials is simple to obtain, even from experts in another country. But finding the right consultant/teacher for a

Table 1
Pathology Milestones with significant informatics components

Milestone	Guiding Competency	Specific Statement	Pathology Informatics Curriculum Area
PC1	Analyzes, appraises, formulates, generates, and effectively reports consultations	Understands and applies EMR to obtain added clinical information (L1)	LIS; clinical information systems
PC2	Interpretation and reporting: analyzes data, appraises, formulates, and generates effective and timely reports	Proficient in using health care records and clinical information to develop a limited and focused differential diagnosis (L5)	Clinical information systems; data analysis; search engines
PC3	Interpretation and diagnosis: demonstrates knowledge and practices interpretation and analysis to formulate diagnoses	Analyzes complex cases, integrates literature, and prepares a full consultative written report with comprehensive review of medical records (L4)	Databases; search engines; data analysis
PC4	Reporting: analyzes data, appraises, formulates, and generates effective and timely reports	Able to complete synoptic report accurately (L4) Keeps current with evolving standards of synoptic reporting (L5)	Databases; data analysis
PC5	Procedure: surgical pathology grossing—demonstrates attitudes, knowledge, and practices that enable proficient performance of gross examination (analysis and appraisal of findings, synthesis and assembly, and reporting)	Produces reports that contain all the necessary information for patient management; edits transcribed reports effectively (L3)	Fundamentals of computing; word processing, databases
MK1	Diagnostic knowledge: demonstrates attitudes, knowledge, and practices that incorporate evidence-based medicine and promote lifelong learning	Performs scientific literature review and investigation of clinical cases to inform patient care (evidence-based medicine) and improve diagnostic knowledge of pathology (L3)	Databases, search engines, data analysis
SBP1	Patient safety: demonstrates attitudes, knowledge, and practices that contribute to patient safety	Explores other resources, such as EMR and radiology (L2) Trouble-shoots patient safety issues (including preanalytical, analytical, and postanalytical, as needed, without supervision (L4)	Laboratory and clinical information systems; connectivity; interfaces and networks Data analysis, graphic tools; data protection and backup

SPB2	Laboratory management: regulatory and compliance	Understands coding and the need to document appropriately in reports (L3) Uses best practices for billing compliance (L5) Understand and apply/teaches others policies and procedures in PHI as defined by HIPAA (L2/L3/L4)	Security, privacy, and confidentiality of laboratory data
SBP3	Laboratory management: resource utilization	Recognizes different budget types (L2) Develops and manages a laboratory budget (L5)	Fundamentals of computing; spreadsheets
SBP4	Laboratory management: quality, risk management, and laboratory safety	Interprets quality data and charts and trends (L3) Has completed a quality improvement project (L4) Utilizes continuous improvement tools, such as lean and Six Sigma (L5)	Databases, user interface; spreadsheets
SBP5	Laboratory management: test utilization	Organizes basic data for utilization review (L2) Able to create charts and graphs that demonstrates utilization patterns (L4) Demonstrates a broad portfolio of analyses for UR in complex scenarios and team management to drive change in areas both within and outside of the department (L5)	Presentation graphics; spreadsheets
SBP6	Laboratory management: technology assessment	Able to perform a cost-benefit analysis (L3) Participates in new instrument and test selection, verification, implementation and validation (including reference range analysis) (L4)	Data analysis; spreadsheets
SBP7	Informatics		See text and **Fig. 1**
PBLI1	Recognition of errors and discrepancies	Participates in RCA (L3)	Various
PROF1	Licensing, certification, examinations, credentialing	Begins assembling portfolio of experiences, including case log and participation in administrative tasks (L2)	Fundamentals of computing; database
ICS2	Interdepartmental and health care clinical team interactions	Prepares and presents cases at multidisciplinary conferences (L3)	Image management; presentation graphics

Abbreviations: EMR, electronic medical record; HIPAA, Health Insurance Portability and Accountability Act; ICS, interpersonal communication skills; L, level; MK, medical knowledge; PBL, practice-based learning; PC, patient care; PHI, personal health information; PROF, professionalism; RCA, root cause analysis; SBP, systems based practice; UR, utilization of resources.

Table 2
Residency-level curriculum for pathology informatics

Core Area	Terms and Concepts	Applications
Computing fundamentals	Hardware Software Networks Internet related	Storage selection System performance Interfaces Languages Architecture
LIS	LIS components Data standards System management Software customization	Critical feature selection Implementation process RFP process Integration Service model selection Trade-offs between types
Data analysis	Databases Transactions Analytics	Expert systems Architecture and type Data mining
Security, privacy, and confidentiality	HIPAA Audits Firewalls Encryption	Selection of security methods Data backup options Compliance planning
Regulatory issues	Audits and standards Compliance planning Accreditation bodies	Inspection planning Documentation Risk avoidance
Digital imaging and telepathology	Pixel, resolution, bits Compression Image analysis Storage Streaming	Scanning options Storage planning Clinical solutions Integration
Additional technologies	Voice recognition Artificial intelligence -Omics Multiplex data streams	

Abbreviations: HIPAA, Health Insurance Portability and Accountability Act; LIS, laboratory information system; RFP, request for proposal.

Adapted from Henricks WH, Boyer PJ, Harrison JH, et al. Informatics training in pathology residency programs: proposed learning objectives and skill sets for the new millennium. Arch Pathol Lab Med 2003;127:1009–18.

longer-term informatics problem is harder, given (1) the limited number of known well-trained practitioners and (2) the lack of a readily available reimbursement structure to gain access to or interest from the consultant/teacher. National meetings of pathology-related organizations often include informatics topics, although some attendees have contended that the relative quantity of programs has diminished over the past decade whereas the need has been increasing. Several excellent textbooks covering the full range of PI have been published, partially filling the IT learning gaps as far as the foundational core is concerned, but these tend to offer little when it comes to solving a particular IT problem.

LABORATORY INFORMATICS TRAINING AT THE UNIVERSITY OF OKLAHOMA

The authors' informatics core rotation consists of 14 1-week blocks (as shown in **Table 5**). In block A, initial lectures focus on laboratory information systems (LIS) and include an overview of the different areas of computerization required for modern laboratory practice: LIS for the clinical laboratory, LIS for the anatomic pathology laboratory, laboratory billing systems, and office automation computing and networking. Possible stand-alone subsystem computers for more specialized laboratory sections are also discussed, which may

PIER Essentials 1

- Informatics in Pathology Practice
- Fundamentals of Information Systems
- Importance of Databases
- Introduction to Data Representation & Communication Standards
- Data Availability and Security

Entry-Level Proficiency
ACGME Milestone Level 1
Workable Timing: PGY 1
Instructional Hours: 6-8

PIER Essentials 2

- LIS Components & Functions
- Specialized LISs & Middleware
- Patient Data Security & Regulatory Standards
- Data & Communication Standards Use in Pathology
- Digital Imaging & Informatics
- Basics of Health Care Information Ecosystem

Basic Proficiency
ACGME Milestone Level 2
Workable Timing: PGY 2
Instructional Hours: TBD

Pathology **I**nformatics **E**ssentials for **R**esidents

PIER Essentials 3

- Role of Pathologist in LIS & EHR Projects
- LIS Installation & Upgrades
- LIS Customization
- Patient Data Security & Privacy Requirements
- Information Systems & Laboratory Performance
- Health Care IT Regulatory Environment & the Clinical Laboratory
- Laboratory Integration into the Healthcare Information Ecosystem

Intermediate Proficiency
ACGME Milestone Level 3
Workable Timing: PGY 3
Instructional Hours: TBD

PIER Essentials 4

- Role of Pathologists in LIS Management
- Regulatory & Accreditation Requirements
- Computerized Provider Order Entry (CPOE) Troubleshooting
- Result Reporting Management &Troubleshooting
- Data Sources for Quality Improvement & Research
- Informatics Tools & Laboratory Utilization /Performance Monitoring

Advanced Proficiency
ACGME Milestone Level 4
Workable Timing: PGY 4
Instructional Hours: TBD

Fig. 1. Informatics core curriculum for residency training as proposed by API, APC, and CAP to meet Milestone SBP7. EHR, electronic health record; PGY, post-graduate year; TBD, to be determined. (*From* Association of Pathology Chairs. Pathology Informatics Essentials for Residents instructional resource guide. Available at: http://www.apcprods.org/pier/documents/PIERIRG_Release0_July2014_v1.pdf; with permission).

Table 3
Didactic curriculum content for postresidency training

Major Area	Topics Covered
Information	Information theory, information architecture, information quality, information manipulation, human-computer interaction, design principles, special information domains
Information systems	Infrastructure fundamentals, LIS, interfaces, system life cycle, health information systems, imaging systems
Workflow and process	Process and quality improvement, business process management, workflow analysis methods, automation, special process domains
Leadership and management	Leadership, management, regulation, teams, cross-organizational project issues

include Food and Drug Administration–approved transfusion medicine applications, molecular pathology systems, so-called big data–associated applications, middleware for point-of-care testing outreach program, and middleware for total track automation systems in the core clinical laboratory. These preliminary lectures include the types of computer hardware and software required for the various topographies of systems available: (1) local area networks deploying intelligent client workstations, (2) central mainframe computers deploying intelligent workstations running emulation software, and (3) central mainframe computers using a central core database deploying essential thin clients with so-called dumb workstations. A discussion is included of the type of equipment required in the traditional laboratory computer center, the specialized ambient environmental and security requirements, fire protections, system backup devices and media and media security/storage, daily central computer maintenance and management requirements, system updates including procedures for tracking new versions and changes, maintaining a test environment for evaluation/testing of new or modified applications prior to implementation on the live system, and disk maintenance routines including compression and elimination of disk fragments. It is stressed that (1) the continuous availability of all computer systems is essential for the operation of the laboratory and (2) a knowledgeable well-trained pathologist in IT has the overall responsibility of maintaining the full function, reliability, and security of all IT systems critical to the patient care mission of the laboratory.

The various staffing requirements of the LIS section as part of block A are discussed, including (1) laboratory data center managers, (2) database specialists, (3) system programmers, (4) system security officer, and (5) system operations personnel. Requirements for bench-level computer experts in each laboratory section are also focused on, with technologists assigned responsibility for (1) operation systems software on laboratory instruments and associated interface software; (2) middleware software for system monitoring, interfacing, and autovalidation; and (3) tracking automation software and associated interfaces and

Table 4
Sample resident informatics projects

Project Synopsis	Estimated Time Frame	Comments
Closing the loop with critical action results—project to ensure that significant LIS-generated results triggered EMR response, including follow-up visit scheduling and/or risk management notice	3–6 mo	The number of stakeholders, critical partners, or institutions involved tends to multiply the time required
Standardizing evidence-based care and appropriate utilization of esoteric hematopathology testing—project involving redesign of ordering tools and processes to optimize specimen procurement and test ordering, applying decision-support tools at the appropriate stage	9 mo (multiple iterations required)	Savings provided to institution and payers helped support further projects
Implementation of a decision support tool to optimize IHC utilization	3 mo	Accrued benefits to health system required 6 mo to 1 y to measure meaningfully
Revision of processes and tools for enhanced accuracy of surgical case coding	2–4 mo	

Table 5
Organization of core lectures in laboratory informatics at University of Oklahoma pathology training program—1 week per block

Block A	Introduction to laboratory computers
	Clinical laboratory computerization
	Anatomic pathology computerization
	Business computing
	Office computing and networking
Block B	Use of computers in laboratory statistics
	Statistics of quality control
	Statistical tests of significance
Block C	Use of spreadsheets for statistics
	MediCalc and other statistics programs
	Receiver operator curves
	Integration of graphs with laboratory statistics
Block D	Bits and bytes
	Programming a laboratory computer
	Operating system/system tools
	Job control languages, scripts
	Application programming
	Screens, navigation tools, graphic user interfaces
Block E	Database concepts/file design
	PC database tools for design, creation, and maintenance
	Requisite files in APLIS
	Query tools, sorting, control breaks, record selection criteria
	Reporting tools and graphics
Block F	Selection of an LIS/replacement of LIS
	Implementation issues
	Connectivity and interfaces
	Backup and maintenance
	System support and data recovery issues
	Security, firewalls, HIPAA requirements
Block G	Operation of an LIS
	Required functionality and programs
	Core clinical laboratory computerization
	Point-of-care testing computerization
	Blood bank system
	Microbiology system
	AP system
Block H	Business computing
	Coding, billing, and compliance issues
	Web-based computing
	Process/project management and simulation tools
Block I	Presentation tools
	PowerPoint and other presentation software
	Animation tools
	Multimedia and PowerPoint
	Digital presentation issues
Block J	Imaging and computerization
	Image capture, slide scanning, digital photography
	Merging images and text in presentations
	Image storage
	Voice recognition
Block K	Office automation
	Word processing tools
	Scheduling and time management tools
	E-mail
	Mobile computing—PDAs, laptops, other mobile devices

(continued on next page)

Table 5 (continued)	
Block L	Internet or Web-based activity in the laboratory or clinic Creating and maintaining a Web site Medical reporting using online submission Internet search for educational materials Citation management software
Block M	Laboratory computer standards—ASTM, HL7, LOINC, CIC Interfacing of laboratory equipment Total laboratory automation and connectivity issues EDI (?) interfacing vs scripted approach Scripting and emulation tools Web portals for order entry and results reporting
Block N	LIS management issues Software and hardware support, internal and external Personnel issues—training and competency Table and file maintenance Clinical issues and system requirements Paperless printing and electronic reporting Expert systems and decision support; evidence-based medicine support

Abbreviations: ASTM, American Society for Testing Materials; CIC, connectivity industry consortium; EDI, electronic data interchange; HL7, health level 7; LOINC, logical observation identifiers names and codes.

networking. Personnel required for laboratory billing applications are discussed as well, including (1) charge capture and coding personnel; (2) accounts receivable and payments posting; (3) audits for billing compliance and accounting purposes and associated accounts management; (4) billing statements, cycles, reporting, delinquent accounts, and collections referrals; and (5) billing compliance personnel. Also, paperless middleware support for ongoing documentation of CLIA'88, the Joint Commission, and CAP compliance is essential for efficient laboratory practice and accreditation. Staffing for this application must be considered as part of a laboratory IT team.

During the first blocks, the rotation focuses on the so-called language of computers, which begin with the basis of computer operation at the bit and byte levels and then progresses to terms essential for describing and understanding the disk operating system software, associated hardware, computer memory, binary coding systems for numbers and text, and the unique nature of different types of data (numerical, text, alphanumeric, floating point data, integers, coded hex, ASCII codes, binary vs decimal, and conversions), documents, images, and space requirements for data storage in memory and disk storage. Computer programming languages are described along with concepts of compilers, job control language, scripting languages, macros, and interpretive computer languages. Early sessions (block D) include exercises in software development using off-the-shelf tools and freeware, such as the Basic computer language.

Each resident is required to develop and test at least 5 different programs, with each project solving specific laboratory-based problems. These exercises include the use of programming approaches to use for (1) decision loops, (2) user-interactive screen prompts, (3) calculations using structured language approaches, (4) variable types including subscripted variables and arrays, (5) subroutines and branching, and (6) results output displays and printing including formatting with captions and headings. The authors' experience with the programming exercises suggests that these exercises facilitate a better understanding of how computers actually work in terms of hardware, terms, and functions. They also assist pathology residents' understanding of the limitations of various computer functions and tools.

For interactive programming, screen design programming tools are also discussed as part of block D. Graphic interface tools are included in this section and include concepts of program calls with command lines, program menu screens, and graphic user interface icons/object–oriented approaches. Keyboard tools and mouse functions are included in this discussion as well. After discussions and exercises covered in blocks A through D, the residents are assigned security passwords with more capability and permissions, which allow them to be trained more thoroughly on the LIS systems.

Blocks E and F focus on issues that must be considered prior to the acquisition of an LIS. These blocks include concepts of file design with a focus on tools that allow access into various data elements stored therein. Structured query tools are covered along with exercises to create databases that can be sorted, searched, and processed. These topics include data extraction along with migration of data into various PC-based applications, including spreadsheets and local databases. Record layouts with various file organization, including sequential and indexed files, are covered. Various types of data fields for laboratory applications are discussed, along with the required characteristics of various data fields in databases, in these blocks. Boolean logic and decision support concepts are included in these blocks, with specific examples of structured query approaches using the appropriate data extraction and processing logic. System selection and system replacement criteria are included with emphasis on project risk, especially those risks pertaining to uncontrollable project variables, which may include system interfacing, overall system reliability, total system costs, and system capacity/speed.

Blocks G though K of the Oklahoma resident IT training program focus mostly on the day-to-day operational aspects of the LIS (see **Table 5**). These sessions drill down into the details of the operation of each type of LIS used in the laboratory, with emphasis on the unique role of each LIS system deployed. These blocks also include more detail on the power of the individual workstations and deployed emulation software thereon. Some of these workstation tools have very useful capability, including scripting tools for specialized applications.

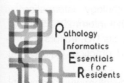

**PIER Essentials 1 –
Outcomes Achievement Checklist**

Pathology
Informatics
Essentials
for
Residents

Resident Name: Click here to enter text.

ACGME Milestone Level 1
Demonstrates familiarity with basic technical concepts of hardware, operating systems, and software for general purpose applications

Informatics in Pathology	
Outcome Statement	**Results**
Understand the relevance of informatics in pathology practice.	☐ Achieved
Describe the difference between IT and Informatics and recognize how pathologists contribute to informatics initiatives.	☐ Achieved
Explain the differences and similarities among pathology informatics, bioinformatics, public health informatics, health care information technology and health knowledge informatics.	☐ Achieved
Comments: Click here to enter text.	

Fundamentals of information Systems	
Outcome Statement	**Results**
Use correct terminology to describe the major types and components of computer hardware, software, and computer networks.	☐ Achieved
Comments: Click here to enter text.	

Importance of Databases	
Outcome Statement	**Results**
Conversant in the fundamentals of databases, including data types, fields, records, database structure, and mechanisms for querying data; understands how data storage affects data retrieval options.	☐ Achieved
Comments: Click here to enter text.	

Introduction to Data Representation and Communication Standards	
Outcome Statement	**Results**
Understand the basics of the standards development process (includes ISO organizations like HL7 and also other processes important in standards development like IHE and ONC).	☐ Achieved
Comments: Click here to enter text.	

Data Availability & Security	
Outcome Statements	**Results**
Understand the elements of data availability as a key part of security.	☐ Achieved
Comments: Click here to enter text.	

Fig. 2. PIER outcomes achievement checklist tool for documentation. (*From* Association of Pathology Chairs. Pathology Informatics Essentials for Residents instructional resource guide. Available at: http://www.apcprods.org/pier/documents/PIERIRG_Release0_July2014_v1.pdf; with permission.)

Block L focuses on Web-based programming and applications on mobile devices, including a discussion of Java programming and cloud-based computing. Various devices can be used in this block for exercises, including Android smartphones and tablets. Laboratory interface standards are covered in block M: American Society for Testing Materials (ASTM) and Health Level Seven International (HL7) standards for data interchange between instruments and the LIS. Interfacing between hospital information systems and electronic medical records (EMR) systems and LIS systems using the HL7 standards are also covered. The final block, block N, of the rotation reviews the main points covered in the entire resident IT program, again with an emphasis on daily operations and system reliability issues. The focus is on the overall responsibility of IT-trained pathologists in the success of a laboratory, which, going forward, is largely determined by the success of the IT deployment and day-to-day operations.

Long-term resident project conceptualization, development, implementation, and monitoring have yet to be entirely successfully structured into the program for every resident, although there have been several individual successes on these components of training, such as those listed in **Table 4**. The model covers the core content well but is faculty intensive. Resources, such as those newly assembled and packaged by API, CAP, and APC as the PIER resource guide, seem to make the acquisition of the core didactic content more readily available to more residents[17] and to facilitate documentation of progress (**Fig. 2**).

SUMMARY

This article presents an overview and considerable detail of the curriculum that the authors and others deem essential for trainees in pathology. These are closely tied to the competencies desired for pathology graduates and ultimately practitioners. The value of case (problem)-based learning in this realm is emphasized, in particular the kind of integrative experience associated with hands-on projects, to cement knowledge gained in the lecture hall or online and to expand competency.

REFERENCES

1. Naritoku WY, Alexander CB, Bennett BD, et al. The pathology milestones and the next accreditation system. Arch Pathol Lab Med 2014;138:307–15.

2. Nasca TJ, Philibert I, Brigham T, et al. The next GME accreditation system—rationale and benefits. N Engl J Med 2012;366:1051–6.

3. Swing SR, Clyman SG, Holmboe ES, et al. Advancing resident assessment in graduate medical education. J Grad Med Educ 2009;1:278–86.

4. Henricks WH, Boyer PJ, Harrison JH, et al. Informatics training in pathology residency programs: proposed learning objectives and skill sets for the new millennium. Arch Pathol Lab Med 2003;127:1009–18.

5. The pathology milestone project. J Grad Med Educ 2014;4:183.

6. Tischler AS. Pheochromocytoma: time to stamp out "malignancy"? Endocr Pathol 2008;19:207–8.

7. Gabril MY, Yousef GM. Informatics for practicing anatomical pathologists: marking a new era in pathology practice. Mod Pathol 2010;23:349–58.

8. Gilbertson JR, McClintock DS, Lee RE, et al. Clinical fellowship training in pathology informatics: a program description. J Pathol Inform 2012;3:11.

9. Pantanowitz L, Tuthill JM, Balis UG, editors. Pathology informatics: theory and practice. Chicago, IL: ASCP Press; 2012.

10. Sinard J. Practical pathology informatics: demystifying informatics for the practicing anatomic pathologist. New York, NY: Springer; 2006.

11. Park S, Parwani A, MacPherson T, et al. Use of a wiki as an interactive teaching tool in pathology residency education: Experience with a genomics, research, and informatics in pathology course. J Pathol Inform 2012;3:32.

12. Kang HP, Hagenkord JM, Monzon FA, et al. Residency Training in Pathology Informatics A Virtual Rotation Solution. Am J Clin Pathol 2009;132:404–8.

13. Kohli MD, Bradshaw JK. What is a wiki, and how can it be used in resident education? J Digit Imaging 2011;24:170–5.

14. ASCP/APF, Lab Management University. Available at: http://www.ascp.org/PDF/LMU/FAQs-v4.pdf. Accessed August 6, 2014.

15. Quinn A, Klepeis V, Mandelker D, et al. The ongoing evolution of the core curriculum of a clinical fellowship in pathology informatics. J Pathol Inform 2014;5:22.

16. Levy BP, McClintock DS, Lee RE, et al. Different tracks for pathology informatics fellowship training: Experiences of and input from trainees in a large multisite fellowship program. J Pathol Inform 2012;3:30.

17. Henricks W, Pantanowitz L, Powell SZ, et al. PIER Instructional Resource Guide. 2014. Available at: http://www.apcprods.org/pier/documents/PIERIRG_Release0_July2014_v1.pdf. Accessed August 18, 2014.

Role of Informatics in Patient Safety and Quality Assurance

Raouf E. Nakhleh, MD

KEYWORDS

- Quality assurance • Quality improvement • Informatics • Patient safety • Surgical pathology

ABSTRACT

Quality assurance encompasses monitoring daily processes for accurate, timely, and complete reports in surgical pathology. Quality assurance also includes implementation of policies and procedures that prevent or detect errors in a timely manner. This article presents uses of informatics in quality assurance. Three main foci are critical to the general improvement of diagnostic surgical pathology. First is the application of informatics to specimen identification with lean methods for real-time statistical control of specimen receipt and processing. Second is the development of case reviews before sign-out. Third is the development of information technology in communication of results to assure treatment in a timely manner.

OVERVIEW

This article discusses the application of informatics to patient safety and quality assurance. It is not possible to write a comprehensive overview in this brief report; instead, this article focuses on recent developments in how informatics is being applied to quality assurance.[1–4]

Quality assurance may be separated into 2 arms. The first is ongoing monitoring to evaluate the extent of possible problems and work to control them over time,[1,2] this is usually divided among the 3 phases of the test cycle. But other monitors of quality assurance include turnaround time (TAT) and customer satisfaction. These monitors do not necessarily relate to patient safety concerns but are important aspects when it comes to the overall success of a laboratory. A list of

quality monitors is shown in **Table 1**. The second arm of quality assurance is implementation of tools and changes to help address the shortcomings of any process.

One of the main principles of quality assurance is to identify risk and then try to mitigate that risk.[1,2,5,6] In surgical pathology there are 3 main areas that present risks: first and most significant is the risk of making the wrong diagnosis, second is delivering the result for the wrong patient, and third is somehow not communicating the result (**Table 2**). As such, most quality assurance activities focus on these 3 areas: (1) interpretive diagnoses, (2) specimen identification, and (3) communication of the result. These areas also correspond to the preanalytical (specimen identification), analytical (interpretive diagnoses), and postanalytical (communication of results) phases of the test cycle.

This article addresses the application of informatics in the traditional 3 phases of the test cycle (**Table 3**). This structure is particularly well suited for devising, implementing, and reporting quality assurance monitors. This structure is equally suited for describing the introduction of procedural changes that ultimately lead to improvement of performance.

Currently, most anatomic pathology laboratory information systems (APLISs) are inflexible and lack interoperability.[3,4] This situation makes it difficult to automate much of the data collection necessary to maintain a vibrant laboratory focused on continuous improvement. It is the authors' hope that with newer generations of systems these functionalities will be routinely and easily used.[4]

In an ideal system, it can be imagined what is possible. Specimen processing and reporting in many respects are similar to manufacturing

Department of Laboratory Medicine and Pathology, Mayo Clinic Florida, 4500 San Pablo Road, Jacksonville, FL 32224, USA

E-mail address: Nakhleh.Raouf@mayo.edu

Surgical Pathology 8 (2015) 301–307

http://dx.doi.org/10.1016/j.path.2015.02.011

Table 1
Quality assurance monitors listed within the test cycle phases and global measures (turnaround time and customer satisfaction)

Quality Assurance Subsections	Monitors
Preanalytical	Specimen identification
	Specimen integrity
	Adequate clinical history
	Accessioning problems
Analytical	Block and slide labeling errors
	Amended report rate
	Rate of case review before sign-out
	Rate of case review for specific organs/diagnoses
	Frozen section/permanent section correlation
Postanalytical	Synoptic reporting and completion rate
	Report delivery
	Critical results
TAT	Frozen section TAT
	Small biopsy TAT
	Complex specimen TAT
	Cytology TAT
	Autopsy preliminary and final TAT
Customer satisfaction (physicians, midlevel providers, administration)	Overall customer satisfaction
	Component customer satisfaction (TAT, ancillary staff, pathologist, communication)
	Customer complaints

Table 2
Highest risk areas to address in surgical pathology

Test Cycle Phase	Risk
Preanalytical	Specimen identification[a]
Analytical	Accurate diagnosis
	Specimen identification[a]
Postanalytical	Communication of results
	Specimen identification[a]

[a] Specimen identification is primarily a problem of the preanalytical phase but identification problems can occur at any phase of the test cycle.

Table 3
Informatics applications used in surgical pathology and test cycle phase and other functions

Informatics Application	Process
CPOE	Preanalytical
Specimen tracking	Preanalytical
	Analytical
	Biorepository
	Postanalytical
	Send-outs
Assignment of cases for quality assurance pre- and postanalytical review	Analytical, cytopathology
	Analytical surgical pathology
	Analytical autopsy
Monitoring and data extraction	All phases, mislabeling
	Postanalytical, amended reports
	Volume indicators
	TAT
Survey tools	Customer satisfaction
Inclusion of image in report	Specimen identification
	Analytical diagnostic check
Whole-slide imaging	Analytical case reviews
	Access for conference cases and clinical correlation
	Facilitates consultation
	More accurate staging
Synoptic reports	Analytical report completeness

operations and can be controlled, like most factories, with few differences.

PREANALYTICAL PHASE

The process begins with the acquisition of the specimen; this step is perhaps the most problematic, because in most instances it is well beyond the control of a laboratory. As such, the laboratory has less power to effect change at this step than most others. One of the keys to successfully implementing change to improve specimen acquisition and proper identification requires that pathologists reach beyond the laboratory to clinical colleagues and ancillary staff to help implement change.[7] The application of informatics has a key role.

SPECIMEN LABELING

The problems occurring in the preanalytical phase are dominated by problems of specimen identification and to some extent tracking of specimens outside the laboratory. Specimen identification starts with specimen order and acquisition. A tool that is often implemented to reduce specimen identification problems is computer physician order entry (CPOE).[8–10] CPOE has been implemented in many surgical pathology departments and offers several advantages over traditional requisition slips received with the specimen. The first benefit of remote order is it provides a check on receipt of the specimen on a particular patient. The computer order is typically placed before a specimen arrives in the gross room. The laboratory knows that a specimen is coming and can prepare and track its arrival. Specimens that are not received in a timely fashion can be traced and found in a timely manner. Specimens that arrive without corresponding computer orders are investigated for possible identification errors.

Computer order entry also offers some advantages that may be built into a system, such as forcing functions that may address the inclusion of useful clinical information. With increasingly more sophisticated systems, it may be possible to attach a clinician's relevant clinical note that clearly defines the clinical question accompanying the specimen. Some systems exist that can generate the order directly from an electronic health record while a physician dictates clinical notes. Because clinical correlation is often cited as a cause of diagnostic error or discrepancy, the ability to force the inclusion of clinical information is a notable improvement to patient care.[11]

Interoperability between electronic health records and an APLIS is a key to adoption of this technology.[4] For example, in most institutions the bar code system used for blocks and slides is different from the system that hospitals or clinics use for patient identification. When CPOE is implemented in most institutions, patient identification information has to be transferred into the ordering system. More ideally, the information should be generated within the electronic health record and transferred seamlessly to the APLIS. Building an electronic requisition can offer greater advantages beyond reducing specimen identification errors. Clinics or operating rooms where specimens are generated can create customized requisitions that include drop-down menus for specimen sites and for frequent clinical questions. Menus for specimen sites have the advantage of using standardized designations for uniform use throughout a department. Forcing functions could also be used to assure capture of these data for use in the current problem and for future investigations.

SPECIMEN TRACKING

FedEx and UPS are well known delivery service companies. They have a remarkable record of delivering all types of packages to their destinations in a timely and safe fashion. Most laboratories should have specimen delivery services that are comparable those of these companies. Anything less seems inadequate. The optimal situation is to have tracking and control of specimens beginning at the source, with patient side labeling and CPOE followed by specimen tracking to receipt in the laboratory and accessioning. Any labeling errors should be tracked, quantitated, and analyzed for possible problems that need to be addressed. With CPOE and advanced specimen tracking technology, maintaining a specimen labeling error monitor is easily done. **Table 4** lists the advantages of specimen tracking with CPOE.

ANALYTICAL PHASE

Within the past 10 years there have been 2 major analytical phase developments in the application of informatics.

Table 4 Benefits of specimen tracking and computer physician order entry	
Informatics Application	**Desired Functionality and Benefits**
Specimen tracking with CPOE	Alerts laboratory of specimen in transit
	Provides a check on specimen identity
	Real-time knowledge of specimen processing
	Processing reports at set points
	Flags delinquent or missing assets
	Improved specimen identification
	Generation of labeled blocks and slides
	Initiates appropriate levels and ancillary studies
	Directs cases to appropriate laboratory or pathologists
	Tracks cases for biorepository
	Tracks case sendouts

SPECIMEN TRACKING

Lean methodology has taken hold with the use of informatics to control all aspects of specimen tracking and quality control.[8,9] Although some investigators proclaim the beginning of the analytical phase at accessioning, others herald the analytical phase with the examination of specimens. Regardless of this overlap in the definition of phases, specimen tracking within the laboratory is more easily accomplished with the aid of informatics. The most important aspect of a tracking system is its ability to account for all assets (specimens, blocks, and slides) in real time. This ability is key to successfully assuring that all specimens are processed and reported in a timely fashion. Tracking specimens in real time gives managers the ability to be proactive rather than reactive.

As specimens are accessioned, informatics can assist in multiple ways. With assignment of a specimen to a particular category (eg, liver biopsy), a host of functions may be unleashed. In cases of liver biopsy, special stains, number of levels, and pathologist assignment may be initiated. In turn, a specimen may be placed in the queue of a histotechnologist for cutting and for special stains as well as pathologists to read the case. If the system is accessible to pathology reception and questions are coming from clinicians regarding the specimen, questions can be easily directed to the appropriate pathologist or that the specimen is being processed and when availability for review is expected may be able to be relayed. In a sophisticated system, a note may be generated to deliver to the pathologists with the specimen to contact the clinician with the result.

From a quality assurance monitoring perspective, the ability to track specimens at every point in the process (accessioning, gross room, embedding, cutting, slide distribution, pathologists' table, and block and slide files) gives managers the ability to find problems when and where they occur and immediately address them.[12] From a documentation standpoint, managers have the ability to accumulate data on mishaps and are able to focus and tackle problematic areas. With sophisticated systems and sufficient time, they may be able to analyze their data by point in the process, physical station, or specific personnel. These abilities can be translated into statistical control.

DIAGNOSTIC ACCURACY

Another analytical intervention that has become the norm is to have a targeted review of cases by a second pathologist. The University of Pittsburgh has pioneered a unique method to conduct reviews of up to 8% of cases in a blinded fashion using the APLIS to flag, distribute, and document review of cases in surgical pathology and cytopathology.[13,14] At the time of sign-out, this tool automatically informs the case pathologist that a case will be reviewed. So the case is not finalized; it is moved to a different work list in the APLIS where it is accessed and review by a second pathologist. The second pathologist has 24 hours to review the case and input a diagnosis into the APLIS system, which is forwarded back to the original pathologist for completion of the case. The reviewing pathologist may agree, disagree minor, disagree moderate, or disagree major. Any disagreements are then worked out between the pathologists and the case is finalized by the original sign-out pathologist. This program was initially used for surgical pathology and decreased diagnostic edits by 55% and has since been adapted for cytopathology. As this program has progressed, the University of Pittsburgh has reported ongoing reduction of amended reports over several years of operation.[15]

Traditional monitors of surgical pathology include monitors of TAT (frozen section, small biopsies, and specific types of cases), amended diagnoses, frozen section/permanent section correlation, and case volumes. Monitors that have become more popular recently include demonstration of adherence to policy regarding review of cases as well as adherence to policy, such as the use of synoptic checklists for cancer reports (see **Table 1**).

As discussed previously, many departments have instituted review of specific types of cases to be reviewed by a second pathologist. Tracking the percent of cases a pathologist signs out that are reviewed is an indicator that demonstrates adherence to policy. This monitor is easily performed with the use of informatics by building a tracking mechanism into the report format. A recent study demonstrated that cases from 45 institutions were tracked at an aggregate rate of 6.6% with a median of 8.2%. Institutions that had review policies tracked cases at a 9.6% rate.[16] The appropriate rate is not clearly defined and is dependent on individual institutional case types and review policies. From this study, a review target of 5% to 15% seems reasonable.

The other aspect of monitoring reviews can be focused on review of specific organ systems or diseases. For example, if a policy states that all initial diagnoses of breast cancer are to be confirmed by a second pathologist, then this should be monitored. Most reporting systems have functionality to identify and check that all initial diagnoses of breast cancer have had a second pathologist review. The extent of review could be assessed for the entire department and can also be monitored for individual pathologists in ongoing professional practice evaluation. Although the University of Pittsburgh describes its experience using a system of random case reviews, a similar system could be set up to review cases for specific organ system or diagnosis. Raab and colleagues[17] have demonstrated that targeted case reviews detect discrepancies at a much higher rate than random case reviews.

COMPLETE REPORTS

The use of synoptic reports has been greatly enhanced with the use of informatics. In 2004, for cancer center designation, the Commission on Cancer mandated that greater that 90% of cancer resections should have complete reports as dictated by the College of American Pathologists cancer checklists. This requirement greatly boosted the use of cancer checklists. Multiple studies have demonstrated that synoptic reports significantly improve the completeness of cancer reports.[18,19] They have also been applied to noncancer conditions with similar results. Although barriers still exist to complete implementation, the use of informatics can facilitate the auditing function of cancer reporting. The barriers include the inconsistent need to include specific information in reports based on the types of specimens taken. For example, lymph node status is a required element for most cancer resection cases. For some organs, however, lymph nodes may not be taken. Accounting these differences in specimen content typically has to be addressed manually and is not automated in most systems.

POSTANALYTICAL PHASE

The inclusion of images in reports is one application of informatics that helps prevent diagnostic errors and misidentification. Many laboratories have developed a practice of taking an image of a significant finding and embedding that image into the report of a case. Most commonly this finding is of a newly diagnosed cancer and is particularly effective if the slide bar code is used to label the image and embed into the report. Pathologists typically dictate cases and verify reports at a different time. The inclusion of an image serves as an additional quality check on the accuracy of the diagnosis. For Example, a pathologist reads a diagnosis of "adenocarcinoma" and then correlates with the image, which hopefully also represents an adenocarcinoma. Although this is a good check that a positive finding correlates with the diagnosis, it is also an opportunity to correlate the finding with the clinical history for congruence. This method, however, does not pick up any false-negative results so should not be relied on as the only diagnostic check of the system.

Over time, it is anticipated that whole-slide imaging will become the norm for pathology microscopic examination.[20] As such, images of specimens will be stored digitally, more easily facilitating review of cases because the steps of slide identification, retrieval, and distribution are eliminated. It would also facilitate a pathologist's ability to consult with others regarding the diagnosis or some aspect of a case by more easily being able to deliver images digitally. Quality assurance review of cases will be much easier as will review of cases for any other reason, such as tumor board meeting or simply to discuss a case with a clinician. Furthermore, digital images could allow more accurate staging (eg, depth of invasion) with the advent of digital tools to measure or quantitate various aspects of a case (eg, tumor volume, infiltrating lymphocytes, or cells positive for specific markers).

Critical result notification is an important aspect of quality. Clinical Laboratory Improvement Amendments mandates that "critical" results be reported to the clinical care team within a predetermined time frame. This is a requirement of The Joint Commission and the Laboratory Accreditation Program of the College of American Pathologists. Recently the College of American Pathologists and the Association of Directors of Anatomic and Surgical Pathology released a guideline addressing critical results in anatomic pathology.[21] They classify these results into 2 groups, urgent and significant unexpected findings. Urgent findings are cases where a life-threatening condition exists and communication should occur as soon as possible. Significant unexpected results are those where a condition exists that should be addressed but is not immediately life threatening. It has been suggested and demonstrated in the clinical laboratory that informatics has a role in the delivery of critical results. Electronic result delivery has become far more feasible with the development and use of handheld devices and the ability to deliver information in multiple modalities. Elegant solutions can also be designed to assure delivery of the message. Monitoring of urgent results delivery failures is a frequently recommended quality monitor. If laboratories have a predetermined list of urgent diagnoses, then those diagnoses can be audited and a determination of the extent of urgent communication of those results can be done.

Monitoring of significant unexpected findings are more problematic because there is no defined list of diagnoses to be tabulated. One possible solution is to code these reports in some unique way when they occur so that they may be tracked and documented. Manual tracking is cumbersome and time consuming. Determining the denominator of possible cases of significant unexpected results is not possible without extensive study of all cases. It may be sufficient to continuously document the practice of notification of significant unexpected results, to be able to demonstrate active implementation of the policy and also to encourage it ongoing use.

Report corrections and amendments are an excellent source of quality assurance data.[22,23] Several studies have used altered reports to evaluate problems in surgical pathology. These studies divide the problems into 4 general categories: specimen defects, misidentification defects, misinterpretation defects, and report defects. Report corrections are a good source of data if corrections are done in a uniform and consistent manor. Standardization of definitions and application of those definitions are critical to having good data.

Corrected or amended reports should be used when there is a change to any part of a report. Addendum reports have been used to correct a report. Addendum reports add information but do not change any information in the original report, which is dangerous because the original false information remains and there is a potential that someone will act based on that information. That is why a corrected or amended report is recommended to change any erroneous information.

The appropriate coding of report corrections and any modifiers can greatly enhance the collection of quality assurance data. At the time of corrections, information regarding the specific correction should be coded and can be classified as to its significance (no harm, harm, and so forth). This information can be used to modify practices to reduce future errors. When applied uniformly and equitably, it can also be used to effectively evaluate processes and individuals.

The final application of informatics in quality assurance has yet to happen but should occur with the next wave of APLIS installations.[20] Soon, surgical pathology data will be managed in computer systems as discrete data elements that are stored in relational databases, which will enable a whole new level of quality assurance where pathology data can be correlated with clinical findings in a dynamic and real-time way. Imagine if pathologists could in an instant review radiographic, gross, and microscopic images side by side. Clinical correlations would become much easier and more definitive, allowing surgical pathology quality assurance data to actually correlate with treatments and outcomes, facilitating the delivery of data and analysis of cancer registries and other public health records.

REFERENCES

1. Nakhleh RE, Fitzgibbons PL, editors. Quality management in anatomic pathology: promoting patient safety through systems improvement and error reduction. Northfield (IL): College of American Pathologists; 2005.
2. Nakhleh RE. Patient safety and error reduction in surgical pathology. Arch Pathol Lab Med 2008;132:181–5.
3. Park SL, Pantanowitz L, Parwani AV. Quality assurance in anatomic pathology. Diagn Histopathol 2013;19(12):438–46.
4. Park SL, Pantanowitz L, Sharma G, et al. Anatomic pathology laboratory information systems: a review. Adv Anat Pathol 2012;19:81–96.
5. Kornstein MJ, Byme SP. The medicolegal aspect of error in pathology; a search of jury verdicts and settlements. Arch Pathol Lab Med 2007;131:615–8.
6. Troxel DB. Medicolegal aspects of error in pathology. Arch Pathol Lab Med 2007;130:617–9.
7. Nakhleh RE. Lost, mislabeled and unsuitable surgical pathology specimens. Pathol Case Rev 2003;8: 98–102.
8. Zarbo RJ, Tuthill M, D'Angelo R, et al. The Henry Ford production system; reduction of surgical pathology in-process misidentification defects by bar code-specific work process standardization. Am J Clin Pathol 2009;131:468–77.
9. D'Angelo R, Zarbo RJ. The Henry Ford production system; measures of process defects and waste in surgical pathology as a basis for quality improvement initiatives. Am J Clin Pathol 2007;128:423–9.
10. Spath PL. Reducing errors through work systems improvement. In: Spath PL, editor. Error reduction in health care. San Francisco (CA); Chicago: Jossey-Bass Publisher; AHA Press; 1999. p. 199–234.
11. Nakhleh RE, Gephardt G, Zarbo RJ. Necessity of Clinical Information in Surgical Pathology: a college of American pathologists Q-probes study of 771,475 surgical pathology cases from 341 institutions. Arch Pathol Lab Med 1999;123:615–9.
12. Pantanowitz L, Mackinnon AC, Sinard JH. Tracking in anatomic pathology. Arch Pathol Lab Med 2013; 137:1798–810.
13. Owens SR, Wiehagen LT, Kelly SM, et al. Initial experience with a novel pre-sign-out quality assurance tool for review of random surgical pathology diagnoses in a subspecialty-based university practice. Am J Surg Pathol 2010;34:1319–23.

14. Kamat S, Parwani AV, Khalbuss WE, et al. Use of a laboratory information system driven tool for pre-signout quality assurance of random cytopathology reports. J Pathol Inform 2011;2:42.

15. Kelly SM, Wiehagen LT, Yousem SA, et al. The impact of pre-signout random review of surgical and cytology cases on error rate in anatomic pathology. Mod Pathol 2014;27(supplement 2):506A.

16. Nakhleh RE, Bekeris L, Souers R, et al. Surgical pathology case reviews before sign-out: a college of American pathologists' Q-probes study of 45 laboratories. Arch Pathol Lab Med 2010;134:740–3.

17. Raab SS, Grzybicki DM, Mahood LK, et al. Effectiveness of random and focused review in detecting surgical pathology error. Am J Clin Pathol 2008; 130(6):905–12.

18. Branston LK, Greening S, Newcombe RG, et al. The implementation of guidelines and computerized forms improves the completeness of cancer pathology reporting. The CROPS project: a randomized controlled trial in pathology. Eur J Cancer 2002;38: 764–72.

19. Ruby SG, Henson DE. Practice protocols for surgical pathology: a communication from the Cancer committee of the college of American pathologists. Arch Pathol Lab Med 1994;118:120–1.

20. Daniel C, Macary F, Carcia Rojo M, et al. Recent advances in standards for collaborative digitial anatomic pathology. Diagn Pathol 2011;6(suppl 1):S17.

21. Nakhleh RE, Myers JL, Allen TC, et al. Consensus statement on effective communication of urgent diagnoses and significant unexpected diagnoses in surgical pathology and cytopathology from the college of American pathologists (CAP) and association of directors of anatomic and surgical pathology (ADASP). Arch Pathol Lab Med 2012; 136:148–54.

22. Volmar K, Idowu M, Meier F, et al. Surgical pathology report defects: a college of American pathologists Q-probes study of 73 institutions. Arch Pathol Lab Med 2014;138:602–12.

23. Meier FA, Varney RC, Zarbo RJ. Study of amended reports to evaluate and improve surgical pathology processes. Adv Anat Pathol 2011;18:406–13.

Moving?

Make sure your subscription moves with you!

To notify us of your new address, find your **Clinics Account Number** (located on your mailing label above your name), and contact customer service at:

Email: journalscustomerservice-usa@elsevier.com

800-654-2452 (subscribers in the U.S. & Canada)
314-447-8871 (subscribers outside of the U.S. & Canada)

Fax number: 314-447-8029

Elsevier Health Sciences Division
Subscription Customer Service
3251 Riverport Lane
Maryland Heights, MO 63043

*To ensure uninterrupted delivery of your subscription,
please notify us at least 4 weeks in advance of move.

Printed and bound by CPI Group (UK) Ltd, Croydon, CR0 4YY

03/10/2024

01040374-0001